A HOLISTIC AND INTEGRATED APPROACH TO LIFESTYLE DISEASES

A HOLISTIC AND INTEGRATED APPROACH TO LIFESTYLE DISEASES

Edited by

Jesiya Susan George
Anne George, MD
Sebastian Mathew, MD
Nandakumar Kalarikkal, PhD
Sabu Thomas, PhD

AAP | APPLE
ACADEMIC
PRESS

First edition published 2022

Apple Academic Press Inc.
1265 Goldenrod Circle, NE,
Palm Bay, FL 32905 USA

4164 Lakeshore Road, Burlington,
ON, L7L 1A4 Canada

CRC Press
6000 Broken Sound Parkway NW,
Suite 300, Boca Raton, FL 33487-2742 USA

2 Park Square, Milton Park,
Abingdon, Oxon, OX14 4RN UK

© 2022 by Apple Academic Press, Inc.

Apple Academic Press exclusively co-publishes with CRC Press, an imprint of Taylor & Francis Group, LLC

Library and Archives Canada Cataloguing in Publication

Title: A holistic and integrated approach to lifestyle diseases / edited by Jesiya Susan George, Anne George, MD, Sebastian Mathew, MD, Nandakumar Kalarikkal, PhD, Sabu Thomas, PhD.
Names: George, Jesiya Susan, editor. | George, Anne, 1961- editor. | Mathew, Sebastian editor. | Kalarikkal, Nandakumar, editor.
Description: First edition. | Includes bibliographical references and index.
Identifiers: Canadiana (print) 20210328894 | Canadiana (ebook) 20210328959 | ISBN 9781774630143 (hardcover) | ISBN 9781774639719 (softcover) | ISBN 9781003180609 (ebook)
Subjects: LCSH: Holistic medicine. | LCSH: Lifestyles—Health aspects.
Classification: LCC R733 .H58 2022 | DDC 610—dc23

Library of Congress Cataloging-in-Publication Data

CIP data on file with US Library of Congress

ISBN: 978-1-77463-014-3 (hbk)
ISBN: 978-1-77463-971-9 (pbk)
ISBN: 978-1-00318-060-9 (ebk)

About the Editors

Jesiya Susan George, MSc

Jesiya Susan George is currently a PhD student in the School of Chemical Sciences at Mahatma Gandhi University, Kottayam, Kerala, India. Her area of research includes epoxy nanocomposites, polymer blends, polymer nanocomposites, and anticorrosive coatings. She has published several chapters and presented papers in various international conferences. She received a prestigious INSPIRE fellowship from the Department of Science and Technology (DST), Ministry of India, and is a first rank holder in her MSc degree in Biopolymer Science from Cochin University of Science and Technology, Kochi, India. She completed Bachelor of Science in Chemistry at Mahatma Gandhi University.

Anne George, MD, MBBS

Anne George, MD, is Associate Professor at Government Medical College, Kottayam and Kerala, India. She has organized several international conferences, is a fellow of the American Medical Society, and is a member of many international organizations. She has several publications to her credit and has edited several books. She did her MBBS (Bachelor of Medicine, Bachelor of Surgery) at Trivandrum Medical College, University of Kerala, India. She acquired a DGO (Diploma in Obstetrics and Gynaecology) from the University of Vienna, Austria; Diploma Acupuncture from the University of Vienna; and an MD from Kottayam Medical College, Mahatma Gandhi University, and Kerala, India.

Sebastian Mathew, MD, MBBS

Sebastian Mathew, MD, has a degree in surgery (1976) with specialization in Ayurveda. He holds several diplomas in acupuncture, neural therapy (pain therapy), manual therapy, and vascular diseases. He was a missionary doctor in Mugana Hospital, Bukoba in Tanzania, Africa (1976–1978) and underwent surgical training in different hospitals in Austria, Germany, and India for more than 10 years. Since 2000, he is the doctor-in-charge of the Ayurveda and Vein Clinic in Klagenfurt, Austria. At present, he is a Consultant Surgeon at Private Clinic Maria Hilf, Klagenfurt, Austria. He is a member of the scientific advisory committee of the European Academy for Ayurveda, Birstein, Germany, and TAM advisory committee (Traditional Asian Medicine, Sector Ayurveda) of the Austrian Ministry for Health, Vienna. He conducted an International Ayurveda Congress in Klagenfurt, Austria, in 2010. He has several publications to his name.

Nandakumar Kalarikkal, PhD

Nandakumar Kalarikkal, PhD, is Director of the School of Pure and Applied Physics and International and Inter University Centre for Nanoscience and Nanotechnology at Mahatma Gandhi University, Kottayam, Kerala, India. He is the recipient of research fellowships and associateships from prestigious organizations such as the Department of Science and Technology and Council of Scientific and Industrial Research of the Government of India. His research activities involve nanotechnology and nanomaterials, sol-gel synthesis of nanosystems, semiconducting glasses, ferroelectric ceramics, and nonlinear and electro-optic materials. He has collaborated with national and international scientific institutions in India, South Africa, Slovenia, Canada, and Australia, and is co-author of several books chapters, peer-reviewed publications, and invited presentations in international forums.

Sabu Thomas, PhD

Professor Sabu Thomas is currently Vice Chancellor of Mahatma Gandhi University. He is also a full professor of Polymer Science and Engineering at the School of Chemical Sciences of Mahatma Gandhi University, Kottayam, Kerala, India, and the Founder Director and Professor of the International and Inter University Centre for Nanoscience and Nanotechnology. Prof. Thomas is an outstanding leader with sustained international acclaims for his work in nanoscience, polymer science and engineering, polymer nanocomposites, elastomers, polymer blends, interpenetrating polymer networks, polymer membranes, green composites, and nanocomposites and nanomedicine. Professor Thomas has received a number of national and international awards. Recently, he has been selected as a member of prestigious European Academy of Sciences. Professor Thomas has published over 800 peer-reviewed research papers, reviews, and book chapters. He has co-edited 100+ books published by the Royal Society, Wiley, Woodhead Publishing, Elsevier, Apple Academic Press, CRC Press, Springer, and Nova, etc. He is the inventor of 15 patents. The *h*-index of Prof. Thomas is 116, and his work has more than 60,000 citations. Prof. Thomas has delivered over 400 plenary/inaugural and invited lectures in national/international meetings in over 30 countries.

Contents

Contributors

K. Anumol
Department of Physiology, Little Flower Institute of Medical Sciences and Research, Angamaly, Kerala, India

Ajay Chaudhary
Department of Biotechnology, Faculty of Life Sciences, Institute of Applied Medicines and Research, Ghaziabad, Uttar Pradesh, India

Hong Chi
Shandong Provincial Key Laboratory of Molecular Engineering, School of Chemistry and Pharmaceutical Engineering, Qilu University of Technology (Shandong Academy of Sciences), | Jinan 250353, China

Jesiya Susan George
International and Inter University Centre for Nanoscience and Nanotechnology, Athirampuzha, Kerala, India

A. Helen
Department of Biochemistry, University of Kerala, Thiruvananthapuram, Kerala, India

Ann Holaday
Mahatma Gandhi University, Kerala, India

Stefan Jackson
Amity College of Engineering, Noida, New Delhi, India

Abhimanyu Kumar Jha
Professor and Head in Department of Biotechnology, School of Engineering and Technology, Sharda University, Greater Noida, Uttar Pradesh, India

K. P. Jibin
School of Chemical Sciences, Mahatma Gandhi University, Kottayam, India

Neetha John
CIPET: IPT-Kochi, HIL Colony, Edyar Road, Udyogamandal PO, Eloor, Cochin 683501, India

Haritha Therese Joseph
Department of Surgery, Regional Institute of Medical Sciences, Imphal, India

K. S. Joshy
Shandong Provincial Key Laboratory of Molecular Engineering, School of Chemistry and Pharmaceutical Engineering, Qilu University of Technology (Shandong Academy of Sciences), Jinan 250353, China

S. K. Kavitha
National Institute of Malaria Research Field Unit, ICMR, Bangalore, India

B. Swathy Krishna
Central Institute of Plastic Engineering and Technology, Institute of Plastic Technology, Kochi, Kerala, India

M. L. Aadithya Lakshmi
Government Ayurveda Medical College, Kottar, Nagercoil, Kanyakumari District, Tamil Nadu, India

Runjhun Mathur
A P J Abdul Kalam Technical University, Lucknow, Uttar Pradesh, India

C. R. Meera
Department of Microbiology, St Mary's College, Thrissur, Kerala, India

Parin N. Parmar
Pediatric Allergology and Integrative Medicine Consultant, Rajkot, Gujarat, India

V. Prajitha
School of Chemical Sciences, Mahatma Gandhi University, Kottayam, India

V. R. Remya
Intenational and Inter University Centre for Nanoscience and Nanotechnology, Athirampuzha, India

Gaurav Saini
Department of Civil Engineering, Sharda University, Greater Noida, Uttar Pradesh, India

Aiswarya Satian
Mount Carmel College, Palace Road, Bangalore, India

Arun M Shankregowda
Faculty of Biosciences and Aquaculture, Nord University, N-8026 Bodø, Norway

Mahek Sharan
Department of Biotechnology, Faculty of Life Sciences, Institute of Applied Medicines and Research, Ghaziabad, Uttar Pradesh, India

R. Shelma
Department of Chemistry and Polymer Chemistry, KSMDB College, Kollam, Kerala, India

Sheo Prasad Shukla
Rajkiya Engineering College, Banda, Uttar Pradesh, India

Sabu Thomas
Intenational and Inter University Centre for Nanoscience and Nanotechnology, Athirampuzha, India

K. Vandana
Quality Department, Quess Group of Companies, Bengaluru, India

Surya M. Vijayan
Department of Surgery, Wayanad Institute of Medical Sciences, Wayanad, India

Abbreviations

15-LOX	15-lipoxygenase
5-LOX	5-lipoxygenase
AIA	adjuvant-induced arthritis
AIDS	acquired immunodeficiency syndrome
AMPs	antimicrobial peptides
ART	antiretroviral treatment
BDL	below detection limit
BHC	benzene hexachloride
BMI	Body Mass Index
BRM	biologic response modifiers
BSA	bovine serum albumin
CAB	cellulose acetate butyrate
CAD	computer-aided design
CIA	collagen-induced arthritis
CII	type II collagen
COX	cyclooxygenase
CRC	colorectal cancer
CS	chitosan
DDD	dichlorodiphenyldichloroethane
DDE	dichlorodiphenyldichloroethylene
DDI	didanosine
DDSs	drug delivery systems
DDT	dichlorodiphenyltrichloroethane
DLP	digital light projection
DMDs	digital micromirror devices
DOPA	3,4-dihydroxy-L-phenylalanine
DSST	Digit Symbol Substitution Test
EAC	Ehrlich ascites carcinoma
EBV	Epstein–Barr virus
EC	electrical conductivity
EGCG	epigallocatechin-3-gallate
EHD	electrohydrodynamic
FAP	familial adenomatous polyposis
FAS	Fatigue Assessment Scale

FDA	Food and Drug Administration
FDM	fused deposition modeling
GNPs	gold NPs
GPX	glutathione peroxidase
GSH	glutathione
HBV	hepatitis B virus
HCH	hexachlorocyclohexane
HIV	human immunodeficiency virus
HPV	human papilloma viruses
I3C	indole-3-carbinol
IDU	injection drug use
IHNV	infectious hematopoietic necrosis virus
IN	integrase
IPH	interpenetrating hydrogel
JRM	*Justicia gendarussa*
LHRH	leutinizing hormone releasing hormone
LOX	lipoxygenase
LTRs	long tandem repeats
MCP	major capsid protein
MDA	malondialdehyde
MDR	multidrug resistant
MMPs	matrix metalloproteinases
MMSE	Mini-mental State Examination
MMSL	mask projection stereolithography
MPO	myeloperoxidase
MWCNT	multi-walled carbon nanotube
NBE	*o*-nitrobenzyl ether
NEP	needle exchange program
NIR	near-infrared
NK	natural killer
NOS	nitric oxide synthase
NPs	nanoparticles
NSAIDs	nonsteroidal anti-inflammatory drugs
OCPs	organochlorine pesticides
PAHs	polycyclic aromatic hydrocarbons
PCA	principal component analysis
PCL	polycaprolactone
PDEAEMA	polydiethylaminoethyl methacrylate
PDLGA	poly(D,L-lactide-co-glycolide)
PEA	phenylethylamine alkaloids

PEG	poly(ethylene glycol)
PGA	polyglycolic acid
PGS	polyglycerol sebacate
PHBV	poly(3-hydroxybutyrate-co-3-hydroxyvalerate)
PHEMA	polyhydroxyethyl methacrylate
PICs	preinitiation complexes
PL	polysaccharide
PLA	polylactic acid
PLGA	poly(lactic-*co*-glycolic acid)
PLLA	poly-L-lactic acid
PM	peritoneal macrophages
PMMA	polymethyl methacrylate
PSP	polysaccharopeptides
PSQI	Pittsburgh Sleep Quality Index
QAS	quaternary ammonium salt
QOL	quality of life
QPEI	quaternary ammonium PEI
RA	rheumatoid arthritis
Rb	retinoblastoma
RNS	reactive nitrogen species
ROS	reactive oxygen species
RP	rapid prototyping
RT	reverse transcriptase
RTCs	reverse transcription complexes
SDGs	Sustainable Development Goals
SLA	stereolithography
SLCT	Six Letter Cancellation Test
SLS	selective laser sintering
SOD	superoxide dismutase
TDF	tenofovir disoproxil fumarate
THMs	trihalomethanes
TLC	total lymphocyte count
TPP	tripolyphosphate
TPU	thermoplastic polyurethane
TWTPs	tap water treatment plants
UV	ultraviolet
VEGF	vascular endothelial growth factor
WSSV	White Spot Syndrome Virus
ZDV	zidovudine

Preface

Holistic medicine is a form of healing in which the affected individual's body, mind, spirit, and emotions are considered for his or her wellness. A holistic doctor may use all forms of healthcare, from conventional medication to alternative therapies, to treat a patient, underpinned by the concept that there is a strong correlation between physical health and general "well-being." However a major misconception toward holistic medicine is that it is treated as an alternative or complementary medicine, but holistic medicine utilizes a wide range of treatment approaches together and encourages open-mindedness for these different approaches.

This book is a collection of contributions from scientists, doctors, researchers, and healthcare experts working enthusiastically to provide complete wellness to every person. Chapters in this book deal with basics of holistic medicine that give detailed explanations regarding the novel lifestyle diseases such as various types of cancers, health problems due to overnight mobile usages, AIDS, and asthma, etc. In addition, effective strategies for therapies using new techniques and effective utilization of various plant extracts are also covered in the book.

This book aims to cater to the needs of scientists, doctors, researchers, and other healthcare experts all over world; it provides knowledge that will help them take an effective holistic approach to contemporary lifestyle diseases.

We are especially gratefully indebted to everyone for their support and tolerance which made this book possible. Editors would like to acknowledge and thank Apple Academic Press, Inc., for the permission to publish this book and their support and help throughout the process.

CHAPTER 1

AIDS: Control and Possible Cure by Using Gene Therapy and Gene Editing Technology

MAHEK SHARAN,[1] AJAY CHAUDHARY,[1] and ABHIMANYU KUMAR JHA[2*]

[1]*Department of Biotechnology, Faculty of Life Sciences, Institute of Applied Medicines and Research, Ghaziabad, Uttar Pradesh, India*

[2]*Professor and Head in Department of Biotechnology, School of Engineering and Technology, Sharda University, Greater Noida, Uttar Pradesh, India*

[*]*Corresponding author. E-mail: abhimanyu2006@gmail.com*

ABSTRACT

Human immunodeficiency virus (HIV) is a retrovirus that causes acquired immunodeficiency syndrome (AIDS). This syndrome has raised global mortality rate from December 1999 to 2016. The number of patients suffering from AIDS increased to 36.7 million, resulting in 1 million deaths per year. HIV contains single-stranded RNA (ssRNA), integrase enzyme and reverse transcriptase that allows the conversion of its ssRNA into dsDNA, formation of long tandem repeats, integration of viral DNA into host DNA. Development of provirus and antibodies neutralization is by gp120 and gp41 utilization. This metabolism and protein expression by T-cell hijacking involves *gag*, *tat*, *pol*, *env*, and *art* genes, reducing the immunity. Depression is more prevalent among people living with HIV (PLWHIV) than that in general population at clinical stages II and III of HIV. The treatment of AIDS available, single receptor targeted/antiretroviral technology, viral eradication, and kick and kill strategy, only halt the disease or have major drawbacks but gene therapy and gene editing technology can possibly cure it. Protein VRCO7-αCD3 inhibits the activation and killing of latently infected T cell. CCR5 protein-encoding gene, devoid of virus adherence surface and stem cell transplantation, might cure AIDS completely by gene therapy. The alteration of CCR5 and direct cut of viral gene targeting provirus by gene editing technology may cure AIDS. Different approaches in this technology include blockage of *pol* and *tat* genes, blockage of long tandem repeats process with location and research on gene, and preparation of HIV vaccine.

CURRENT TREATMENTS AVAILABLE WITH MAJOR DRAWBACKS	FUTURE POSSIBLE TREATMENTS
• KICK AND KILL STRATERGY	• VACCINE WITH ALTERED CCR5 GENE PREVENTING THE DISEASE
• ANTI RETROVIRAL THERAPY	
• CCR5 TARGETTED THERAPY	• REVERSE TRANSCRIPTASE INHIBITOR
• **DRAWBACKS**	• BLOCKAGE OF pol and tat GENE
• VIRUS REACTIVATE AFTER TREATMENT	
• MUTATION RESULTS IN THE RESISTANCE TO MULTIPLE DRUGS	
• ALLOGRAFT REJECTION	

1.1 INTRODUCTION

The disease which is often referred to as a slow poison for the body causing serious infections, tumors, and even certain cancer is acquired immunodeficiency syndrome (AIDS). The virus causing this deadly disease is human immunodeficiency virus (HIV), a type of a retrovirus enfold in a capsid, protein coat possessing two copies of ssRNA. It has enzymes, which help the virus to infect host cell and construct new viruses such as reverse transcriptase, the characteristic enzyme of retrovirus which converts its ssRNA to dsDNA and protease, an enzyme which cuts the host DNA and integrase (IN), which helps the virus dsDNA to bind to the host DNA.

The spread of this menacing disease started during the pre-1980s when HIV emerged in Kinshasa which is the largest city of Democratic Republic of the Congo in 1920 where HIV jumped from the chimpanzees to humans [2], marking the beginning of the epidemic of AIDS in 1980s. According to the UNAIDS global statistical data of 2017, around 36.9 million patients were infected and 940,000 patients were died, where there was occurrence of 1.8 million new infected cases. In the initial stage of AIDS, the patients experience a normal influenza-like symptoms such as body ache, fever, and many more followed by the final stage of infection where the immune system of the patient becomes completely nonfunctional along with unwanted weight loss, resulting in new infections and diseases such as tuberculosis that can lead to patient's demise.

AIDS, which is commonly transmitted through the liquid exchange and from mother to newborn, requires a large investment in basic and clinical research with aim of developing safe, affordable, and ascendible cure for it. As no permanent cure, but only temporary treatment such as sustained viral remission and viral eradication such as antiretroviral treatment (ART) and kick and kill strategy to eradicate viral reservoir resulting in only cessation of disease. According to the UNAIDS global statistical data of 2017, ART for AIDS was received by 21.7 million.

The major drawbacks observed in the available current treatments for AIDS are the rebound of the disease once the treatment is stopped. Therefore, new techniques of biotechnology including gene therapy by mutation and stem cell transplantation [8] along with gene editing could serve as the permanent cure for this deadly disease and its epidemic by complete eradicating the virus, resulting in the rise of a healthy world.

1.2   EPIDEMIOLOGY

After the first case of AIDS was reported, millions of people have died because of it since then. AIDS was first reported in United States in 1981 and in 1983, in Central and East Africa, it was recognized among heterosexual men [2].

Approximately 3.7 million new infections were estimated from 1980 to 1987 and from 1984 to 1991, there was a decrease in new infections from 130,000 to 60,000 [3]. In year 2012, approximately 2.3 million new infections were reported which showed decline by 34% since 2000 [1]. Approximately 9.7 million of people had accessed antiretroviral drugs and the death rate of AIDS declined to 28% from 2006 to 2012 [1].

AIDS increased the mortality rate in some countries of sub-Saharan Africa with high prevalence of HIV with more than 10% of infected adults [3]. In the year 2012, there were 780,000 people living with HIV in China, out of which 46.5% were infected through heterosexual HIV transmission and 28.4% were the case of injection drug use (IDU) infection [1].

In 2012, India was reported to have largest number of people living with HIV among the countries of Asia which was 2.1 million people living with AIDS infection [1]. Since 2007, there was a decline in the number of people living with HIV from 2.23 million to 2.12 million in 2012 [4]. In India, the number of new infection was 300,000 in 1998, which decreased to 120,000 in 2012 [4].

1.2.1   *UNAIDS GLOBAL STATISTICS ON THE AIDS EPIDEMIC [30]*

Since the commencement of the epidemic of AIDS, 77.3 million people have become infected with HIV and killed around 35.4 million people from

AIDS-related illnesses. In 2017, there were 36.9 million people living with HIV in which 1.8 million were children and 35.1 million were adults. Around 7,000 young women aged between 15 and 24 years become infected with HIV every week.

TABLE 1.1 Number of Human Immunodeficiency Virus (HIV) Patients in 2000 and 2012 in Different Regions

Regions	Number of HIV Patients		References
	2000	2012	
Asia	3,800,000	4,800,000	Fettig et al. [1]
Latin America and The Caribbean	1,600,000	1,750,000	Fettig et al. [1]
North Africa and Middle East	130,000	260,000	Fettig et al. [1]
North America	940,000	1,300,000	Fettig et al. [1]

TABLE 1.2 UNAIDS Global Statistics on the AIDS Epidemic

	2000	2013	2017
People living with HIV (PLWHIV)	27.4 million	34.3 million	36.9 million
New HIV infections	2.8 million	2.0 million	1.8 million
AIDS-related death	1.5 million	1.2 million	940,000

The regional statistics showed that in sub-Saharan Africa, three out of four new infections were reported, among adolescents girls aged 15–19 years. In 2016, around 10.4 million people developed tuberculosis and 1.2 million people were living with HIV. It was estimated that 49% of people living with HIV and tuberculosis are unaware of their coinfection. Only 47% of all people living with HIV are virally suppressed but not permanently cured.

1.3 CAUSE, SYMPTOMS, TRANSMITTANCE, AND PREVENTION OF AIDS

AIDS is still a major concern of all countries in the world. Even though there are treatments that control the disease but still are not able to cure it permanently, thus, raising the mortality rate.

1.3.1 CAUSE

HIV jumped from African chimpanzees having a similar strain like that of simian immunodeficiency virus. It is a virion that consists of enveloped particle of 100 nm diameter along with the nucleic matter that comprises of two ssRNA molecules of 7–10 kb in size. The virus structure has the envelope that enables it to infect the host and direct enters into its cell. 5′ end capping component, R gene which ensures correct end-to-end transfer and 3′ end component, PPT gene which is used as primer for DNA synthesis and U3 gene as signal in reverse transcriptase. The proteins such as protease and the genes such as *pol* which are responsible for proteolytic cleavage and integration of viral DNA into host and by the usage of all these components, the HIV is able to enter into host and converts its RNA to DNA by using the enzyme reverse transcriptase (RT) and integrates it in the host genome. The CD4+ T cells are the targets of HIV, which gradually destroys it as an indication. The research revealed that total lymphocyte count (TLC) can be considered as surrogate marker for CD4+ cell count in individuals infected by HIV [31]. TLC along with its percentage in HIV-infected persons can also be used as an absolute CD4+ count predictor [9] and TLC as CD4- T cell surrogate to initiate ART [10].

1.3.2 SYMPTOMS

The symptoms of AIDS have been categorized into four stages (Figure 1.1). Initially, after infection, the patient may experience the influenza-like illness in which the symptoms include fever, shivers, chills, dry cough, body aches, and more. The second stage is the window period (the no symptoms phase where the virus would be replicating inside without any observable symptoms) followed by the commencement of the third-stage phase which is interference with the immune system increasing the risk of infection of tuberculosis and tumors. The fourth stage is the final stage, which includes the unwanted weight loss and ultimately death. This lethal disease is transmitted from person to person in very unusual way which is very different from a normal pathogen. HIV cannot be spread by casual contact with these body fluids, as the virus is unable to survive for a long time period outside the human body because it dies as soon as the body fluid dries up. This is the only relief as it stops the furthermore severe transmittance of disease [21].

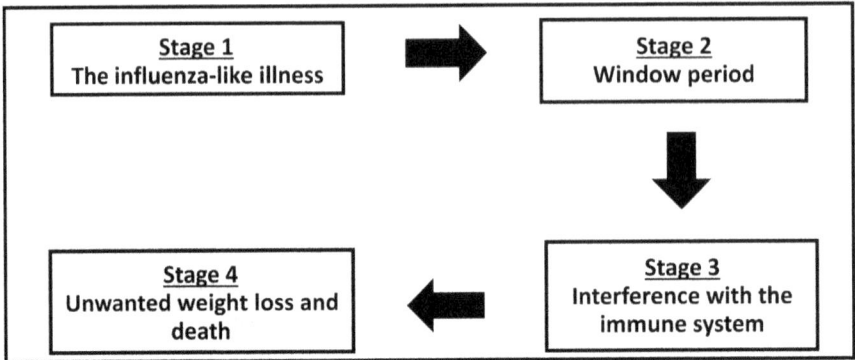

FIGURE 1.1 Four stages of HIV infection.

1.3.3 TRANSMITTANCE

AIDS transmittance takes place through unprotected intercourse (lack of precaution and prevention during the intercourse). Another major transmittance medium is contaminated blood transfusion that is the unchecked transfer of the blood for the presence of HIV. The third reason is the infected hypodermic needle use, which enters the skin of the healthy patient infecting him. Even during pregnancy, delivery, and breastfeeding from a mother to child by the vertical transmitted infection, AIDS occurs.

1.3.4 PREVENTION

Prevention is better than cure and a life saver method in the case of AIDS. The precaution taken during the intercourse against any STD is best prevention. The needle exchange program (NEP) is a social service protecting injecting drug users protection from AIDS. Exclusive use of the no relay NEP provides greater HIV protection than NEP use involving syringe relay [12]. The right treatment of those who are infected will indirectly prevent the infection. It can be prevented in babies by giving mother and child antiretroviral medication, which acts on HIV cycle and acts on different viral targets by use of multiple drugs; highly active antiretroviral therapy (HAART) markedly decreases HIV transmission risk [11]. But, treatments do not change the reality of this life-threatening disease as medications for this are very expensive and despite many successful programs running to treat individuals infected with HIV still many people in this world are living with AIDS.

1.4 RETROVIRUS CYCLE

The HIV belongs to Lentivirus subgroup. It is a member of Retrovirus family. In mature form, it is round in shape and has a diameter of 100 nm with an envelope of membrane made of lipid. The icosahedral envelope (100–120 nm), composed of trimers of gp120 (a surface protein) and gp41 (a transmembrane protein), covers the capsid and the capsid contains inside the two identical molecules of viral genomic linear 35S ssRNA of 7–10 kb which are present with viral enzymes, RT and IN. It is composed of three major internal protein gp30, gp70, and structure proteins inducing antibodies. Some regulatory proteins regulate the production rate of HIV are *tat, rev, nef, vif, vpr,* and *vpu* [5].

Life cycle of a retrovirus occurs in several steps (Figure 1.2). It starts with the recognition of CD4 receptor by the glycoprotein g120, which is present as gp41 and gp120 trimers [4]. An additional site is formed for gp120, after conformational changes in CD4 and gp120, binding with coreceptors CCR5 and CXCR4, which leads to the fusion of cell membrane and viral envelope, which forms a channel into plasma membrane of the target host cell [5].

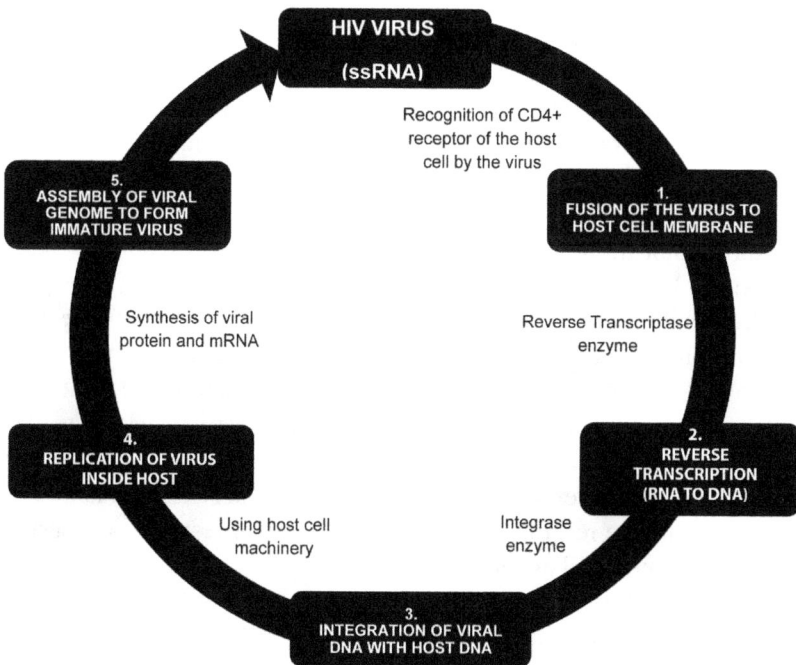

FIGURE 1.2   Different steps of retrovirus cycle.

The viral RNA of virion undergoes a process of reverse transcription to synthesize a linear double-stranded DNA molecule by the enzyme packaged by virion called RT. Reverse transcription complexes (RTCs) and preinitiation complexes (PICs) are generated after partial and progressive disassemble of viral core (uncoating of viral core) [4].

PIC (composed of IN and proviral DNA) is transported into nucleus through nucleopores and after transportation of proviral DNA, IN enzyme facilitates the integration of DNA proviral genome into host cell genome. During cell division, proviral genome replicates with target host cell genome [5].

A cellular DNA-dependent RNA polymerase binds to the long-tandem repeats of promoter of proviral genome to form viral mRNA and genomic RNA, which cause infection to the host cells [5].

1.5   PROPOSED MECHANISMS OF TREATMENT

1.5.1   KICK AND KILL STRATEGY

A strategy which scientists have been working onto cure AIDS is "kick and kill", which has a prime aim to activate inactive HIV cells hiding inside reservoirs and killing them while a person is under treatment. In kick and kill strategy, HIV-infected mice are injected with a synthetic compound **SUW133** to activate the mice's inactive HIV cells concurrently treated with antiretroviral drugs to kill them [13]. Large latent reservoirs observed to get reactivated by many agents. Thus, it is clear that this autoreactivation of this reservoir cannot be treated by the immune system of organism (Stanford University). Later, a discovery showed that nearly 25% of the inactive cells died within 24 hours. *Bryostatin 1*, a natural compound (extracted from a marine animal called *Bugula neritina*) which is less toxic than the natural ones, is previously used [14]. Without including kill strategy, the clinical trials were identified and reviewed which only promise on surrogate measures activating latent T-cells but negative effects on cure and during vaccine immune booster, the proportion of patients of ART with neutralizing antibodies, immune response regulators, and similar result was observed in clinical trials where kill agents were tested [15].

A trial referred to as the RIVER (Research In Viral Eradication of HIV Reservoirs) was performed to develop a cure for HIV, which did not find any difference in effect between those who were given standard ART and those who received the kick and kill therapy ("CHERUB", a UK collaboration of five universities). According to a research conducted in 2018, two therapies, using *vorinostat* (cancer managing drug) to activate the reservoir CD4+ T cells to force HIV against immune system and two vaccines, which help to recognize and cure HIV but still had comparable level of CD4+ T cells [16].

- HIVconsv vaccine vectored by ChAdV63, delivers the HIV's DNA pieces into the cells whose genetic information is used to produce immune response by the body against the virus—*ChAdV63.HIVconsv*.
- Modified Vaccinia virus Ankara, a viral vector which is replication deficient that could be used as an efficient platform for vaccine production—*MVA*.

A randomized phase II trial was run for a period of 3 years by investigators starting from 2015 to 2018, in Brighton and London, where they applied kick and kill strategy on a total of 60 men, having HIV and being treated by ART [17]. On the other hand, a test on mice was conducted by using the shock and kill treatment inducing the hidden or latent viruses to resurface by using a combination of four drugs that can destroy the HIV reservoir [19]. Safety was also a concern along with treating the disease [18].

Despite all the new approaches of kick and kill strategy to cure AIDS and an understanding of the efficacy of each person component is necessary. In most people, within 2–3 weeks of stopping ART, the virus will reactivate. Although infrequent at one in 100,000 cells, these latently-infected cells contain infectious virus that can reactivate upon ART cessation [20].

1.5.2 ANTIRETROVIRAL THERAPY

Since the discovery of AIDS in the 1980s, the HIV research has been proliferated. Even though antiretroviral therapy was one of the biggest achievement in treatment of AIDS, but still the main focus is to find a permanent cure before 2020.

The medicines that treat HIV are called antiretroviral drugs; under this category, drugs fall into six main types treating in different ways. Combination of drugs is known to be the best way to control HIV as well as to lower the chances of virus converting into a resistant one. Combination antiretroviral therapy and HAART recommend medicines in different combinations like three different medicines from two of the groups prescribed depend on factors like how many pills the patient should take each day. The HAART stops the virus from making copies of itself in the body thus, helping to prevent transmission of HIV including from mother to child during pregnancy.

ART treats HIV but mutation results in the resistance to multiple drugs, which limit the treatment. In UK, according to HIV drug resistance database, 30% of the treated patients received resistant tests followed by the virological failure in 2014, in which drug resistance was observed as compared to 72% in 2002. T69 insertion and associated mutation in RT confer high level resistance to nucleotide RT inhibitor and Q151M mutation cause high level resistance to zidovudine (ZDV), didanosine (DD1), and stavudine and low level resistance to tenofovir and lamivudine. T69 mutation is linked to DD1 and Q151M mutation is linked to D4T stavudine. In the mutation of T69i, any insertion in *beta3-beta4* loop of RT occurs between codons 66 and 70 [22].

ART guidelines have a protocol for switching patients who fail nonnucleotide RT inhibitor-based first-line regimen to second-line regimen which is based on the protease inhibitor which opened the door for third line which is based on significant viremia while being on second-line ART. Therefore, patients now switch to third-line ART and are observed being able to suppress viral load along with adherence counseling and have early treatment outcomes along with resistance testing in which patients show poor response and are at risk of failure to second-line ART among which 57.3% of cell is on third line. Suppression of viral load by ART during first intercourse months prevents this therapy [23].

ART patients require regimens encompassing multiple drug classes. TRIO regimen is effective and is used in patients harboring multidrug-resistant HIV in which the dose is six pills twice daily and even more. Treatment fatigue among HIV-infected patients is due to the major role played by high pill burden due to a lot of medicines prescribed in ART.

First-line regimen includes four different drugs:

1. Integrase inhibitor 150 g
2. Pharmacologic boosting agent 150 mg
3. Emtricitabine or FTC 200 mg
4. Nucleotide tenofovir disoproxil fumarate (TDF) 300 mg.

Elvitegravir/cobicistat/emtricitabine (E/C/T/TDF) allows consumption of two pills daily and compact once-daily multidrug regimen and the steady state concentration with low concentration of darunavir can result in viral suppression by 94% of 89 participants [24]. HIV disrupts the function of monocytes, its phenotype, and some functional and phenotypic abnormalities associated, which are persistent to the disruption caused by ART. The antiretroviral therapy leads to viral suppression, improvement in the immune system, and better outcomes [25].

1.5.3 CCR5 TARGETED THERAPY

HIV cell entry depends on binding to the CD4 receptor and chemokine coreceptors CCR5 which is the main receptor for HIV cell entry and CXCR4. Individuals having a homozygous CCR5-D32 deletion are highly protected from HIV-1 infection and in 2008, a sustained virus control and eradication of HIV were achieved by CCR5-D32 allogeneic transplantation in an HIV-infected patient possessing homozygous stem cells. Two ways are there to treat, which is to use a CCR5-negative cell source such as hematopoietic stem cells to copy the initial finding or to knockdown CCR5 expression by gene therapy. The five approaches in recent scenario proposed for treatment are: short hairpin RNA; transcription activator-like effectors nuclease also referred as TALEN; a ribozyme; CRISPR/Cas9 stands for CRISPR-associated protein 9 nuclease or clustered regularly interspaced palindromic repeats also called CRISPR and zinc finger nucleases referred as ZFN, among which three are currently being clinically tested [7].

The CCR5 is one of the main coreceptor, which is responsible for infection caused by macrophage-tropic R5 HIV-1. A receptor protein which shows nonexpressing behavior at the surface of the cell is due to the deletion of 32 bp in the gene which codes for CCR5 (CCR5Δ32). Homozygous individuals having CCR5Δ32 are resistant to R5 HIV-1 infection. CCR5 targeting antibodies have been identified, which specifically bind to the surface of cell line expressing CCR5. The CCR5 recognizing human antibodies were identified causing allograft rejection that made individuals face a mismatch situation even when they had no history of any kind of drug abuse or blood transfusion [29].

1.6 FUTURE ASPECTS

Since the epidemic of AIDS, millions of people have been infected and died due to HIV. Though available, AIDS treatment can halt and control the further infection of HIV but cannot cure it completely. One of the major reasons of HIV transmission might be the unawareness of people about HIV/AIDS and their HIV status. So, people should keep themselves aware and take preventive measures, if they are infected, to control and stop its transmission. Since the starting of the treatment of AIDS, various mechanisms are used to cure it such as the antiretroviral therapy which includes various combination of drugs and viral eradication by kick and kill strategy, but the common drawbacks in all the current treatments are that once the patient stops taking the pill, the disease rebounds, as HIV is stored in latent reservoirs inside host cells which lead to the need for permanent cure. The novel biotechnological approaches may cure AIDS by gene editing technology and gene therapy.

CCR5 is a coreceptor of CD4 cells, which is responsible for HIV binding and infection; therefore, deletion of 32 base pairs in CCR5 coreceptor causes inhibition of its expression on cell surface, making it a nonfunctional gene product which makes cells resistant to HIV and its infection. The deletion of 32 bp by gene therapy in which it can be mutated as well as dysfunction induced. The use of engineered chemokines induces receptor downregulation, therefore preventing the binding of CCR5 to HIV [28].

HIV latent reservoir precursors are the hematopoietic cells [27] and cure for AIDS can only be achieved if the virus is eradicated from reservoirs itself in the resting T-cells along with other hematopoietic cells [26]. Since CCR5 is responsible for adherence of virus to the cell surface, the transplantation of stem cell with *CCR5* gene mutation into bone marrow of patient may completely cure people infected with HIV/AIDS.

There is no vaccine approved by the CDC yet, but vaccines may have the ability to cure AIDS. A vaccine can be prepared with HIV-RNA or DNA altered through gene editing technology by the deletion of long tandem repeats (LTRs) (code for promotor viral genes transcription). Another vaccine can be prepared by gene editing technology where the immune cells from an HIV-positive patient can be inserted with an altered *CCR5* gene and administered in whole population thus, preventing this disease. Anti-CCR5 vaccination is an innovative anti-HIV strategy, which could provide effective protection or safe containment of the spread of the virus [28].

The provirus can be directly targeted by a RT inhibitor, which should be given with a complementary HIV-RNA strand that can bind to ssRNA of HIV thus, ceasing replication by making it unstable and killing it by drugs as well as targeting the provirus to locate and reverse the gene for reservoir eradication by inhibitory enzyme causing DNA slicing of genome. Blockage of *pol* (codes for enzymes protease, RT along with IN) and/or *tat* gene (codes for transactivator protein) can be blocked thus, blocking its functions. Apart from it, the LTR process can be blocked or deleted leading to nonconversion of ssRNA into dsDNA thus, inhibiting the infection. So, the detailed knowledge of HIV gene and its function, clinical trials, and research are needed for more ways to permanently cure AIDS.

1.7 CONCLUSION

AIDS has been killing millions of people since pre-1980s and no permanent cure has been found till date since the commencement of the AIDS epidemic. In today's scenario, AIDS is a major concern as it is a big barrier in achieving the goal of a healthy and disease-free world. By the help of biology and chemistry, the HIV structure has been studied and many drugs and their combinations have been setup to inhibit this infection. The biotechnology is a boon as by this, the molecular level structure of HIV has been studied and the function of different genes has been decoded which can completely cure AIDS. The treatments such as antiretroviral therapy (use of combination of drugs to treat AIDS) and viral eradication following kick and kill strategy, treating AIDS by vaccines such as ChAdV63.HIVconsv and MVA, are able to only pause this disease and once the medications are stopped, virus rebound as they live in latent reservoirs; also, the combination of different medicines have various side effects and taking more than half a dozen pill hampers the health as well as are very expensive thus, limiting the treatment to only rich strata of society. The treatment should be accessible to all, so different gene therapies such as mutation of *CCR5* gene and stem cell transplantation with defective CCR5, gene edit technologies by removing immune cells from patient and alter *CCR5* gene and inject again or targeting the provirus to locate and reverse the gene for reservoir eradication by inhibitory enzyme causing DNA slicing of genome, gene silencing such as *pol* and *tat* gene as well as vaccines of glycoproteins which have complementary HIV-RNA or altered HIV-DNA, and gene deletion of LTRs region are various approaches toward a permanent and cheap cure for the patients.

KEYWORDS

- **HIV**
- **AIDS**
- **reverse transcriptase**
- **CCR5**
- **ART**
- **kick and kill**
- **gene editing**
- **protein VRCO7-αCD3**

REFERENCES

1. Fettig, J., Swaminathan, M., Murill, C. S. and Kaplan, J. E. (2014) Global epidemiology of HIV. *Infect Dis Clin North Am.* 28(3): 327–337.
2. Faria, N., Rambaut, A., Suchard, M. A., Baele, G., Bedford, T., Ward, M. J., Tatem, A. J., Sousa, J. D., Arinaminpathy, N., Pepin, J., Posada, D., Peeters, M., Pybus, O. G. and Lemey, P. (2014) The early spread and epidemic ignition of HIV-1 in human population. *Science.* 346(6205): 56–61.
3. Smith, J. H. and Whiteside, A. (2010) The history of AIDS exceptionalism. *J Int AIDS Soc.* 13: 47.
4. Paranjape, R. S. and Challacombe, S. J. (2016) HIV/AIDS in India: an overview of the Indian epidemic. *Oral Dis.* 22(Suppl 1): 10–14.
5. German Advisory Committee Blood (Arbeitskreis Blut), Assessment of pathogen transmissible by blood. (2016) Human immune deficiency virus (HIV). *Transfus Med Hemother.* 43(3): 203–222.
6. Nisole, S. and Saïb, A. (2004) Early steps of retrovirus replicative cycle. *Retrovirology.* 1: 9.
7. Hütter, G., Bodor, J., Ledger, S., Boyd, M., Millington, M., Tsie, M. and Symonds, G. (2015) CCR5 targeted cell therapy for HIV and prevention of viral escape. *Viruses.* 7: 4186–4203.
8. Hütter, G. (2016) Stem cell transplantation in strategies for curing HIV/AIDS. *AIDS Res Ther.* 13: 31.
9. Blatt, S. P., Lucey, C. R., Butzin, C. A., Hendrix, C. W. and Lucey, D. R. (1993) Total lymphocyte count as a predictor of absolute CD4+ count and CD4+ percentage in HIV-infected persons. *JAMA.* 269: 622–626. doi: 10.1001/jama.1993.03500050100034.
10. Sreenivasan, S. and Dasegowda, V. (2011) Comparing absolute lymphocyte count to total lymphocyte count, as a CD4 T cell surrogate, to initiate antiretroviral therapy. *J Global Infect Dis.* 3(3): 265–268.
11. Hull, M. W. and Montaner, J. (2011) Antiretroviral therapy: a key component of a comprehensive HIV prevention strategy. *Curr AIDS/HIV.* 8(2): 85–93. doi: 10.1007/s11904-011-0076-6.
12. Valente, T. W., Foreman, R. K., Junge, B. and Vlahov, D. (2001) Needle-exchange participation, effectiveness, and policy: Syringe relay, gender, and the paradox of public health. *J Urban Health.* 78(2): 340–349.
13. Marsden, M. D., Loy, B. A., Christina, X. W., Ramirez, M., Schrier, A. J., Murray, D., Shimizu, A., Ryckbosch, S. M., Near, K. E., WookChun, T., Wender, P. A. and Zack J. A. (2017) In vivo activation of latent HIV with a synthetic bryostatin analog effects both latent cell "kick" and "kill" in strategy for virus eradication. *PLoS Pathogens.* 13(9): e1006575. doi: 10.1371/journal.ppat.1006575.
14. Kortmansky, J. and Schwartz, G. K. (2003) Bryostatin-1: a novel PKC inhibitor in clinical development. *Cancer Invest.* 21(6): 924–936.
15. Thorlund, K., Horwitz, M. S., Fife, B. T., Lester, R. and Cameron, D. W.(2017) Landscape review of current HIV "kick and kill" cure research—some kicking, not enough killing. *BMC Infect Dis.* 17(1): 595. doi: 10.1186/s12879-017-2683-3.
16. Fidler, S., Stohr, W., Pace, M., Dorrell, L., Lever, A., Pett, S., Kinloch, S., Fox, J., Clarke, A., Nelson, M., Khan, M., Fun, A., Kelly, D., Kopycinski, J., Johnson, M., Hanke, T., Yang, H., Howell, B., Kaye, S., Wills, M., Barnard, R., Babiker, A. and Frater, J. (2018) A randomised controlled trial comparing the impact of antiretroviral therapy (ART) with

a 'Kick-and-Kill' approach to ART alone on HIV reservoirs in individuals with primary HIV infection (PHI); RIVER trial. *J Int AIDS Soc.* 10: 21.

17. Imperial College London. (2018). First randomized trial of 'kick and kill' approach to HIV cure leaves puzzles to be solved. https://www.sciencedaily.com/releases/2018/07/180724110046.htm.

18. Cooper, D. (2018) Brought HIV research and treatment to resource-poor settings. *BMJ.* 3: 361. doi: https://doi.org/10.1136/bmj.k1567.

19. Lewin, S. (2014) Sharon Lewin: guiding us towards a cure for HIV. *Lancet.* 384(9939): 223. doi: 10.1016/S0140-6736(14)61198-3.

20. Pitman, M. C. and Lewin, S. R. (2018) Towards a cure for human immunodeficiency virus. *Intern Med J.* 48(1): 12–15. doi: 10.1111/imj.13673.

21. Tjotta, E. (1991) Survival of HIV-1 activity after disinfection, temperature and pH changes or drying. *J Med Virol.* 35(4): 223–227.

22. Stirrup, O. T., Dunn, D. T., Tostevin, A., Sabin, C. A., Pozniak, A., Asboe, D., Cox, A., Orkin, C., Martin, F. and Cane, P. (2018) The UK HIV Drug Resistance Database and the UK Collaborative HIV Cohort: Risk factors and outcomes for the Q151M and T69 insertion HIV-1 resistance mutations in historic UK data. *AIDS Res Ther.* 15: 11. doi: 10.1186/s12981-018-0198-7.

23. Evan, D., Hirasen, K., Berhanu, R., Malete, G., Ive, P., Spencer, D., Faesen, S. B., Sanne, I. M. and Fox, M. P. (2018) Predictors of switch to and early outcomes on third-line antiretroviral therapy at a large public-sector clinic in Johannesburg, South Africa. *AIDS Res Ther.* 15: 10. https://doi.org/10.1186/s1298-018-0196-9.

24. Harris, M., Ganase, B., Watso, B., Harrigan, R. P., Montaner, J. S. G. and Hull, M. W. (2017) HIV treatment simplification to elvitegravir/cobicisat/emtricitabine/tenofovir disproxil fumarate (E/C/F/TDF) plus darunavir: a pharmacokinetic study. *Res Ther.* 14: 59. doi: 10.1186/s12981-017-0185-4.

25. Nabatanzi, R., Cose, S., Joloba, M., Jones, S. R. and Nakanjako, D. (2018) Effects of HIV infection and ART on phenotype and function of circulating monocytes, natural killer and innate lymphoid cells. *AIDS Res Ther.* 15(1): 7. doi: 10.1186/s12981-018-0194-y.

26. Zou, S., Glynn, S., Kuritzkes, D., Shah, M., Cook, N., Berliner N. and NHLBI AIDS Blood Session Working Group. (2013) Hematopoietic cell transplantation and HIV cure: where we are and what next? *Blood.* 122(18): 3111–3115. doi: 10.1182/blood-2013-07-518316.

27. McNamara, L. A. and Collins, K. L. (2011) Hematopoietic stem/precursor cells as HIV reservoirs. *Curr Opin HIV/AIDS.* 6(1): 43–48.

28. Lopalco, L. (2010) CCR5: From natural resistance to a new anti-HIV strategy. *Viruses.* 2(2): 574–600. doi: 10.3390/v2020574.

29. Ditzel, H. J., Rosenkilde, M. M., Garred, P., Wang, M., Koefoed, K., Pedersen, C., Burton, D. R. and Schwartz, T. W. (1998) The CCR5 receptor acts as an alloantigen in CCR5Δ32 homozygous individuals: identification of chemokine and HIV-1-blocking human antibodies. *Proc Natl Acad Sci USA.* 95(9): 5241–5245.

30. Factsheet—Latest global and regional statistics on the status of the AIDS epidemic. (2018) *UNAIDS* http://www.unaids.org/sites/default/files/media_asset/UNAIDS_FactSheet_en.pdf.

31. Wondimeneh, Y., Ferede, G., Yismaw, G. and Muluye, D. (2012) Total lymphocyte count as surrogate marker for CD4 cell count in HIV-infected individuals in Gondar University Hospital, Northwest Ethiopia. *AIDS Res Ther.* 9: 21. https://doi.org/10.1186/1742-6405-9-21.

CHAPTER 2

Health Hazards of Overnight Mobile Phone Usage: A Comparative Study

K. ANUMOL

Department of Physiology, Little Flower Institute of Medical Sciences and Research, Angamaly, Kerala, India; E-mail: anulobomariya@gmail.com

ABSTRACT

Smartphone usage has become highly increasing among the teens and the youth over the past decade. They give prior importance to this media than their health and academics. Sleep is a crucial aspect for healthy cognitive and physical functioning. Looking intently at phone, television, etc., until bedtime, it has been reported as a cause for insomnia. The emitting radiations along with the sleep loss may contribute to wide range of health disorders. The present study was undertaken to compare the sleep pattern disturbances and associated physiological and cognitive variations in students with overnight smartphone usage and controlled smartphone usage. The study groups were comprised a total of 60 samples and they were examined for four consecutive months and the data was collected at the end of each month and data analysis was done. Our study results showed that overnight smartphone users had significant sleep pattern disturbances (p value of 0.02%) and most of the students were reported of having hypertension, hyperglycemia, excess fatigue, obese problems, cognitive sagging, etc., while comparing with the controlled users. Hence, this pilot study put forth valid evidence about the probable future health threats among the youth who uses smartphones during night in an uncontrolled manner.

2.1 INTRODUCTION

Exposure to the modernized technologies contributes a positive effect on social prosperity of man. But, as it is rapidly reshaping into the newer forms by creating a stream of electronic pleasures, there rises a critical and contemptible circumstance in young grown-ups by the irresponsible handling of mobile phones. It creates a psychological dependency among youngsters toward mobile phones [1]. Recently "Brain in the News by Dana Foundation" presented an article of Alice G Walton (copyright Forbes, 2017) that unveils the present status of youngsters in terms of their mobile usage. Moving into the depth of this topic, they incorporated a series of findings related to mobile phones and concluded that youngsters are addicted to the phone to a great extent and most of the time, they are dealing with the social medias rather than any other things through the phone. Shockingly, the suicidal behavior is getting higher among these in overtime users [2]. When these phones held on head side while sleeping, it brings about several risks to the human brain, which include variations in sleep and cognition and is examined and proved in a series of studies [3, 4]. But, how much extent the usage is incorporated with the adverse effects in terms of different physiological and cognitive variables are yet unknown. Thus, this study intended to compare the effects on sleep pattern and associated physiologic and cognitive parameters due to overnight smartphone usage through regular follow-ups for 4 months.

2.2   MATERIALS AND METHODS

The study was conducted among the students of Little Flower Institute of Medical Sciences and Research, Angamaly, Kerala for a period of 4 months (August 2018 to November 2018). After obtaining institutional ethical clearance, the student population of 300 aged between 18 and 25 years were screened based on their smartphone usage pattern by means of a predesigned questionnaire (consisting of demographic details, problematic mobile phone use scale, and details regarding pattern of usage such as hours, night usage, and purpose).

Based on the scores obtained, the samples were assigned into two different groups randomly: the overnight users and the controlled users. The overnight usage time of the users was about 1.30–3 h and beyond after bedtime. The controlled users were reported of having no usage or negligible use (maximum duration of 15 min). The students, who have met the inclusion criteria for the overnight and controlled smartphone usage, were selected by simple random sampling. Thus, 30 samples per each group have been recruited. After obtaining an informed written consent from the students, the sleep pattern and associated physiological and cognitive variations were assessed for four consecutive months and compared using standardized techniques.

2.2.1   ASSESSMENT OF SLEEP DISTURBANCES BY PITTSBURGH SLEEP QUALITY INDEX (PSQI)

Pittsburgh Sleep Quality questionnaire was a standard 19-item self-rated scale with seven subscales estimating subjective experience of quality and patterns of sleep over the earlier month. There are seven domains which are 'subjective sleep quality, sleep latency, sleep duration, habitual sleep efficiency, sleep disturbance, use of sleeping medication, and daytime dysfunction' and the absolute score varied as 0–21. The higher scores demonstrating the worse sleep quality and scores less than 5 indicate excellent sleep quality [5].

2.2.2   ASSESSMENT OF PHYSIOLOGICAL VARIABLES

2.2.2.1   ASSESSMENT OF BODY MASS INDEX (BMI)

It is measured by checking anthropometric measurements. BMI indicates the nutritive status of a person [3, 5]. It can be calculated using the formula:

$$BMI = \frac{Weight\ (kg)}{Height\ (m^2)}$$

2.2.2.2   ASSESSMENT OF BLOOD PRESSURE

Blood pressure is measured by using digital sphygmomanometer. Time points for BP measurement were during afternoon hours (2–3 pm) and this chosen time was maintained for whole 4 months. It was measured in the right hand by keeping the client in sitting posture by using digital BP apparatus.

2.2.2.3   ASSESSMENT OF BLOOD GLUCOSE LEVEL

Blood glucose level is measured using an electronic glucometer. The blood glucose was measured by applying a drop of blood to a test strip, which is then inserted to a glucose meter and the reading is noted.

2.2.2.4   ASSESSMENT OF FATIGUE—FATIGUE ASSESSMENT SCALE (FAS)

The FAS is a valid self-reported questionnaire to assess the degree of fatigue. The score range of 10–21 indicates normal and a range above 22 indicates substantial fatigue [6].

2.2.3   ASSESSMENT OF COGNITION

Cognition levels were checked by the following measures.

2.2.3.1   IMMEDIATE OBJECT RECALL

Subject was presented to 20 objects that were set on a table. The subjects were given 15 seconds to look at the objects before they were removed. The subjects were then instructed to record whatever number of items as could be allowed from memory within the given time of 60 s [7, 8].

2.2.3.2   DIGIT SYMBOL SUBSTITUTION TEST (DSST)

This is the test which examines sustained concentration and response speed. Rapid processing of information is required to substitute the symbols precisely and rapidly. A hundred numbers will be arbitrarily printed out on a paper. The subject will be instructed to sketch a circle over even numbers and a triangle over odd numbers. The time taken to substitute a symbol for all the 100 digits will be recorded [8].

2.2.3.3   SIX LETTER CANCELLATION TEST (SLCT)

The 26 letters of the English alphabet were rumpled and written in black shade on a white paper. The test consists of a "test worksheet" in which opted six target letters to be dropped. The students were asked to cutoff as many of the six target letters within the predefined duration of 1 min and 30 s [9].

2.2.3.4   MINI-MENTAL STATE EXAMINATION (MMSE)

The MMSE is a questionnaire used for the systematic and thorough assessment of mental status. It contains 11 segments that analyze different domains of cognitive function: orientation to time and place, immediate memory (retention), attention and calculation, short-term memory recall, and language with a maximum score of 30 and the score equal or below 23 shows cognitive impairment [10].

2.2.4   STATISTICAL ANALYSIS

All data was entered into Statistical Package for the Social Sciences (SPSS 16.0 version) for analysis. The results were expressed as mean ± SD of each variable and in percentage form. The comparison was performed by ANOVA, Fischer's exact test, independent sample *T*-test, and chi-square test. *p* value of 0.05 or less was interpreted as significant for the analysis.

2.3 RESULTS AND DISCUSSIONS

2.3.1 *ASSESSMENT OF SLEEP DISTURBANCES BY PITTSBURGH SLEEP QUALITY INDEX*

PQSI score was higher in the overnight mobile user group indicative of poor sleep. Among the students, 83.3% of the controlled mobile users were having good sleep whereas almost all the students in the overnight mobile usage group were having poor sleep. The differences among these two groups were showed to be statistically significant with a *Pp* value of 0.020 as shown in Table 2.1 and Figure. 2.1.

TABLE 2.1 Comparison of PSQI Scores Among Students

Pittsburgh Sleep Quality Index Scores	Controlled Mobile Users (N = 30)	Overnight Mobile Users (N = 30)	Chi-Square Analysis	*p* value
(Mean ± SD)	8.0 ± 2.4	15.6 ± 2.0	Test score 5.455	0.020

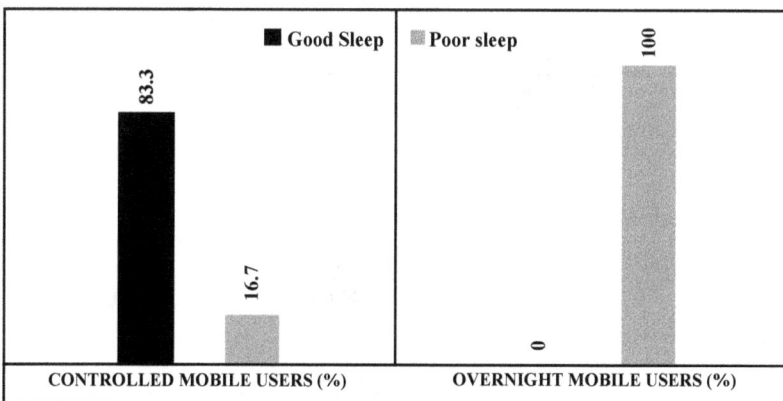

FIGURE 2.1 Sleep pattern variation among students.

2.3.2   ASSESSMENT OF PHYSIOLOGICAL VARIATIONS

2.3.2.1   BODY MASS INDEX

Anthropometric measurements among the two groups were similar, with BMI being slightly higher in the overnight mobile users' group which is not statistically significant (*p* value 0.611). Overweight and obese were higher in the overnight mobile users' group (*p* value < 0.001*)* compared to the controlled user group as depicted in Tables 2.2 and 2.3 and Figures 2.2 and 2.3.

TABLE 2.2   Assessment of Body Mass Index in Students

Body Mass Index	Controlled mobile users (N=30)	Overnight mobile users (N=30)	ANOVA test
Height(m) (Mean ± S.D)	1.56 ± 0.05	1.56 ± 0.05	*p* value 1.000
Weight (kg) (Mean± S.D)	59.6 ± 29.2	62.5 ± 4.9	*p* value 0.567
BMI (kg/m²) (Mean ± S.D)	24.4 ± 12.1	25.5 ± 1.2	*p* value 0.611

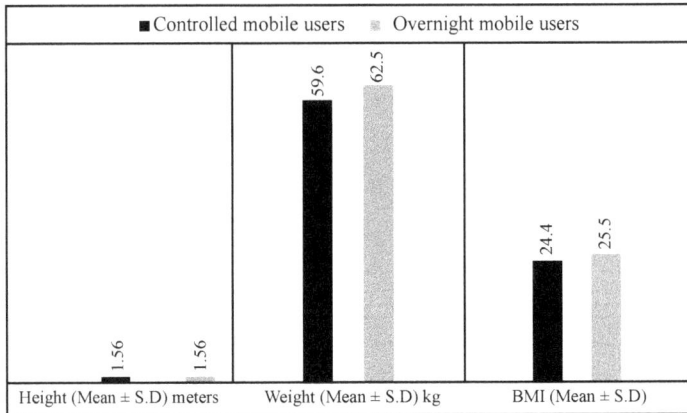

FIGURE 2.2   Assessment of Body mass Index among the students.

TABLE 2.3   Body Mass Index Classification

BMI Classification	N (%)	N (%)	Fischer's Exact test
Normal	28 (93.3)	09 (30.0)	*p* value <0.001
Overweight	00 (0.0)	20 (66.7)	
Obese	02 (6.7)	01 (3.3)	

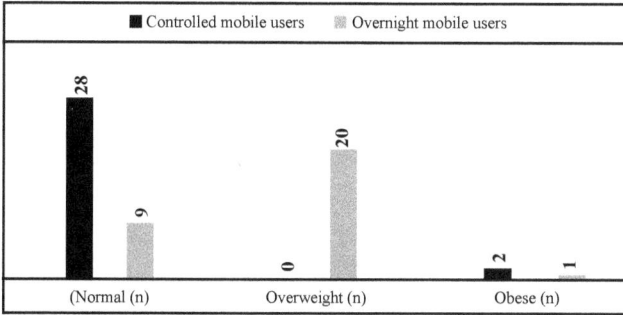

FIGURE 2.3 Body mass index classification among two groups.

2.3.2.2 ASSESSMENT OF BLOOD PRESSURE

The systolic blood pressure and diastolic blood pressure values among the students showed a comparable mean difference. The overnight users have a higher systolic blood pressure with a mean value of 130.1 ± 3.7 compared to controlled mobile phone users (p value < 0.001). The diastolic blood pressure was also comparably high among the overnight mobile phone users than controlled users (p value 0.041) as depicted in Table 2.4 and Figure 2.4.

TABLE 2.4 Assessment of Blood Pressure Among Students

Blood pressure (mm of Hg)	Controlled mobile users ($N = 30$)	Overnight mobile users ($N = 30$)	ANOVA test
Systolic blood Pressure (Mean ± S.D)	113.5 ± 10.3	130.1 ± 3.7	*p value < 0.001
Diastolic blood pressure (Mean ± S.D)	77.3 ± 5.6	80.7 ± 6.7	**p value of 0.041

*p value<0.001 and **p value of 0.041 as significant for systolic and diastolic blood pressure.

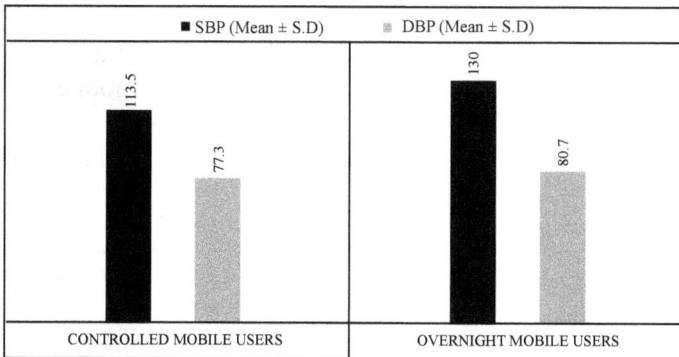

Values represented as Mean ± of systolic and diastolic blood pressure

FIGURE 2.4 Blood pressure variations among students.

2.3.2.3   BLOOD GLUCOSE LEVEL

Table 2.5 and Figure 2.5 show a comparable difference of Random blood glucose (RBS) levels among students in the two groups. The overnight mobile user group shows higher blood glucose level compared to controlled user group (p value < 0.001).

TABLE 2.5   Assessment of Blood Glucose Level in Students

Random Blood Glucose (RBS) levels (mg/dl)	Controlled mobile users ($N = 30$)	Overnight mobile users ($N = 30$)	ANOVA test
BG levels (Mean ± S.D)	83.0 ± 9.5	117.8 ± 7.9	p value < 0.001

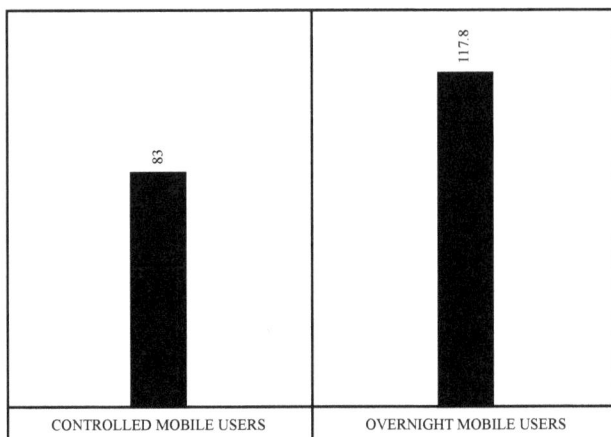

FIGURE 2.5   Random blood glucose variations among students.

2.3.3   FATIGUE ASSESSMENT

Table 2.6 and Figure 2.6 show a comparable difference of fatigue assessment score among the two different groups. The overnight mobile users had a fatigue score of 28.6 ± 3.4 when compared to the controlled users 14.04 ± 1.9. This difference was statistically significant with a p value of <0.001.

TABLE 2.6   Assessment of Fatigue Among Students

Fatigue Assessment Score	Controlled Mobile Users (N = 30)	Overnight Mobile Users (N = 30)	Chi-square test
FAS (Mean ± SD)	14.04 ± 1.9	28.6 ± 3.4	Test score 56.12 (df 1)
No fatigue	30 (100)	01 (3.3)	p value < 0.001
Fatigue present	00 (0.0)	29 (93.7)	

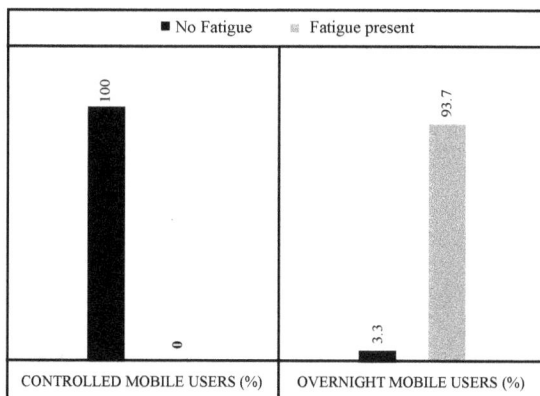

FIGURE 2.6   Comparison of fatigue among students.

2.3.4   ASSESSMENT OF COGNITIVE FUNCTIONS

2.3.4.1   MINI-MENTAL STATUS EXAMINATION

The MMSE score was generally higher in controlled mobile users (27.4 ± 0.8) when compared to overnight users (23.9 ± 1.9). This difference was statistically significant with a p value of <0.001 as shown in Table 2.7 and Figure 2.7.

TABLE 2.7   Mini-mental Status Examination Scores among Students

MMSE	Controlled Mobile Users (N = 30)	Overnight Mobile Users (N = 30)	Independent Sample T-test
MMSE (Mean ± SD)	27.4 ± 0.8	23.9 ± 1.9	*Test score 18.26 (df 1)*
No cognitive impairment	30 (100)	16 (53.3)	*p value < 0.000*
Mild cognitive impairment	00 (0.0)	14 (46.7)	

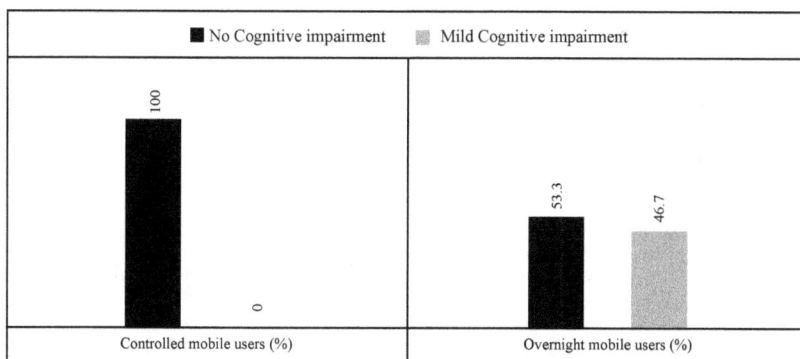

FIGURE 2.7   Comparison of Mini Mental Status Examination scores among students.

2.3.4.2 SIX LETTER CANCELLATION TEST

The SLCT scores were showed a better score for controlled mobile users than overnight users and this was statistically significant with p value of <0.001 as shown in Table 2.8 and Figure 2.8.

TABLE 2.8 Six Letter Cancellation Test Scores among Students

Six Letter Cancellation Test	Controlled Mobile Users (N = 30)	Overnight Mobile Users (N = 30)	Independent Sample *T*-Test
SLCT (Mean ± SD)	49.3 ± 5.1	25.8 ± 4.3	Test score 19.232 (df 58) p value < 0.001

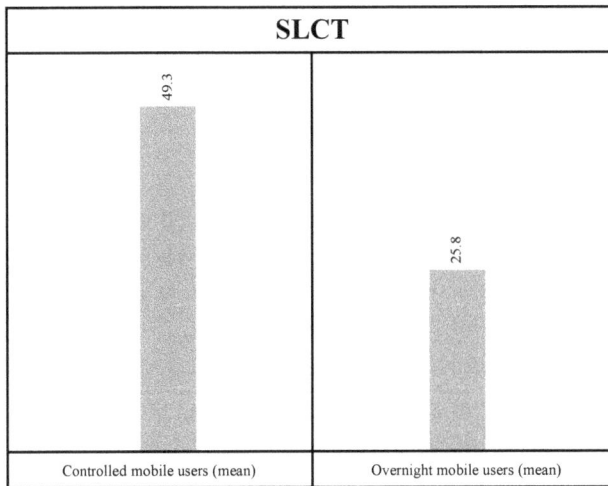

FIGURE 2.8 Comparison of Six Letter Cancellation Test scores among students.

2.3.4.3 DIGIT SYMBOL SUBSTITUTION TEST

The DSST scores showed that controlled mobile users were on average faster in substituting the numbers and this difference was not statistically significant as shown in Table 2.9 and Figure 2.9.

TABLE 2.9 Digit Symbol Substitution Test Scores among Students

Digit Symbol Substitution Test	Controlled Mobile Users (N = 30)	Overnight Mobile Users (N = 30)	Independent Sample *T*-test
DSST (Mean ± SD)	4.6 ± 9.5	5.0 ± 0.9	Test score 0.210 (df 58) p value 0.834

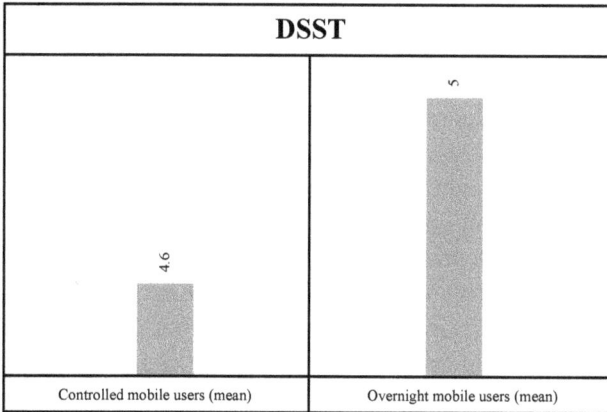

FIGURE 2.9 Comparison of Digit Symbol Substitution test scores among students.

2.4 DISCUSSION

Varieties of studies have been employed to find out the cause for the sleeplessness in mobile phone users and theorize that reduced melatonin production in relative to the emitting radiation during hours of dark time [4]. Overtime use of mobile phones may lead to reduced melatonin production [11]. Jarupat S et al. (2002) again supports the above findings and confirmed that electromagnetic radiation discharged from the mobile phone reduce the concentration of blood melatonin in humans [12].

In 2015, Shobha and Deepali have conducted a study in a group of medical students to know the effect of mobile usage on sleep quality and daytime sleepiness. The results showed that students with mobile phone usage more than 2 hours show poor sleep quality and increased daytime sleepiness [13].

Mobile-phone usage after lights out shown significant relation with sleep-pattern disturbances in a study conducted in Japanese adolescents [14].

In my study, the comparison is done between overnight mobile users and controlled mobile users. My study also validated the content that overuse of overnight mobile usage causes much sleep deprivation in students with the help of PSQI.

The fatigue range in the mobile phone users is not yet analyzed; hence, with the help of fatigue assessment scale, it has been made clear that an increase in bedtime mobile phone use was associated with more fatigue compared to the normal users.

Cognitive variation in mobile phone users has been analyzed by variety of studies. Studies reported that much cognitive disabilities are happening in overtime mobile phone users. The reported effects were reduced short-term memory, poor decision-making ability, diminished learning capacities, etc. [15, 16].

In my study, overnight mobile users are compared with the controlled users in terms of certain cognitive variables such as orientation, immediate memory retention, attention, short-term memory recall, and rapidity of responsiveness. Cognitive variations are evident in overnight mobile phone users than in controlled users. The study does not point that the users are cognitively disabled, but to state that the range of cognitive variations is high comparing with the normal users. The speed of responsiveness and recalling is slower compared to the controlled users.

Not much study has been put forward yet about the physiological variations happening in the overnight mobile phone users. In the present study, the BMI level of overnight mobile phone users found to be high compared to the controlled users. Hence, much of the overnight users were overweight and obese. Sedentary lifestyle with mobile phone dependence can account for the development of obese feature in constant users described by Kapdi et al. [17]. Similar evidence is also put forth by Spiegel et al. [18].

Electromagnetic radiation coming out of the phones can be the root cause for this health effects.

Reported cases of recall problems, lack of focus, sleep disturbances, etc., have identified again in users [19]. Thermal effects due to holding posture of mobile phones close to the body cause complaints of headache, sleep-wake problems, memory loss, poor attention, discomfort, high blood pressure, and even brain tumors too [15]. Recently, Stalin et al. (2016) had performed a study, which claims that constant mobile usage causes visual and auditory problems, fatigue, sleep disturbances, etc., but the hypertension was inversely correlated in terms of mobile usage. Although certain studies have suggested obesity in persons with poor sleep, the variation in blood pressure was not significantly identified in this study [20]. In our study, both systolic and diastolic blood pressure were found to be higher in overnight users (p value < 0.001 and p value of 0.041). Most of them were at borderline range of developing hypertension.

No study yet worked on blood glucose level variations among mobile phone users. In our study, the blood glucose levels were found to be high in overnight mobile phone users (p value < 0.001)

Thus, our study figure out and validate the fact that mobile phone use has decremental effects on one's own health.

2.5 CONCLUSION

Results of present study show overnight mobile phone using students that have disturbed and poor sleep quality. Most of them become fatty due to lack of activities and are tired almost all the time. Majority of them are having high blood pressure with borderline values comparing with controlled users. High blood glucose levels are also identified in them. Even though they are responding to the cognitive tests, they are slow in responding in certain aspects; sometimes, same rapidity as of controlled users, but the results were inaccurate. The students could not maintain concentration for much time.

Thus, the study gives a valid basis for the probable health threats for similar youth who uses mobile phone in an uncontrolled manner during the nighttime. The study enunciates possible future health problems such as cognitive disabilities, overweight problems, diabetes, hypertension, and memory problems in those with overnight time usage.

Thus, the study gives a valid basis for the probable future health threats such as sleep disorders, overweight problems, and hyperglycemic complications among similar youth who uses mobile phone in an uncontrolled manner during the nighttime.

2.6 RECOMMENDATION

The inference of present study findings emphasizes and recommends further research on possible health threats of overnight mobile phone usage, so that the people, especially teens and youth, can be made aware about it with scientific evidence.

KEYWORDS

- **smart phone usage**
- **sleep**
- **cognition**
- **blood pressure**
- **blood glucose**

REFERENCES

1. Balakrishnan, V. and Raj, R. G. (2012). Exploring the relationship between urbanized Malaysian youth and their mobile phones: A quantitative approach. *Telematics and Informatics*, 29(3), 263–272.
2. Walton, A. G. (2018). Phone addiction is real and so are its mental health risks (copyright Forbes). Brain in the News Dana Foundation. 25: 1–2. Available from http://bit.ly/2CtKjMH.
3. Preece, A. W. (1999). Effect o f a 915-MHz simulated mobile phone signal on cognitive function in man. *International Journal of Radiation Biology*, 75(4), 447–456.
4. Koivisto, M., Revonsuo, A., Krause, C., Haarala, C., Sillanmäki, L., Laine, M. and Hämäläinen, H. (2000). Effects of 902 MHz electromagnetic field emitted by cellular telephones on response times in humans. *Neuroreport*, 11(2), 413–415.
5. Buysse, D. J., Reynolds III, C. F., Monk, T. H., Berman, S. R. and Kupfer, D. J. (1989). The Pittsburgh Sleep Quality Index: a new instrument for psychiatric practice and research. *Psychiatry Research*, 28(2), 193–213.
6. Michielsen, H. J., De Vries, J., Van Heck, G. L., Van de Vijver, F. J. and Sijtsma, K. (2004). Examination of the dimensionality of fatigue. *European Journal of Psychological Assessment*, 20(1), 39–48.
7. Vajravelu, H. R., Gnanadurai, T. K., Krishnan, P. and Ayyavoo, S. (2015). Impact of quantified smoking status on cognition in young adults. *Journal of Clinical and Diagnostic Research*, 9(12), CC01.
8. Lezak, M., Howieson, D. and Loring, D. (2012). Neuropsychological assessment. 5th edition. Oxford University Press. *Oxford, New York, ISBN, 10*, 9780195395525.
9. Pradhan, B. and Nagendra, H. R. (2008). Normative data for the letter-cancellation task in school children. *International Journal of Yoga*, 1(2), 72.
10. Fulop, G., Strain, J. J., Fahs, M. C., Schmeidler, J. and Snyder, S. (1998). A prospective study of the impact of psychiatric comorbidity on length of hospital stays of elderly medical-surgical inpatients. *Psychosomatics*, 39(3), 273–280.
11. Adams, S. K., Daly, J. F. and Williford, D. N. (2013). Article commentary: adolescent sleep and cellular phone use: recent trends and implications for research. *Health Services Insights*, 6, 99–103. HSI-S11083.
12. Cao, M. and Guilleminault, C. (2012). Acute and chronic sleep loss: implications on age-related neurocognitive impairment. *Sleep*, 35(7), 901–902.
13. Deepali, A., Shobha, M. and Reddy, S. P. (2015). A study of mobile phone usage on sleep and stress among first year medical students. *Research Journal of Pharmaceutical Biological and Chemical Sciences*, 6(5), 720–723.
14. Carskadon, M. A., Acebo, C. and Jenni, O. G. (2004). Regulation of adolescent sleep. *Annals of the New York Academy of Sciences*, 10(21), 276–291.
15. Al-Khlaiwi, T. and Meo, S. A. (2004). Association of mobile phone radiation with fatigue, headache, dizziness, tension, and sleep disturbance in Saudi population. *Saudi Medical Journal*, 25, 732–736.
16. Van den Bulck, J. (2007). Adolescent use of mobile phones for calling and for sending text messages after lights out: results from a prospective cohort study with a one-year follow-up. *Sleep*. 30(9): 1220–1223.
17. Kapdi, M., Hoskote, S. Joshi, S. R. (2008). Health hazards of mobile phones: an Indian perspective. *Journal of the Association of Physicians of India*, 56, 893–897.

18. Spiegel, K., Tasali, E., Penev, P. and Van Cauter, E. (2004). Brief communication: sleep curtailment in healthy young men is associated with decreased leptin levels, elevated ghrelin levels, and increased hunger and appetite. *Annals of Internal Medicine*, 141(11), 846–850.

19. Alhola, P. and Polo-Kantola, P. (2007). Sleep deprivation: Impact on cognitive performance. *Neuropsychiatric Disease and Treatment*, 3(5), 553–567.

20. Stalin P, Abraham S. B., Kanimozhy K., Prasad R. V., Singh Z. and Purty A. J. (2016). Mobile phone usage and its health effects among adults in a semi-urban area of southern India. *Journal of Clinical and Diagnostic Research*. 10(1), LC14.

CHAPTER 3

Individualized and Integrative Management of Pediatric Asthma: A Health Promoting Approach for Clinical Practice

PARIN N. PARMAR

Pediatric Allergology and Integrative Medicine Consultant, Rajkot, Gujarat, India; Email: parinmnparmar@gmail.com

ABSTRACT

Pediatric asthma is the most common pediatric chronic disorder, which contributes significantly to morbidity in children. Most treatments for pediatric asthma in modern medicine are safe and aim at control of the disease, but only a few of them can change natural course of the disease. The model presented in this chapter aims to integrate principles of several complementary/alternative medicine systems into evidence-based conventional treatment of pediatric asthma. Most important components of the model are individualization in treatment approach, lifestyle changes, and overall health promotion, so that the personalized treatment plan for an asthmatic child aims at improved quality of life, decreased medicine requirement, minimization of risk of adverse effects both from conventional and alternative treatments, and improved overall health.

3.1 INTRODUCTION

Pediatric asthma is the most common chronic disease in children and its incidence and prevalence have been increasing in most countries over several decades. Advances in modern medicine and availability of quality emergency care have been able to decrease mortality due to acute attacks of asthma.

However, for long-term management of asthma, except for allergen-specific immunotherapy (for selected asthmatic children with allergic etiology only), there is no disease-modifying therapy available and role of pharmacological treatment is mainly limited to prevention and control of symptoms and exacerbations. As controller medications cannot change natural course of asthma and have to be continued for unpredictable duration, side effects of controller medications, drug compliance, and drug default are important problems in management of many asthmatic children.

The present model has been inspired from famous quote by Sir William Osler, "The good physician treats the disease; the great physician treats the patient who has the disease." The key components of the model include individualization, rational integration of complementary/alternative medicine systems, and overall health promotion of an asthmatic child.

3.2 INDIVIDUALIZATION IN MANAGEMENT OF PEDIATRIC ASTHMA

With recognition of multiple phenotypes, endotypes, and comorbidities, it is possible to think of pediatric asthma as a multifactorial, multifaceted disorder caused by complex interactions between multiple modifiable factors (such as environment, nutrition, and psychosocial factors) and nonmodifiable factors (such as genetics). If it is possible to identify unique modifiable factor/s that trigger, aggravate, or sustain airway inflammation in an individual child, it is possible to modify such factors positively; such modification is to reduce airway inflammation, to improve asthma symptoms, and thereby to reduce medicine requirements in a child with asthma. Of course, a detailed history of a child's environment, diet, triggers, and psychosocial factors is necessary for suspecting and/or identifying such factors.

In modern medicine, allergy interventions (allergy diagnosis, allergen avoidance, and allergen-specific immunotherapy) are best examples of individualization. Inhaled corticosteroids and leukotriene antagonists are important asthma preventer medications; however, they are helpful to control airway inflammation, but they do not treat "allergy," which is an immunological abnormality. If "allergy" is addressed by allergen avoidance or allergen-specific immunotherapy, need of preventer medications decreases. Role of individualization in allergy interventions is self-explanatory—a child with milk allergy would require milk reduction/avoidance, while a child with wheat allergy would require wheat reduction/avoidance. A child with house dust mite allergy would be benefitted by environmental measures and immunotherapy for the specific house dust mite, while the one with allergy to *Cynodon dactylon* (a pollen) would be benefitted by environmental measures and immunotherapy for the specific pollen. Thus, for example, for 10 same-aged children with same severity of asthma, preventer medications would be same, but allergy interventions would be different, specific, and individualized to each of them. Also, based on allergy diagnosis, diet changes and environmental modifications would also be different for each of them.

Common aeroallergens in children include house dust mites, molds, pollens, insect allergens, and pet danders, while common food allergens in children include proteins in milk and milk products, peanut, soy, wheat, Bengal gram, tree nuts, egg, fish, and shellfish.

Irritants in a child's environment can aggravate both allergic and nonallergic asthma, while aeroallergens usually aggravate symptoms in children who are allergic to specific allergen/s only. Detailed environmental history helps to identify exposure to a known or possible irritant/s in a child's environment. Important irritants in one's environment include cigarette smoke, biomass fuel smoke, vehicle emissions, industrial air pollutants, indoor sprays (for various uses such as insect control or fragrance), etc. Before suggesting environmental measures, it is important to know the patient's environment in detail, otherwise important details about presence of irritants in one's environment could be missed.

The next step is to educate parents about role of environmental factors in pediatric asthma, especially in terms of increased medication requirements and increased frequency of acute episodes. Avoidance of unnecessary use of irritants inside home could also be emphasized to build environmental literacy [1], especially because indoor air quality is important not only for asthmatic patients but also for other healthy family members [2]. Even if environmental history does not suggest exposure to a known irritant "among all rooms in the house, an asthmatic child's bedroom should be the best one in terms of exposure to sunlight, air circulation, and ventilation" can be a practical advice. It is also reasonable to educate all family members to quit smoking completely considering effects of second-hand and third-hand smoke exposure [3].

Role of diet in pediatric asthma is interesting as most pediatric asthma guidelines do not suggest specific dietary interventions, except for avoidance of food allergens for children with known food allergy. However, for an individual patient, emphasis on a balanced diet, avoidance of food additives, and correction of micronutrient deficiencies (whether contributing to asthma or not) could improve overall health.

For example, if a 4-year-old asthmatic child's diet consists of 50%–60% of milk products, it is reasonable to educate the parents about balanced diet, irrespective of the fact that role of milk products in asthmatic children without milk protein allergy is unproven. Similarly, intolerance to specific food additives (such as benzoate, tartrazine, etc.) has reported to cause asthma in a few individuals only, but for a specific asthmatic child whose diet includes daily packed foods, it is reasonable to consider a "trial" of freshly cooked food in home for a few weeks. These are examples of dietary interventions, which are individualized to a child and which are aimed at restoring healthy and balanced nutrition for improvement and maintenance of overall health, irrespective of diagnosis of asthma. Again, detailed diet history is essential before making such suggestions.

Considering diversity of foods and dietary habits across the world and complexities of immunological and digestive processes involved in processing of food in human body, it appears too ambitious to find a "universally proven" diet strategy for asthmatic children. Therefore, the fact that there are no "universal dietary guidelines for pediatric asthma" cannot change the fact that diet is cornerstone of health and a balanced diet has to be emphasized in every patient, irrespective of diagnosis.

Micronutrients are important in health and disease. Deficiencies of vitamin D, vitamin C, magnesium, zinc, selenium, etc., have been implicated in pediatric asthma, but their exact roles are unknown. However, if a micronutrient deficiency is suspected on the basis of other clinical clues, its correction could be part of health promoting approach and may benefit an asthmatic child indirectly or via unknown mechanisms.

For example, until exact role of vitamin C in pediatric asthma is proven, correction of vitamin C deficiency is likely to benefit asthmatic children by reducing respiratory infections [4], which are known to trigger asthmatic attacks. Similarly, correction of vitamin D deficiency may not "cure" pediatric asthma, but if it is detected on basis of laboratory investigations, its correction is important as a health promoting approach also.

Whether biochemic cell salt remedies are nutritional supplements or homeopathic medicines is a debate, however, if they are considered as nutritional supplements, detailed history of some asthmatic children may clearly point to indication of deficiency/-ies of one or more biochemic cell salts [5, 6]. For example, aggravation of symptoms by emotional stress may suggest deficiency of kali phosphoricum, while presence of white tongue may suggest deficiency of kali muriaticum or calcarea phosphorica.

As per theory of biochemic medicine, symptoms and signs in a patient result from cellular deficiency/-ies of specific salt/s and supplementation of the specific salt/s should restore the health. For selection of appropriate cell salt, detailed history and examination of the child are necessary, which include all the symptoms and signs (not only those related to asthma), their modalities (diurnal variations, seasonal variations, etc.), aggravating factors, improving factors, type of nasal discharge/expectoration, tongue examination, skin examination, etc.

If detailed history and examination of the child suggest deficiency of one or more salt/s, supplementation of them as per biochemic theory can be considered as a health promoting measure, if the physician thinks so. Use of biochemic cell salts as adjunct to conventional medicine requires consideration of possible pros and cons because of lack of clinical trials evaluating effectiveness and safety of biochemic cell salts in children. It also requires basic knowledge of homeopathy and biochemic cell salts on part of the clinician.

Physical activity and exercise are important modifiable factors. Obesity has complex relationship with asthma and weight reduction has shown to benefit obese asthmatic children [7]. Low physical activity has shown to increase risk of childhood asthma in some studies, while exercise is a known trigger of asthma [8]. Thus, knowing various factors such as lifestyle (sedentary versus active), triggers (exercise), specific needs (such as obesity, other comorbidities), and personal preferences are important to plan a personalized exercise program.

Regular practice of Yogic interventions has shown to improve control of pediatric asthma in several studies [9]. Examples of Yogic practices that benefit an asthmatic child include (but are not limited to) Surya Namaskar, Nadi Shodhana Pranayama, Kapalbhati Pranayama, Bhastrika Pranayama, Jala Neti, Kunjal Kriya, and various asanas. Again, like all other holistic systems, a Yoga program for a child is individualized to his/her present age and health status (not only focusing on asthma, but considering overall health such as respiratory health, cardiovascular health, digestive health, and mental/emotional health).

When considering integration of Yoga in conventional medicine, availability of a qualified Yoga instructor, age of child, and parental preferences should be considered.

Among modifiable factors, psychosocial factors need specific mention. Negative life events can source of both acute and chronic stress in children and can adversely affect asthma via both immunologic and nonimmunologic mechanisms [10]. For an asthmatic child, consideration of parental mental health is also important as parental stress, especially maternal stress has shown to be associated with poor prognosis of the child's asthma [11]. Thus, an appropriate psychological intervention should be done when a physician suspects role of stress in a child with asthma. Stress reducing measures can reduce stress-related aggravations and, therefore, can reduce overall medication requirements of the patient.

In modern medicine, childhood asthma is known to be associated with multiple comorbidities (allergic rhinitis, chronic sinusitis, gastroesophageal reflux disease, food allergy, obesity, atopic dermatitis, depression, behavioral disorders, etc.) [12]. As different asthmatic children have different comorbidities, it is important to diagnose and manage them simultaneously in every asthmatic child. For example, in a child with allergic rhinitis with asthma, simultaneous appropriate management of allergic rhinitis is likely to reduce need of asthma preventer medications, while in an obese asthmatic child, weight reduction is likely to improve asthma control.

3.3 RATIONAL INTEGRATION OF COMPLEMENTARY/ ALTERNATIVE SYSTEMS

The present model allows integration of Yoga in long-term management of pediatric asthma. There is also scope for integration of "nutritional homeopathy" if use of biochemic cell salts is considered a nutritional intervention.

Integration of Ayurveda requires specific mention. Ayurveda is a traditional system of medicine originated in India, which emphasizes the importance of individual unique "prakriti" (in English, word "constitution" can be best used to explain the concept of "prakriti") of a person. There are three "doshas"—kapha, pitta, and vata; doshas are abstract humors, which give rise of the unique "prakriti" of a person. Balance between three doshas is equivalent to optimum health, while imbalance between three doshas gives rise to a disease.

Identification of deficiency or excess of a dosha requires evaluation of physical and psychospiritual characteristics of a person in both healthy and diseased states, based on which appropriate lifestyle measures and Ayurvedic medicines can be suggested. As the present model focuses on interventions related to modifiable factors (diet, exercise, environment, and psychosocial factors), it does not include prescription of Ayurvedic medicines, which must be done by a qualified Ayurvedic physician. However, if a physician evaluates a child's pathophysiology from perspective of Ayurveda, it is possible to suggest changes in lifestyle or environment, which may be helpful to improve asthma.

As per Ayurveda, most asthmatic children are characterized by excess of kapha and/or vata doshas; imbalance of pitta dosha is seen in some patients. Thus, if detailed history of environment, diet, and psychosocial factors suggests any modifiable factor/s, which is known to produce imbalances in one or more doshas, appropriate measures can be suggested. For example, living in a warm room is an environmental measure, which balances excess kapha and vata doshas, especially when history suggests aggravation of symptoms in cold climate. Even when a child is not known to be allergic to house dust mites or molds, this simple environmental measures based on Ayurveda concepts could be helpful. Similarly, relaxation could be a practice, which balances excess vata dosha in an anxious asthmatic patient as anxiety is known to aggravate vata dosha. Thus, stress reduction is important for an asthmatic child not only from modern psychoneuroimmunology perspective, but also from Ayurveda perspective. Changes in diet and dietary habits can also be suggested based on principles of Ayurvedic nutrition. However, for making such suggestions, a clinician requires to have knowledge of basic principles of Ayurveda.

As core concept in the present model is "individualized" approach, which is aimed at decreasing requirement of controller medicines and emphasizing overall improvement of a child's health, there is also scope for integration of other complementary systems (such as music therapy, acupuncture, and acupressure) without increasing medicine requirement in the child. Of course, safety is priority while considering integration of complementary/ alternative systems; other important factors being knowledge of basics of the system, availability of expertise, legislations of the country, etc.

A proposed model for rational and safe integration of complementary/ alternative systems in clinical practice is shown in Figure 3.1.

3.4 HEALTH PROMOTION BY EDUCATION

The present model incorporates one or more measures that involve lifestyle modifications. For some of these measures, specific benefits in pediatric asthma may not be known, but they can be integrated if they have other health benefits (e.g., improved indoor air quality, a balanced diet with adequate micronutrients). Some of these measures may be easily acceptable (e.g., weight reduction for an obese child), while some of them may be not-so-easy to accept (e.g., quitting smoking by all family members). Therefore, parental education and patient education, when possible, are an essential component of the present model. Parental motivation and involvement in the child's long-term management are necessary and the clinician must discuss pros and cons of lifestyle modification/s that is/are suggested to the child, with clear mention of availability as well as nonavailability of scientific evidence.

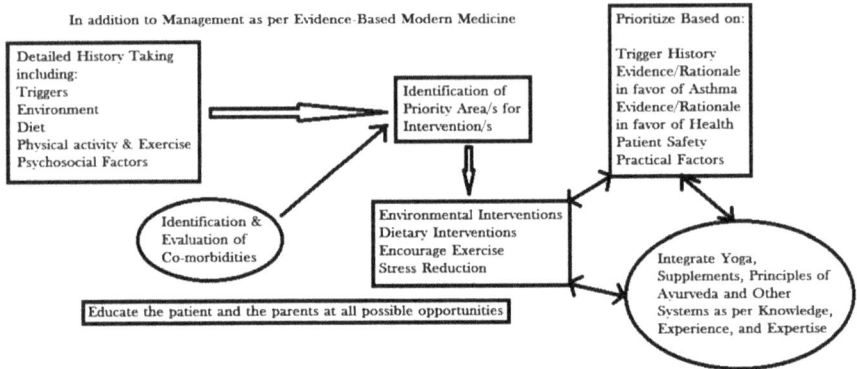

FIGURE 3.1 Model for rational and safe integration of complementary/alternative systems in clinical practice in management of pediatric asthma.

Detailed history taking is very important for identification of triggers, risk factors, comorbidities, and negative lifestyle factors, which also guide selection of health promoting measures that are important for an individual child. As emphasis is on individualization, the model does not recommend a "flowchart"-based strategy and is flexible to rationalized thinking, practical factors, and parental preferences. For example, for an adolescent who presents with asthma exacerbation before every examination, stress management would be the priority, while for an asthmatic child with known milk protein allergy, avoidance of milk products is the most desirable dietary change.

In author's clinical practice, the model has shown to eliminate need of controller medicines in some patients and to decrease dose of controller medicines in many patients, with additional benefits such as improved overall health of the patient, parental satisfaction, parental involvement, and improved drug compliance. The major limitation of this model is that it is difficult to make generalized recommendations because of highly individualized nature of the intervention/s. Another limitation is long time required for detailed history taking and counseling, but a dedicated pediatric asthma clinic can overcome this limitation.

Please note that discussion of proven and unproven environmental measures, dietary interventions, exercise strategies, stress management strategies, and basics of complementary/alternative systems are beyond the scope of this chapter. Interested readers are requested to refer literature related to the specific topic.

3.5 CONCLUSION

Pediatric asthma is a complex and multifactorial chronic disease and recent advances suggest existence of several subtypes and comorbidities. It is rational to consider every asthmatic child as unique and not to adhere to "one-size-fits-all" model. Further research is required in both conventional and complementary/alternative medicine systems to improve long-term prognosis of pediatric asthma.

KEYWORDS

- **childhood asthma**
- **integrative medicine**
- **complementary and alternative medicine**
- **personalized medicine**
- **lifestyle medicine**

REFERENCES

1. Perovich, L. J., Ohayon, L. J., Cousins, E. M., Morello-Frosch, R., Brown, P., Adamkiewicz, G. and Brody, J. G. (2018) Reporting to parents on children's exposures to asthma triggers in low-income and public housing, an interview-based case study of ethics, environmental literacy, individual action, and public health benefits. *Environmental Health*, 17, 48. https://doi.org/10.1186/s12940-018-0395-9 (accessed Jan 26, 2019).
2. Strom-Tejsen, P., Zukowska, D., Wargocki, P. and Wyon, D. P. (2016) The effects of bedroom air quality on sleep and next-day performance. *Indoor Air*, 26, 679–686. https://doi.org/10.1111/ina.12254 (accessed Jan 26, 2019).
3. Drehmer, J. E., Walters, B. H., Nabi-Burza, E. and Winickoff, J. P. (2017) Guidance for the clinical management of third hand smoke exposure in the child health care setting. *Journal of Clinical Outcomes Management*, 24, 551–559.
4. Hemila, H. (2017) Vitamin C and infections. *Nutrients*, 9, 339. https://doi.org/10.3390/nu9040339 (accessed Jan 26, 2019).
5. Boericke, W. and Dewey, W. A. (2014) The 12 tissue remedies of Schussler. New Delhi: B. Jain Publishers.

6. McCabe, V. (2009) The healing echo discovering homeopathic cell salt remedie. New Jersey: Basic Health.
7. Lang, J. E. (2014) Obesity and asthma in children: current and future therapeutic options. *Paediatric Drugs*, 16, 179–188.
8. Lochte, L., Nielsen, K. G., Petersen, P. E. and Platts-Mills, T. A. E. (2016) Childhood asthma and physical activity: a systematic review with meta-analysis and graphic appraisal tool for epidemiology assessment. *BMC Pediatrics*, 16, 50. https://doi.org/10.1186/s12887-016-0571-4 (accessed Jan 26, 2019).
9. Agnihotri, S., Kant, S., Mishra, S. K. and Singh, P. (2017) Role of yoga in childhood asthma. *Indian Journal of Traditional Knowledge*, 16, S21–S24.
10. Bloomberg, G. R. and Chen, E. (2005) The relationship of psychologic stress with childhood asthma. *Immunology and Allergy Clinics of North America*, 25, 83–105.
11. Yamamoto, N. and Nagano, J. (2015) Parental stress and the onset and course of childhood asthma. *Biopsychosocial Medicine*, 9, 7. https://doi.org/10.1186/s13030-015-0034-4 (accessed Jan 26, 2019).
12. Mirabelli, M. C., Hsu, J. and Gower, W. A. (2016) Comorbidities of asthma in US children. *Respiratory Medicine*, 116, 34–40.

CHAPTER 4

Holistic Healing Village: *Where Food Is Medicine*

ANN HOLADAY

Mahatma Gandhi University, Kerala, India

International and Inter University Centre for Nanoscience and Nanotechnology, Mahatma Gandhi University, Kottayam, Kerala, India; E-mail: jivaneesha@gmail.com

ABSTRACT

It is increasingly evident that diet and lifestyle play a pivotal role in chronic disease especially heart disease, diabetes and cancer. Research is now revealing that the quality and lack of diversity of food in the modern diet is a major risk factor in disease. It has proven that the processing of food e.g. additives, preservatives, artificial colorings, caking agents, emulsifiers, etc., interfere with the micro biome of the gut causing inflammation, weakens the immune system which is the cause of chronic illness. The human micro biome is designed to assimilate plant and animal nutrients sourced from unadulterated nature, not from food that has been altered for commercial reasons. Modern agriculture is a major player in the production of food using billions of tons of pesticides, chemical fertilizers, ripening agents and herbicides in particular glyphosate, the active ingredient in "Roundup." Food is grown for weight and appearance not for nutritional value which is severely compromised because soil does not rebuild when chemicals are used. Chemicals, antibiotics and hormones used in factory farming make agriculture a main contributor to water and soil pollution. Recent research has shown that the micro biome of soil is closely related to the human micro biome which gives credence to the theory that health depends on healthy soil to provide healthy food. The "Holistic Healing Village" explores an alternative approach to care by demonstrating an ancient ayurvedic principle "Food as Medicine" in a healing environment for those whose lives are devastated by chronic disease.

4.1   INTRODUCTION

The earth is in great peril due to the corporatization of agriculture, the sudden climate change creates a crisis, and the ever-increasing levels of global poverty, starvation, and desertification on a massive scale. The present condition of global trauma is not "natural," but a result of humanity's destructive actions. According to Masanobu Fukuoka, it is reversible. "We need to change, not only our methods of earth stewardship, but also the very way we think about the relationship between human beings and nature" [1]. Acquiring a good mental and physical health in our day-to-day life is somewhat luxury rather than right. Despite advanced technologies, research, and vast expenditures to achieve health, modern society is plagued with diseases such as cancer, diabetes, obesity, heart disease, allergies, pain, addiction, mental illness, and more. The causes of diet and lifestyle diseases are multifaceted and complex [2] to include stressful lifestyles, the breakdown of family, and most importantly access to real, natural food.

The quality and suitability of industrialized food and modern lifestyles are major factors. Food available to most people is far removed from what the human digestive system is designed to assimilate. Industrialized food is mass produced for weight, shelf-life, and uniformity, it is contaminated by chemicals, and is low in essential nutrition. This is due to modern-day farming practices, which are *monoculture.* Monoculture is the system of industrialized farming where large areas of the same crop are cultivated—even organic farming is mainly monoculture [3]. In monoculture, fertilizers, herbicides, and pesticides are required, along with an overuse of water, increased evaporation, erosion, and is a type of environmental disaster. Furthermore, it does not create soil whereas in sustainable, natural systems of farming, there is diversity, complexity, and positive interactions creating soil, rich in microorganisms necessary to sustain life on earth.

"Holistic Healing Village" offers an art of living in harmony with our mother nature. Principles of Ayurveda are combined with education, experience, and training in the "natural farming techniques" where diet and lifestyle model are created in which health, healing, and disease prevention can thrive [4]. The Holistic Healing Village deals with sustainable production of food, sustainable living, and a stress-free lifestyle. It can be a center of health education where communities can learn simple, sustainable living, natural farming, composting, recycling, and reusing of the natural resources. It can be the driving force behind innovation for living in harmony with nature where real food is the foundation.

Ayurveda recognizes the interconnectivity of body, mind, spirit, and importance of food in the healing process when it states that:

"When the diet is wrong, medicine is of no use"
"When the diet is right, medicine is of no need" [5]

Keywords: diet and lifestyle, agribusiness, climate change, holistic healing village, monoculture, pesticides, herbicides, sustainable living, water conservation, evaporation, erosion, industrialization, chemical farming, multicropping, genetic modification, superbugs, superweeds, Sustainable Development Goals, chronic illness, principle of the five elements, Prakriti, Purusha, Ayurveda, six tastes, Ama, Agni, refined food, gluten intolerance, intensive farming, Keeling curve, Vedic farming, zero budget farming, do-nothing farming, native American farming, fertility farming, self-sufficiency, Green Revolution.

4.2 HOLISTIC HEALING VILLAGE *"Where Food is Medicine"*

"Holistic Healing Village" concept is based on the fundamental right to live the way nature intended, providing pure food and water, pure air, and the freedom to be healthy. However, the current systems of food production and modern healthcare systems are based on economics rather than the welfare and sustainability of life on earth. Modern farming methods over the last 50 years have developed for quantity and appearance of food and the efficiency of production rather than the health-giving quality of food.

The "Green Revolution" began this process of industrialization after the Second World War when monoculture farming became normal farming practice. Chemicals were introduced to stimulate growth, pesticides to eliminate the risk of losing crops from infestations, and herbicides to eliminate weeds to make harvesting easier. More recently, the introduction of genetic modification has created another unnatural evolution in plant life where pesticides, herbicides, and fertilizers become part of the plant itself. Many foods have been genetically modified, so that they do not reseed naturally (terminator seeds); this means that the farmer cannot save seeds from year to year but has to buy every year. This has created great hardship for many farmers worldwide and made them slaves of the producers of seeds, pesticides, herbicides, and fertilizers. These farming methods have crept into the system without fully realizing the long-term effects on the earth and the multitude of living organisms, which have evolved over billions of years to create sustainable natural systems.

The modern healthcare system is a system of procedures to detect and treat disease. Although there is a lot of talk about disease prevention, the only preventative measures which are realistically taken are vaccinations. Research has shown vaccinations can be the cause of disease itself because of the use of aluminum, formaldehyde, and other chemicals used in their production. Scientific developments show that we are largely in the dark in determining the long-term effects of the use of drugs in healthcare and in chemical substances used in food production [6]. As time goes on, future generations will be subjected to chemical substances throughout their lives causing disease and affecting the quality of life.

Modern healthcare is centered around hospitals which are now profit centers where diagnostic and surgical procedures take place. They are places where patients go for a short period of time for acute care to either fight disease or be treated for traumatic conditions. They are expensive places to run, staff, and equip. Technological advancements have made them extremely efficient to do what they do effectively and costs are only going up. Nursing homes and rehabilitation centers are merely extensions of the hospital where people go to recover from procedures and take medication; these are not places intended to promote health, to rejuvenate, or to get well. Healthcare today is, in fact, sickness care where immediate needs are addressed but are not places where long-term treatment and support are effectively delivered or where patients can expect health to improve. In fact, hospitals can indeed be dangerous places as referenced by Gary Null in his book "Death by Medicine" [7]. The upsurge of "superbugs" such as methicillin-resistant *Staphylococcus aureus* caused by the overuse of antibiotics, the overall weak immune systems of present-day populations, and overly sterile conditions in hospitals is alarming.

Indeed, there is an urgent need to address the production of food and more effective ways to deliver long-term care. Modern healthcare and food production are both huge multibillion dollar industries owned by large corporations who can buy their way into governments to further their business goals. Changes in the present systems will have to be driven by grassroots movements worldwide who say "enough is enough, we can do better than this."

The United Nations General Assembly declared in 2015 17 "Sustainable Development Goals (SDGs): An Agenda for Transformation" to be achieved by 2030. "This declaration expresses the firm commitment to health for all, based on the inextricable link between the health of the next generation and the health of the planet." The five Ps were proposed as a framework for the SDGs "people, planet, prosperity, partnership, and peace" [8]. Population should be added to this list, which is incessantly talked about but numbers are only increasing. Humanity is straining the earth by consumerism not by its numbers [9]. The earth is big enough for everybody, there are enough natural resources, but if all we do is pollute the planet with current diet and lifestyles and corporate greed, life on earth is doomed [10].

The human body is a highly tuned machine which, when given the right fuel, performs efficiently and remains healthy but if not, eventually breaks down like any other machine. Advanced systems of modern medicine and holistic medicine cannot solve today's global health problems until the food available to the masses is what nature intends humans to eat. We are at a crossroads where unless we solve the critical issue of diet among the masses, optimum health cannot be achieved regardless of the system of medicine being practiced.

The Holistic Healing Village can initiate a movement to take the current crisis of environmental decline and bring people back to nature to care for themselves and the land. Natural medicine must come to the forefront of care for long-term chronic conditions, where modern medicine offers an acute care and little more than symptom control.

4.3 PRINCIPLES OF AYURVEDA

Ayurveda is an ancient well-accepted ethnic system in the Indian subcontinent since prebiblical era [11]. The core strength of Ayurveda is its integrated holistic approach to health and diseases using natural treatments derived from various medicinal plants. Laying emphasis on self-discipline and modest living with high human values, the system strongly advocates a unique set of assumptions and principles on diet and physical practices for a daily, healthy living. The classical Ayurvedic system was probably driven by insight, intuition, and astute observation of human behavior and of nature. "The soil is more important than the seed" concept underlies Ayurvedic treatment strategies [12].

Ayurveda, based on the "Principle of the Five Elements," is the science of life. The five elements are the energies of all living things and everything in nature. When these energies are balanced, there is optimal health and when out of balance, there is disease.

To truly understand the connection between living beings, food, and nature, it is important to grasp the Vedic view of creation which describes how evolution began. It is based in Samkhya philosophy and is the theory of existence, which recognizes 24 cosmic principles called the Tattvas [13].

First Cosmic Principle: Prakriti described as the base substance of the universe. It is unintelligent, unconscious, and inert but it possesses a potential manifestation power and potential that has three qualities: the quality of purity and balance (Sattva), potential for action (Rajas), and the quality of inertia or resistance to action (Tamas).

Prakriti is the first cause of the universe and accounts for whatever is physical which is matter and energy. As per Albert Einstein's theory of $e = mc^2$ which says that energy and matter are the same thing but are interchangeable; however, Einstein did not recognize Purusha.

Second Cosmic Principle: Purusha is the manifestor or the intelligence principle. It is pure, free, and independent. Puruṣha is neither produced nor does it produce—it just is.

First Stage of Creation: Prakriti is manifested by Purusha and begins to evolve into primal nature made up of the five elements from which all physical bodies derive. These are "earth," the densest element which has the five elements in it such as water, fire, air, and ether. "Fire" contains all the elements, except water earth, "water" contains all the elements, except earth, and "air" has the "ether" element in it [13].

Ayurveda describes the force of the elements not so much by their physical nature, although that is a factor, but by their qualities. Earth is the force of stability, water is the force of cohesion, fire is the force of transformation, air is the force of movement, and ether is the most pervasive element. Everything in nature consists of the five elements and it is the qualities of these elements, which provide characteristic property to a matter. According to the theory of creation, intelligence exists in each and every thing in nature including cells in the body and in every molecule of food. Nature has devised a symbiotic relationship between food and the digestive systems for all living beings, which means that the human digestive system can only derive energy from the food which nature has provided.

4.3.1 AYURVEDA'S CONNECTION TO FOOD

Ayurveda makes a very specific connection between the principle of the five elements and food by describing the six tastes. The modern diet is primarily aimed at taste; we rarely select our food because of its health benefits but rather because we like the taste. The Western diet is overwhelmingly sweet, sour, and salty and very little bitter, astringent, and pungent, which is why there is so much diabetes and obesity today. The tastes are not a one-size-fits-all but react differently in each individual according to digestion.

4.3.1.1 SIX TASTES

Ayurveda uses the tastes as a guide to treatment of various problems. To pacify space and air (Vata), the sweet, sour, and salty tastes are recommended. To pacify fire (Pitta), the bitter, astringent, and sweet tastes are used and to pacify water and earth (Kapha), the pungent, astringent, and bitter tastes are preferred. Herbs are also categorized according to taste and prescribed in the same way.

Sweet Taste (Madura): Sweet promotes the growth of tissues, nourishes, adds bulk to the body, and brings about contentment. But, the excess amount of sweet can cause weakness, laziness, heaviness, and also reduces the digestion rate. The sweet taste will soothe Vata and Pitta, but is aggravating for Kapha. We generally think of sugar as being the sweet taste, but there are many others such as honey, fruits, grains, potatoes, bread, milk, and rice. The refinement of sugar, flour, and rice is the cause of the recent upsurge of diabetes throughout the world. Homogenization of milk renders the fat molecules much smaller and fat is distributed through the milk instead of floating to the top. This may be the cause of many of the food allergies, so prevalent today. In addition, pasteurization destroys valuable bacteria in milk, which renders it more difficult to digest and digestion becomes weaker as a result. Milk, which was once considered to be the elixir of the Gods, today has very little health benefit.

Sour Taste (Amla)—Earth and Fire Elements: The sour taste aids digestion by promoting salivation and increases the digestive fire. Excess amount of sour causes burning sensations on throat, chest, and heart. The sour taste causes the retention of fluid, pacifies Vata but aggravates Kapha and Pitta. Various types of citrus fruit, fermented foods, vinegar, wine, and soy sauce are the main sour foods. The health benefits of wine have been promoted over recent years and as such have increased its consumption considerably. Ayurveda uses herbal and tonic wines as medicine, but only a tablespoon of wine mixed with water as an aperitif to aid digestion is taken.

Salty Taste (Lavana)—Water and Fire Elements: Salt promotes digestion and brings out the taste in food. Excess salt causes water retention, falling and graying of hair, hyperacidity, and infections. Salty pacifies Vata but is aggravating for Kapha and Pitta. Salt is very important to aid digestion but too much causes water retention which is why it is so valuable in the heat when there is a loss of water in the body, leading to dehydration. Ayurveda recommends controlled taking of salt intake; it is in all processed foods, especially canned foods and not recommended at all in home cooking. The best source of salt is mineral and salt from sea because there will be other trace minerals available. Table salt is too processed with decaking and bleaching agents, etc., but table salt contains iodine, which is important for thyroid health. Iodine is best taken as food and is rich in seaweeds, shrimp, etc.

Pungent Taste (Katu)—Air and Fire Elements: The pungent taste is most important for digestion as it helps to discharge oily and sticky waste products which will cause the production of Ama (the toxin produced by undigested food). The pungent taste is germicidal but in excess will cause weakness, thirst, emaciation, and fainting. Pungent pacifies Kapha and aggravates Vata and Pitta. Most diets may not contain adequate amounts of the pungent taste which are in garlic, onions, black pepper, and ginger [14] because of garlic and fresh olive oil. Fresh oils cannot be compared to the oil bought in the West which is old before it gets to the shelf and is why it is good practice to buy small amounts of oil from a good source.

Bitter Taste (Tikta)—Air and Ether Elements: The bitter taste has antibacterial and germicidal properties. If taken in excess, it will cause Vata diseases, dryness, roughness of vessels, and wasting. Bitter pacifies Kapha and Pitta and aggravates Vata. The bitter taste is present in spinach, green cabbage, fenugreek, turmeric, bitter melon, and coffee. The issue of coffee is a controversial one on which there are many opinions. Coffee is consumed in Italy as a cup or two of high quality, freshly ground, strong coffee taken in the morning. This is a lot different than what is commonly consumed in the United States. The bitter taste is very aggravating for Vata which is why we become jittery after too much and cannot sleep. The bitter taste is beneficial for diabetes. In Ayurveda, bitter melon, a vegetable in the squash family, is commonly used to treat diabetes.

Astringent Taste (Kashaya)—Air and Earth Elements: Astringent is a sedative, stops diarrhea and bleeding, promotes healing, and the absorption of fluids. In excess, it causes dryness of the mouth, constipation, retention of gas, and a weakened vitality. The astringent taste causes Vata diseases and pacifies Pitta and Kapha. Legumes or pulses, broccoli, cauliflower, artichoke, cranberries, grains, pomegranate, and radish are the astringent taste. Unripe bananas are eaten for the astringent taste [15].

A complete Indian meal with pickles, bitter melon, and sweet rice pudding is the most healthy of all diets because it has all of the tastes. But, this does not mean that an Ayurvedic diet has to be Indian food; all the tastes can be blended to create a healthy well-balanced diet in any culture.

Of course, there are certain things which the ancients could not have predicted when they devised this system of evaluating food and medicines. The main one is the industrialization of food, which has depleted micronutrients in the soils. The trace elements such as selenium and magnesium found in dark green leafy vegetables and essential for muscle health are found in soil and are seriously depleted. Potassium, a similar element to salt, is vital and many diets are not so much high in salt as low in potassium. The element iron is 1/12 of what it was 50 years ago. Trace elements and micronutrients are severely lacking in the modern diet.

4.3.2   *AYURVEDIC CONCEPT OF AMA AND AGNI*

Ama is the toxin produced by undigested food. Food, which is inappropriate, for example, food which digestion does not recognize, such as preservatives, additives, artificial colorings, flavorings, and chemicals used in processing. Ama circulates in the body and is the coating on the tongue that we often see in the morning. It becomes a slimy substance and the longer is stays in the body the more deeply rooted it becomes. It gets trapped in weak areas where there is inflammation such as the joints causing arthritis, arteries causing cholesterol, and plaques on the brain and tumors. Ama is the cause of disease which is why Ayurveda advocates regular detoxification.

Overeating, eating without hunger when the stomach is not ready to receive food, and a weak digestion cause the production of Ama. Food supplements, vitamins, and minerals will produce Ama as does medication. Genetic modification of food was not an issue in the days when Ayurveda was developed. However, science now determines that these genetic changes enter the system through the digestive tract. Even though there may not be any immediate effect, the long-term consequences of altering food for ourselves and for animals are a very dangerous game to be playing in terms of life on earth.

Modern medicine describes "leaky gut" which is Ama.

Ayurveda describes Agni the digestive fire, which transforms food in the digestive system into energy. Strong Agni is essential to good health and becomes weak when food is inappropriate for digestion. Modern science now describes the microbiome which is Agni indigestion.

4.4   EFFECTS OF PROCESSED FOOD ON HEALTH

Refined Food—creates significant problems in digestion. Bread and baked goods are mostly made of refined flour, which has very little nutritional value compared to whole grains. Jaggery, raw cane sugar, is rich in iron and trace minerals but white, refined sugar is a drug which has no value to the body whatsoever. Refined rice has all nutritional elements removed in the refining process leaving starch, so a bowl of polished rice is like eating a bowl of sugar. The incidence of diabetes throughout the world has reached endemic proportions due to the consumption of refined foods.

Gluten Intolerance—wheat is a heavy, sweet food and it takes a strong digestion to digest it. People, whose diet is high in refined foods, who have a Vata constitution, are in the Vata period of life or have weak digestive systems will have difficulty in digesting wheat. However, wheat has been a staple food since time in memorial and yet gluten intolerance is only a recent phenomenon. Wheat today is heavily genetically modified to resist the herbicide "roundup" so not only has the wheat been altered, it is sprayed with herbicide. Roundup is known to cause mitochondrial impairment, acute membrane damage, DNA damage, and cancer. These are serious consequences just to make farming more efficient. Furthermore, the nutritional value of commercially produced wheat is a fraction of that of heritage wheat and much higher in gluten content. However, it is 16 times more productive.

Gluten intolerance is the canary in the coal mine telling us there is something fundamentally wrong with wheat and yet there has been no attempt to take modified wheat off the market.

4.5   MODERN-DAY FARMING PRACTICES

Monoculture—is the agricultural practice of producing a single crop, plant, or livestock species, variety or breed in a farming system, at the same time. It is widely used in both industrial and organic farming and has allowed increased efficiency in planting and harvesting. Continuous monoculture is when the same species is grown year after year in the same fields, which leads to a rapid buildup and spread of pests and diseases. Most crops have a particular insect, fungus, or blight associated with them. In nature, these will attack weak plants so that the species develops resistance. If only one crop is planted, then the whole crop is wiped out by its specific infestation. A major cause of the potato famine in Ireland in the mid-1800s was caused by growing only one variety of potato, the Irish Lumper. A potato blight infected potato crops across Europe and in Ireland, the potato was the main food of the poor. Over a million, people died of starvation and another million emigrated because of it. Monoculture practice has been widely criticized for its environmental effects and for putting the food supply chain at risk.

Multicropping avoids this tragedy as does crop rotation which is closer to nature's patterning of diversity [16].

Pesticides and Herbicides—crops have specific pests which attack them and modern farming practices include pesticides to protect crops. This results in the gradual erosion of soil, an increase in pest resistance, and the unintended killing of pest's natural predators. Insects and weeds develop a resistance to pesticides and herbicides. Superweeds and superbugs have evolved so farmers are forced to use more and more, increasingly, toxic chemicals to get the same result. Nine of the 12 most dangerous and persistent organic chemicals are pesticides and they are very toxic to humans and other animals to say nothing of birds, worms, microorganisms in the soil, and invertebrates to name just a few. 98% of sprayed insecticides reach a destination other than their target, for example, air, water, bottom sediments.

The biggest issue with monoculture farming is that it does not build soil. The health of soil is crucial to the quality of food produced in terms of its nutritional value. Every time a crop is produced and it extracts nutrients from the soil which have to be restored. Modern farming uses chemicals instead of natural composted material. If this does not happen, the food produced eventually becomes worthless, it may look good, and be very uniform but it has very little nutritional value.

Intensive Factory Farming—as much as we can say that we can care about animal welfare in the modern world, the evidence of blatant cruelty and disregard for animals, birds, and fish in the name of consumption shows that we could not care less as long as we have animal protein and fish to eat. Humans do not have the right to exploit other species to this extent for their own greed. If we just took what we needed and respected the animals that sacrifice their lives to provide food for us as the ancients did would be one thing, but it is not the case in modern farming practices. Billions of animals are slaughtered daily throughout the world for human consumption without any regard for the fact that they too deserve a place on earth. They have the right as we do to breathe fresh air, to eat the food that nature provides, to love and nurture one another, and to raise their young. We seems to be blind to it and yet we get enraged when poachers in another country slaughter elephants for their tusks, when the Orca whale is carrying her young pup after its death as if the animals we eat did not have any feelings.

We are already paying the price for this abuse in diseases related to diet and lifestyle. We learn in Ayurveda that humans do not have the digestive tract to digest meat. The tract of carnivores is short, so that elimination after digestion is very quick. The human tract is designed to digest plant material and is long which means that meat stays in the tract too long and rots in the gut creating toxins (Ama).

Ayurveda tells us that our food has to have life (Prana) in it in order to sustain life. If a piece of meat is put in the ground, it rots but if a seed is put in the ground, it grows because it has life. Ayurveda also tells us that our food has energy and this energy affects us. When an animal has suffered, been deprived of a natural life, and fed unnatural food, it not only gets physically sick but negative energy goes into the meat. It is any wonder that loneliness, isolation depression, fear, and anxiety are a normal part of modern-day living.

Because animals, birds, and fishes are in such unnatural conditions in factory farms, they develop diseases. Antibiotics are routinely given to livestock, which ends up in meat for consumption. Animals are often fed growth hormones, which also contaminate meat. The antibiotics and hormones in manure from factory farmed animals end up in soils and water supply and what should be a benefit to the land is in fact toxic waste. Cows have a ruminant digestive system where the stomach has four compartments to digest grass but are fed grain in intensive farming. Cows are fed genetically modified soy, which affects the milk and meat which ultimately affects the consumer [17].

4.5.1   ENVIRONMENTAL IMPACT OF MODERN FARMING PRACTICES

Modern farming practices do not produce soil; therefore, over time, it becomes depleted and eventually useless resulting in food deficient in nutrients and minerals. Even though inputs such as fertilizers and organic materials produce a short-term gain, the soil does not have the capacity to restore itself. Manure from factory farms, where animals are given antibiotics, will destroy the natural bacteria in soil, which breaks down organic material. Artificial fertilizers, pesticides, and herbicides are not only harmful in food. They are pollutants in water systems getting into wells, aquifers, rivers, and eventually into the ocean. Even though water systems can be purified, eventually the environment suffers resulting in the loss of species. Worms and other living organisms die in soil where there are artificial fertilizers, pesticides, and herbicides. Phosphorus and nitrogen are used to increase plant growth in intensive farming causing pollutants in streams, rivers, and oceans. Only 20% of phosphorus and nitrogen is actually used on the fields, the rest fuels toxic algae blooms destroying coral reefs, seagrasses, and killing fish. At the current rate, it is expected to rise exponentially in the next 10 years.

(A)

(B)

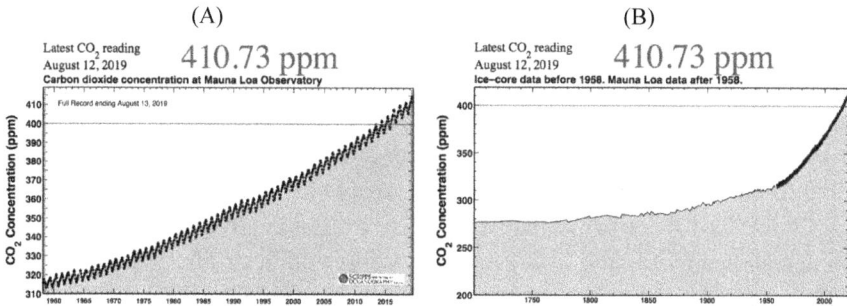

FIGURE 4.1 Effect of *Carbon Dioxide* in the Atmosphere

The major cause of global warming is increased carbon dioxide in the atmosphere much of which is the result of burning fossil fuels. The destruction of plant life and industrialized farming contributes significantly to carbon dioxide levels, which are accelerating at an alarming rate. Charles David Keeling devised a precise measurement of atmospheric carbon dioxide charted in the left-hand graph called the "Keeling curve." The vertical lines show an increase in carbon dioxide during the autumn and winter when leaves and vegetation are rotting and a decrease during the spring and summer when plant life converts carbon dioxide to chlorophyll in photosynthesis. Photosynthesis forms the basis of the food chain and occurs in green plants and algae. It is the process by which sunlight combines with carbon dioxide, water, and chlorophyll to produce energy.

The Keeling curve on the right shows an exponential increase in carbon dioxide levels since the industrial revolution. Up until that time, carbon dioxide levels were constant [18]. The increase is partially due to the burning of fossil fuels but the decimation of plant life particularly trees is a significant factor. Melting permafrost is now contributing significantly and we are approaching dangerous levels of carbon dioxide in the atmosphere [19]. Recent levels are 410 parts per million whereas in 2018, it was 406.70 ppm which is a significant increase in less than 3 years.

The earth is a living organism, which has an abundance of the five elements to support life. What we see in nature today did not appear overnight, it took billions of years to get to the place where the simplest forms of life could exit. The earth is our mother, but we create huge scars on her with mining, we suck her life blood when we take oil from her body, and cover her with concrete so that she cannot breath. Natural systems which sustain life on earth are being pushed to a tipping point.

4.5.2   *CARBON DIOXIDE IN THE ATMOSPHERE AND CLIMATE CHANGE*

The earth is a living organism which has an abundance of the five elements to support life. What we see in nature today did not appear overnight, it took billions of years to get to the place where the simplest forms of life could exits. The earth is our mother, but we create scars on her with mining, we suck lifeblood from her when we take oil from and cover her with concrete so that she cannot breath. Natural ecosystems which sustain life on earth are being pushed to a tipping point to where the earth will be unable to recover.

Our earth is under stress as manifested by global warming of which a major cause is increased carbon dioxide in the atmosphere as a result of burning fossil fuels (emissions). Industrialized agriculture and deforestation contribute significantly to carbon dioxide levels which are accelerating at an alarming rate.

4.5.2.1   *THE KEELING CURVE*

Charles David Keeling devised a precise measurement of atmospheric carbon dioxide, charted in a graph called the "Keeling Curve." Data is collected by Scripts CO_2 program from the Mauna Loa Observatory since 1958. Prior to 1958 was from ice-core data. This graph demonstrates the exponential increase in carbon dioxide levels starting at the time of the industrial revolution with a more dramatic increase since 1958. Before the industrial revolution CO_2 levels were more or less constant between 250 and 300 ppm even when the earth cycled through dramatic climatic changes 18]. The present increase is not only due to emissions but the decimation of plant life particularly old forests and trees. Melting permafrost is a significant contributing factor due to melting ice caps. We are now approaching dangerous levels of carbon dioxide in the atmosphere [19]. Recent levels in May of 2021 418.41ppm whereas in 2018 it was 406.70 ppm which is a significant increase in just four years.

This graph shows a closer view of the curve after 1958 when measurements of CO_2 were taken at regular intervals throughout the year. The vertical lines show an increase in carbon dioxide during the autumn and winter when leaves and vegetation are rotting and a decrease during the spring and summer when plant life converts carbon dioxide to chlorophyll in photosynthesis. Photosynthesis forms the basis of the food chain and occurs in green plants and algae. It is the process by which sunlight combines with carbon dioxide, water and chlorophyll to produce energy.

May 11, 2021

Carbon dioxide concentration at Mauna Loa Observatory

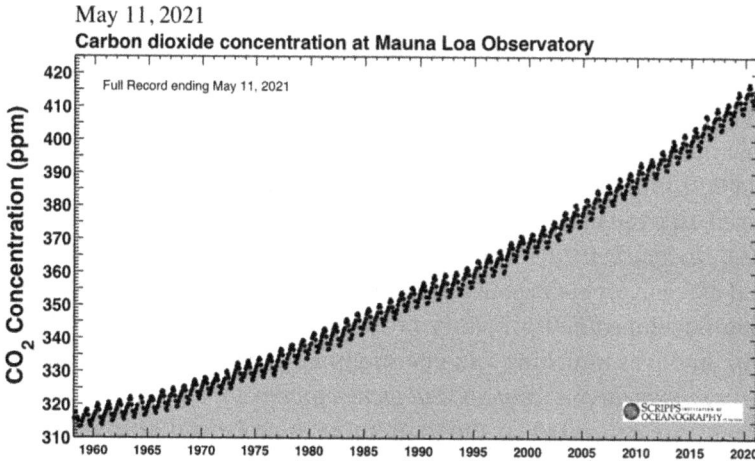

FIGURE 4.2

4.6 NATURAL FARMING

Natural farming supports an ecosystem with diversity, complexity, and positive interactions resulting in on-going building of soil, rich in microorganisms necessary to provide a sustainable food supply which has all the nutrients and minerals necessary for health. Microorganisms breakdown organic material much like digestion, water and heat are required, and there are insects, bugs, worms, small mammals, and manure all working together to create soil. Composted material on the farm becomes the soil for plants grown [20].

It is an on-going process where plants take nutrients from the soil and soil is rebuilt. Roots of trees open up the soil and aerate it as do small mammals such as moles. The process is sustainable creating soil, rich in microorganisms, bacteria, fungi, micronutrients, and trace minerals. A natural farm uses 4% of a monoculture site to grow the same amount of food.

Indigenous peoples have managed the earth with sophisticated agriculture systems up until about 150 years ago when modern farming began to ignore the health of soil and traditional knowledge was lost. We have to reeducate ourselves to understand how natural systems interact to sustain life on earth.

4.6.1 METHODS OF NATURAL FARMING

Rishi Kheti or Vedic Farming: In India, natural farming is also known as "Rishi Kheti" in India, a practice which includes ancient Vedic principles of farming including the use of animal wastes and herbs for controlling pests and promoting growth. The Rishis, sages of ancient India, used products from the cow such as buttermilk, milk, curd, and cow urine for preparing growth promoters. Vedic farming follows the Law of Ahimsa (nonviolence) without the use of chemical fertilizers and pesticides. High quality, organic, and natural food is produced, which has medicinal value. Vedic farming is practiced all over India today [21].

Zero Budget/Spiritual Farming: The Indian agriculturist Subhash Palekar studied extensively on this method of farming which is a variation of natural farming developed and primarily practiced in Southern India. Zero budget farming involves mulching and intercropping [*definition: two or more crops which complement one another and grown together*]. Preparations, including cow dung, are generated on site to promote microbe and earthworm activity in the soil [22].

Native American Farming Practices: Native American tribes worked the land in strikingly similar ways to today's natural farmers and did so for over 10,000 years. According to contemporary Native Americans, it is only through interaction and relationships with native plants that mutual respect is established. Knowledge and the management of California's natural resources by Native Americans who recall what their grandparents told them about how and when areas were burned, which plants were eaten and which were used for basketry, and how plants were tended. The complex picture that emerges from this and other historical source material dispels the hunter-gatherer stereotype long perpetuated in anthropological and historical literature. We come to see California's indigenous people as active agents of environmental change and stewardship. Tending the wild persuasively argues that this traditional ecological knowledge is essential if we are to successfully meet the challenge of living sustainably [23].

Masanobu Fukuoka was trained as a scientist; he rejected both modern agribusiness and centuries of agricultural practice, deciding instead that the best forms of cultivation mirror nature's own laws. Over the next three decades, he perfected his so-called "do-nothing" technique, common sense, sustainable practices that all but eliminate the use of pesticides, fertilizers, tillage, and perhaps most significantly, wasteful effort.

One-straw Revolution: By Masanobu Fukuoka—Fukuoka's inspiring book that was first published in English in 1978. The One-Straw Revolution is an ecological farming method described as "do-nothing farming" avoiding inputs and equipment [24].

Sowing Seeds in the Desert: *Natural Farming, Global Restoration, and Ultimate Food Security*: This book is a summation of many years of travel and research and is Fukuoka's last major work and perhaps his most important work. Fukuoka spent years working with people and organizations in Africa, India, Southeast Asia, Europe, and the United States to prove that you could indeed grow food and regenerate forests with very little irrigation in the most desolate of places. "Only by greening the desert," he said "would the world ever achieve true food security" [1].

Fertility Farming—Fertility Pastures: Newman Turner explored an approach to farming that makes minimal use of plowing, eschews chemical fertilizers and pesticides, and encourages cover cropping and manure application [21]. Newman Turner holds that the foundation of the effectiveness of a fertile soil—and the measure of a fertile soil—is its content of organic matter, ultimately, its humus. Upon a basis of humus, nature builds a complete structure of healthy life—without need for disease control of any kind. In fact, disease treatment is unnecessary in nature, as disease is the outcome of the unbalancing or perversion of the natural order and serves as a warning that something is wrong. The avoidance of disease is, therefore, the simple practice of natural law. Newman Turner's advice for building a productive, profitable organic farming system rings as true today as it did 60 years ago when it was written and details his methods of intensive pasture-based production of beef and dairy cows [25] in this practical guide to profitable, labor-saving livestock production. He developed a system of complex herbal mixtures or blends of pasture grasses and herbs, with each ingredient chosen to perform an essential function in providing a specific nutrient to the animal or enhancing the fertility of the soil. He explains his methods of cultivation, seeding, and management [26, 27].

Permaculture Farming: This type of farming uses the principles described but goes beyond and is more scientific. It integrates food production and the home and/or "hospital" as in the proposed "Holistic Healing Village" to create a sustainable living system that minimizes the impact on the environment [28]. Permaculture is about designing sustainable human settlements. It is a philosophy and an approach to land use, which weaves together microclimate, annual and perennial plants, animals, soils, water management, and human needs into intricately connected productive communities [29]. It promotes the use of natural fertilizers making use of natural carbon cycles, so that waste from plants becomes the fertilizer for another. Permaculture regards the farm as an energy bank and aims to close the energy loop by optimizing what is already there. Minerals are always lost every time produce is sent to market but in permaculture, energy used by one element is passed on for the benefit of other elements. Plants are allowed to reseed and are interplanted for pest control.

Permaculture design maximizes diversity of produce and plant life and all space is used effectively and efficiently. A site looks more like a food-forest with open glades full of herbs and perennials rather than food grown in rows. Nature's methods are imitated by conserving soil and water and optimizing natural energies such as wind, dust, leaves, bird, and animal droppings. Permaculture methods are capable of converting landscapes. For example, plants grown along polluted rivers or roadsides can filter out toxins and break them down to safer levels. A well-designed system is the foundation for nutritious food and habitat for people and animals.

For maximum nutritional value, produce should be eaten less than 3 hours after harvesting. Permaculture reduces the huge transportation costs in the modern system by bringing food production closer to the consumer. It is a complex science where design is important and it can be applied to home gardens, rooftops, community spaces, and commercial enterprises. It has the potential to revolutionize the way plant life is cultivated all over the world. It can provide meaningful work where knowledge is essential to all those who work on the farm. People contribute toward the production of food in their daily lives becoming self-sufficient and as they experience living in harmony with nature, they become excited about sustainable living. Communities naturally develop around the farm and it becomes an ever-evolving process.

Bill Mollison, cofounder of the permaculture movement, stated "permaculture, like a bicycle, is adaptable and has great potential but is only as good as the user." Permaculture (permanent culture) is the conscious design and maintenance of agriculturally productive ecosystems, which have the diversity, stability, and resilience of natural ecosystems. The main objective of permaculture is to create certain living environments, which are sustainable and productive. It is the harmonious integration of landscape and people providing their food, energy, shelter, and other material and nonmaterial needs in a sustainable way. Permaculture design is a system of assembling conceptual, material, and strategic components in a pattern, which functions to benefit life in all its forms. The philosophy behind permaculture is one of working with rather than against nature, of protracted and thoughtful observation rather than protracted and thoughtless action, of looking at systems in all their functions rather than asking only one yield of them, and of allowing systems to demonstrate their own evolutions [30].

4.7   HOLISTIC HEALING VILLAGE FOR CHRONIC ILLNESS

A total of 25% of adults in the USA have at least two chronic conditions and chronic disease constitutes a major cause of mortality. The World Health Organization attributes 38 million deaths per year to noncommunicable disease [31].

The definition of chronic conditions is one that is persistent or longstanding and develops over a long period of time and is distinguishable from acute disease which is recent onset. The course of disease lasts for more than 3 months and often lifelong. It can be a recurrent condition, which can relapse repeatedly with periods of remission. Chronic disease is noncommunicable distinguished by its noninfectious causes. Some chronic diseases such as HIV/AIDS are caused by transmissible infections.

Loneliness is a big issue in modern society, especially for the elderly and those with chronic mental and physical conditions. The family unit has almost disappeared and in ^^the "me" society, people are used to managing their lives alone. This works when young, healthy and financially viable but without good health and/or financial security people become dependent on help from others. In modern society, there is no framework whereby people can support one another. People suffering from chronic, debilitating conditions are often young with their lives ahead of them. They may be alone without support and have difficulty in managing without help; they are often unable to continue working and to support themselves financially. They may end up in an apartment building in one room all day with nothing but the TV and internet for company. They may not be able to go outside and even if they are able, cannot enjoy nature. Depression and suicide are not uncommon.

Modern medicine has little to offer chronic illness other than band-aid solutions, which never get to the root cause of afflictions. However, natural systems of medicine have a great deal to offer but it takes time and long-term results are only effective if the patient maintains the practices as a way of life. Short, intermittent periods of treatment provide a limited benefit.

Holistic health providers believe that each person is an individual and has the capacity to learn how to take care of their own health. Individuals must experience health to be inspired, so that if they leave the village they know what they must do to maintain good health. A loving, caring, welcoming, and mutually supportive environment will be created in the village where everyone not only learns to help themselves, but to help others.

The Holistic Healing Village gives everyone a chance to become a participating member of a community. Once patients become more mobile and their overall strength and well-being improves, they become more active and are able to contribute to the community in whatever capacity they are able. This concept not only provides an opportunity for carers and support staff, but also for patients to learn to look after themselves and be independent.

4.7.1   COMMON CHRONIC DISEASE DIAGNOSES

4.7.1.1   MENTAL DISORDERS

Autism, anxiety, stress, post-traumatic stress disorder (PSD), depression, addictions, insomnia, dementia, and Alzheimer's disease—are all suitable for treatment in a Holistic Healing Village setting.

4.7.1.2   MOTOR NEURONE DISEASES

Amyotrophic Lateral Sclerosis [32]:

- *Common name*—Lou Gehrig's disease.
- *Pathology*—Specific disease which causes the death of neurons controlling voluntary muscles.
- *Incidence*—About 5%–10% of cases are inherited from a person's parents. The disease can affect people of any age, but usually starts around the age of 60 years and in inherited cases around the age of 50 years. The average survival from onset to death is 2–4 years.
- *Prevalence*—In Europe and the United States, the disease affects about two people per 100,000 per year.

Progressive Muscular Atrophy:

- *Common name*—muscular dystrophy
- *Pathology*—affects both the upper and lower motor neurons

Progressive Bulbar Palsy:

- *Pathology*—motor neurone disorder attacking the nerves supplying the bulbar muscles characterized by the degeneration of motor neurons in the cerebral cortex, spinal cord, brainstem, and pyramidal tracts.
- *Incidence*—Slow in onset with symptoms starting in most patients around 50–70 years of age.

Primary Lateral Sclerosis:

- *Pathology*—progressive muscle weakness in the voluntary muscles
- *Primary lateral sclerosis is a rare condition and the incidence is uncertain*
- *Motor neuron disease* also includes hereditary spastic paraplegia, pseudobulbar palsy, and spinal muscular atrophies.

4.7.1.3   AUTOIMMUNE DISEASES

Autoimmune disease is a condition in which the immune system mistakenly attacks normal cells. The immune system normally guards against bacteria and viruses and sends out cells to attack these foreign invaders. The immune system can normally tell a normal cell from a virus or bacteria, but in autoimmune disease, it attacks normal cells. Examples are celiac disease, diabetes mellitus type 1, Graves' disease, inflammatory bowel disease, multiple sclerosis, psoriasis, rheumatoid arthritis, systemic lupus erythematosus, fibromyalgia, and chronic fatigue syndrome [33].

Multiple Sclerosis:

- *Pathology*—The most common immune-mediated disorder affecting the central nervous system. It is a demyelinating disease in which the insulating covers of nerve cells in the brain and spinal cord are damaged
- *Incidence*—In 2015, about 2.3 million people were affected globally with rates varying widely in different regions and among different populations. That year about 18,900 people died from MS, up from 12,000 in 1990
- *Prevalence*—The disease usually begins between the ages of 20 and 50 years and is twice as common in women as in men.

Lupus:

- *Common name*—Systemic lupus erythematosus
- *Pathology*—Aautoimmune disease in which the body's system mistakenly attacks healthy tissue in many parts of the body
- *Incidence*—Rate of systemic lupus erythematosus varies between countries from 20 to 70 per 100,000
- *Prevalence*—Women of childbearing age are affected about nine times more often than men. While it most commonly begins between the ages of 15 and 45 years, a wide range of ages can be affected.

Those of African, Caribbean, and Chinese descent are at higher risk than White People

4.7.1.4 NEUROMUSCULAR DISEASE

Parkinson's Disease:

- *Common name*—Stiff-man syndrome
- *Pathology*—Long-term degenerative disorder of the central nervous system that mainly affects the motor system
- *Incidence*—In 2015, Parkinson's disease affected 6.2 million people and resulted in about 117,400 deaths globally
- *Geographic prevalence*—Typically occurs in people over the age of 60 years, of which about 1% is affected. Males are more often affected than females at a ratio of around 3:2. When it is seen in people before the age of 50 years, it is called young-onset PD

Cerebral Palsy:

- *Pathology*—Group of permanent movement disorders that appear in early childhood
- *Incidence*—It occurs in about 2.1 per 1000 live births. In those born at-term, rates are lower at 1 per 1000 live births
- *Geographic prevalence*—Cerebral palsy is the most common movement disorder in children. The rate is higher in males than in females; in Europe, it is 1.3 times more common in males. The prevalence rates converge toward the average rate of 2:1000

Muscular Dystrophy:

- *Pathology*—Group of muscle diseases that results in increasing weakening and breakdown of skeletal muscles over time. It occurs due to mutations in genes that are involved in making muscle proteins. This can occur due to either inheriting the defect from one's parents or the mutation occurring during early development
- *Incidence*—Affects about one in 5000 males at birth

Spina Bifida [34]:

- *Pathology*—Bbirth defect where there is incomplete closing of the backbone and membranes around the spinal cord

- *Incidence*—Rates of other types of spina bifida vary significantly by country from 0.1 to 5 per 1000 births
- *Prevalence*—On average, in developed countries, it occurs in about 0.4 per 1000 births. In the United States, it affected about 0.4 per 1000 births and in India, about 1.9 per 1000 births

4.8 CHARACTERISTICS OF A HOLISTIC HEALING VILLAGE

4.8.1 PHYSICAL CHARACTERISTICS

Vaidyagrama, in Kerala, India has all the components of a Holistic Healing Village. In fact, many of the concepts in this paper have been inspired by Vaidyagrama [35].

- *Farm*—There should be at least 5–10 acres of land to develop a natural farm with a Holistic Healing Village integrated into it to serve the village and surrounding community. Design of the farm itself is of utmost importance taking into consideration water and waste management, sunlight, slopes, etc., so that all areas are used to their fullest potential and maximized for growing. It may not be possible to develop a new farm, but to work with surrounding farms. In this case, farmers would be guided into natural farming, so that a cooperative effort is achieved. Permaculture farming is a science, which takes training and expertise; it is not a haphazard method and takes time to develop. The farm should be as close as possible to a closed system where all waste stays on the farm, composted, and goes back to the land.
- *Buildings*—Wherever possible, natural materials sourced locally are used. Sustainable power sources and waste management systems are implemented and are part of the plan. Buildings should be placed according to Vastu and constructed in such a way as to trap breezes to avoid air conditioning and minimize the need for heat. In some cases, there may already be a building which has to be used initially and worked into the plan, but in most cases, it is easier and less expensive to start from scratch rather than adapt existing buildings mainly because of the handicap access issue.
- *Healing Center*—It is of modular construction. Each modular unit carefully designed and replicated throughout. The advantage here is that one can start small and add accordingly. Modules are placed in a square alignment, so that there are large gardens enclosed between the

modules for growing herbs, medicinal plants, trees for shade, edible flowers, and food.

- *Module*—It consists of four units each approximately 700 square feet providing simple accommodation for one or two people. There are two treatment rooms to each module one for men and one for women and a small utility kitchen for making tea and small meals.
- *Unit*—It has a bedroom with two single beds designed, so that they can be together or separate. It has a large bathroom with walk-in shower dressing area and toilet. There is a dining area that can be used as an office and a covered patio off the bedroom for outdoor living
- *Connectivity*—The units are connected by wide-covered pathways interconnecting all areas of the village providing freedom of movement for all residents. The client units are in the central zone of the village with activity facilities, staff housing, on the periphery. Pathways are wide enough for wheelchairs and walkers with sitting areas intermittently placed, so that the whole village is a place for social interaction.
- *Kitchen*—The kitchen is the central focus of operation where pure, simple, and fresh food is prepared. It is also a place large enough for classes for clients to participate. At Vaidyagrama, food is delivered to the rooms in a tiffin (a vacuum, insulated container). This is just one. For example, there could be other ways for food to be managed. As food is the most important aspect of the village, this aspect has to be carefully considered in the plan.
- *Administrative Offices, Laundry, Classrooms, Meeting Rooms, Library, Cafe, and Exercise Rooms* would be on the periphery with covered pathways leading to them. A wide pathway surrounds the central zone, wide enough for a golf cart for delivery of heavy items and supplies.
- *Traffic*—There are no motorized vehicles within the village. Only a water-permeable pathway surrounding the units for delivery purposes, golf carts could be used. The village is completely self-sustainable with water purification and sewage systems. Plastic is not allowed in the village and everything used is reused or recycled. Only renewable sources of energy are available and electromagnetic radiation is minimized. Drugs and alcohol are not allowed on the premises [36].

4.8 "CAMP HILL" PROJECT [37]

It was originally started in Scotland. Camp Hill is an international, intentional community for children with learning disabilities. The main focus of this project is biodynamic farming [38], which is similar to other natural farming methods with a spiritual and astrological component. The "Camp Hill" project is based on the concept of Seva *(sanskrit word meaning service to others)* and is largely run by volunteers. There are many different skills to be learned at Camp Hill including self-sufficiency, care of animals, cooking, and how to contribute to community life. Cottage industries such as pottery are encouraged.

4.10 DOCUMENTATION

A considerable issue that holistic medicine faces is that it does not have a meaningful system of documenting the success (or failure), side effects, and so on, of treatment. There are many modalities in natural healing, which address all aspects of the human condition and its tendency toward complete health. However, standardized documentation should be an integral part of treatment. It takes many years for a disease to develop and so it can take as long to bring the disease to a manageable level. Holistic medicine does not necessarily talk about cure, even though that does happen, the intent is to bring clients with debilitating diseases to a place where they can take an active part in their communities, have a meaningful purpose in life, and be independent.

Documentation is crucial to the ongoing success of this project, so that treatment protocols can be written for specific conditions and replicated in holistic villages throughout the world. What makes it difficult is that Ayurveda treats the individual not the disease neither of which are standard. However, with modern computerized systems, this should not be an obstacle. When treatment protocols are established, this database could be accessed from all over the world providing guidelines for treatment to all those who suffer. It is, therefore, important for the Holistic Healing Village to be connected to university settings where clinical trials can be launched.

4.11 SUMMARY

The principle foundation of "Holistic Healing Village" is the food grown in naturally sustained soil, rich in micronutrients, minerals, and trace elements managed in such a way as to provide an abundance of food for the village and surrounding community. It can be adapted to almost any circumstance combining natural farming and holistic health systems under the umbrella of

Ayurveda. It can be a center for learning the art of growing food, cooking, self-sufficiency, and the care of others. It can be a health education center for pregnancy, baby and child care, addiction, elder care, etc., and a community center to include dancing, yoga, and even schools could be integrated. "Holistic Healing Village" could potentially change the way society views itself giving those without hope and in isolation a purpose. It could transform communities plagued by violence and oppression by providing meaningful work and opportunities to develop skills and express desires and pave the way to a new future.

Modern medicine tells us that we are living longer because of technological advances, but what is the value of longevity when the biggest issues today are loneliness, isolation, mental illness, and poor health. As practitioners, we know that healing will only work when habits which have created the problem are changed to benefit health, rather than causing disease. We know that the natural state of the body and mind is a healthy one. We see remarkable results just from creating a healing environment to include pure food and water and relief from stress when the body and mind are given a chance to heal.

"Holistic Healing Village" revisits old values bringing food production locally and integrating these values into lifestyles, which enable optimal physical and mental health for humans, healthy plant life and trees, healthy animals, birds, insects, etc., providing a sustainable environment in which all life can thrive.

> The law of karma says "if we have the means to create a problem, so do we have the power to correct it"

> "We have the power to change the way we live. We have the knowledge to benefit all living beings and the environment rather than be the problem for them."

KEYWORDS

- **Ayurveda**
- **permaculture**
- **sustainable living**
- **diet and lifestyle**
- **chronic illness**

REFERENCES

1. Fukuoka, M. (2013). Sowing Seeds in the Desert: Natural Farming, Global Restoration, and Ultimate Food Security. United States: Chelsea Green Publishing.
2. Jamison, D. T., Breman, J. G., Measham, A. R., Alleyne, G., Claeson, M., Evans, D. B. and Musgrove, P. (2006). Disease Control Priorities in Developing Countries. United States: The World Bank.
3. https://en.wikipedia.org/wiki/Monoculture.
4. https://en.wikipedia.org/wiki/Natural_farming.
5. Yeung, A. W. K., Mocan, A. and Atanasov, A. G. (2018). Let food be thy medicine and medicine be thy food: a bibliometric analysis of the most cited papers focusing on nutraceuticals and functional foods. *Food Chemistry*, 269, 455–465.
6. Lyons-Weiler, J. and Ricketson, R. (2018). Reconsideration of the immunotherapeutic pediatric safe dose levels of aluminum. *Journal of Trace Elements in Medicine and Biology*, 48, 67–73.
7. Null, G., Carolyn-Dean, M. D., Feldman, M., Rasio, D. and Smith, D. (2011). Death by Medicine (p. 2). United States: Axios Press.
8. United Nations Sustainable Development goals 2015 www.un.org/sustainabledevelopment/ sustainable-development-goals.
9. https://artdary.net/pdf/fertility-p.
10. Cleveland, D. A. (2013). Balancing on a Planet: The Future of Food and Agriculture (Vol. 46). California: University of California Press.
11. Caraka, Sharma, P. V., Jejjaṭa, Agniveṣa and Dṛḍhabala. (1994). Caraka-Saṃhitā: Agniveśa's treatise (text with English translation). 3 Critical notes (Sūtrasthāna to Indriyasthāna). Chaukhambha Orientalia.
12. Chopra, A., Saluja, M. and Tillu, G. (2010). Ayurveda–modern medicine interface: A critical appraisal of studies of Ayurvedic medicines to treat osteoarthritis and rheumatoid arthritis. *Journal of Ayurveda and Integrative Medicine*, 1(3), 190–198.
13. Vedic Theory of Creation. http://ataytv.com/blogs/details/20-vedic-theory-of-creation.
14. Buettner, D. (2012). The Blue Zones: 9 Lessons for Living Longer from the People who've Lived the Longest. United States: National Geographic Books.
15. VPK Maharishi Ayurveda. https://www.mapi.com/ayurvedic-knowledge/food-tips/six-tastes-of-ayurveda.html.
16. The Hidden Costs of Industrial Agriculture. https://www.ucsusa.org/resources/hidden-costs-industrial-agriculture.
17. Animals on Factory Farms. https://www.aspca.org/animal-cruelty/farm-animal-welfare/ animals-factory-farms.
18. The Keeling Curve. www.scripps.ucsd.edu/programs/keelingcurve.
19. Global Monitoring. Library https://www.esrl.noaa.gov/gmd/ccgg/n.
20. Jacoby, R., Peukert, M., Succurro, A., Koprivova, A. and Kopriva, S. (2017). The role of soil microorganisms in plant mineral nutrition—current knowledge and future directions. *Frontiers in Plant Science*, 8, 16–17.
21. Fukuoka, M. (1985). The Natural Way of Farming. Tokyo: Japan Publications.
22. Khadse, A. and Rosset, P. M. (2019). Zero budget natural farming in india–from inception to institutionalization. *Agroecology and Sustainable Food Systems*, 43(7–8), 848–871.
23. Anderson, M. K. (2013). Tending the Wild: Native American Knowledge and the Management of California's Natural Resources. California: University of California Press.

24. Fukuoka, M. (2010). The One-straw Revolution: An Introduction to Natural Farming. New York: New York Review of Books.
25. Mott, G. O. (1960). Grazing pressure and the measurement of pasture production. *Biology*, 2, 132–138.
26. Turner, F. N. and Rateaver, B. (1951). Fertility Farming. United States: Faber Publishing.
27. Turner, F. N. (1955). Fertility Pastures. United States: Acres USA.
28. Mäder, P., Fliessbach, A., Dubois, D., Gunst, L., Fried, P. and Niggli, U. (2002). Soil fertility and biodiversity in organic farming. *Science*, 296(5573), 1694–1697.
29. Mollison, B., Slay, R. M., Girard, J. L. and Girard, J. L. (1991). Introduction to Permaculture. Australia: Tagari Publications.
30. Mollison, B. (1988). Permaculture: A Designer's Manual. Australia: Tagari Publications.
31. World Health Organization. https://www.who.int/chp/about/integrated_cd.
32. Kiernan, M. C., Vucic, S., Cheah, B. C., Turner, M. R., Eisen, A., Hardiman, O. and Zoing, M. C. (2011). Amyotrophic lateral sclerosis. *The Lancet*, 377(9769), 942–955.
33. Autoimmune Disease. https://en.wikipedia.org/wiki/Autoimmune_disease.
34. Spina Bifida. https://en.wikipedia.org/wiki/Spina_bifida.
35. Natural Ayurveda Healing Village. http://www.vaidyagrama.com.
36. Chikukwa Project. https://permacultureprinciples.com/post/the-chikukwa-project/.
37. The Camp Hill Project. https://en.wikipedia.org/wiki/Camphill_Movement.
38. Biodynamic Farming. https://en.wikipedia.org/wiki/Biodynamic_agriculture.

CHAPTER 5

Colorectal Cancer: A Concern for Young Adults

HARITHA THERESE JOSEPH[1] and SURYA M VIJAYAN[2*]

[1]*Department of Surgery, Regional Institute of Medical Sciences, Imphal, India*

[2]*Department of Surgery, Wayanad Institute of Medical Sciences, Wayanad, India*

Corresponding author. E-mail: suryamv89@gmail.com

ABSTRACT

The large bowel is the last part of our digestive system and consists of the cecum, colon, and rectum. Cancers arising from the large bowel are collectively known as colorectal cancers (CRCs) and are the third most common in men, the second most in women, and the fourth most common lethal malignancy, globally. Incidence of CRC is higher in Western countries and is attributed to changing patterns in the way of living and environmental factors, which can be prevented. Many affluent Asian countries also have similar CRC incidence to that in the West. It is more commonly seen in men, and the average age of diagnosis is 68 years for men and 72 years for women.

5.1 INTRODUCTION

The term "neoplasm" is very complicated to define and one of the pathological definitions states that "a neoplasm is an abnormal mass of tissue, the growth of which exceeds and is uncoordinated with that of the normal tissues, and persists in the same excessive manner after cessation of the stimuli which evoked the change" [5].

Neoplasms can be benign and malignant. Benign neoplasms are relatively innocent and these will remain localized, will not spread to other sites, and are amenable to local surgical removal. Malignant neoplasms, collectively referred to as cancers, on the other hand, tend to adhere to any part of that they seize on in an obstinate manner. A malignant neoplasm can destroy adjacent structures and spread to distant sites (metastasize) to cause death. The most important differentiating feature of malignant versus benign is the presence of metastasis or invasiveness [5].

While the incidence of colon cancer is evenly distributed in both sexes, the incidence increases with increasing age. In most of the older studies, colon cancer patients, less than 40 years of age, are uncommon, with this age group accounting for approximately 2%–4% of patients with colorectal cancer (CRC) worldwide. But recent studies from India [6] and latest Colorectal Cancer Facts And Figures 2017–2019 by American Cancer Society are pointing toward the increasing trend of colon cancer below the age of 40 years with a mean age of 42 years at diagnosis and a decreasing incidence in older age groups [7].

5.2   RISK FACTORS

The high prevalence and preventable nature of CRC bring it to the limelight of the oncological community. Colon cancer is considered to be a near preventable disease by many experts because many of its risk factors are related to the lifestyle of the individual. CRCs can be familial or sporadic. Various factors responsible for the development of sporadic (60–85%) CRCs are age beyond 50 years [1], sedentary lifestyle, consumption of highly saturated fat, overcooked and red meat, ionizing radiation exposure and diet deficient in calcium, environmental and industrial pollution including exposure to pesticides, irritable bowel diseases, etc. [2]. Hereditary causes include cancer syndromes that run in family, which is a group of cancers in colon, ovary, breast, uterus, stomach, gallbladder, and brain along family tree [3]. Genetic and familial etiologies account for only around 20% while the remaining 80% is attributed to multiple risk factors.

Recent studies show that the frequency of CRC in younger patients, particularly less than 40 years of age, is increasing in both Asia and the United States. This is attributed to the lack of screening guidelines in young adults routinely.

5.3 GENETICS

Colon carcinogenesis is a multistep process through which a pre-existing adenoma will transform into carcinoma. The strongest evidence for this is the National Polyp Study, in which 1418 patients were followed for an average of 5.9 years after the removal of all identifiable colonic polyps [4]. Even though the exact mechanism of mutation in a sporadic colorectal carcinoma is not identified, various risk factors, which will lead on to these mutations, are well established through several studies.

Risio [9], in his study "The Natural History of Adenomas," says that traditionally, the dominant theory of CRC development has been the adenoma–carcinoma sequence, which posits that carcinomas of the colon evolve from pre-existing and premalignant lesions, such as adenomas. However, only a few adenomas transform into cancer [9]. On the other hand, malignant tumors of the colorectum derived from flat or depressed *de novo* lesions of the mucosa are described in up to 30% of cases without preceding polypous lesions according to some studies [10] and then came genetic model of colorectal tumorigenesis (Figure 5.1) [11].

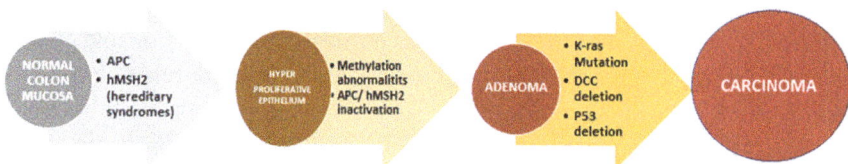

FIGURE 5.1   Genetic model of colorectal tumorigenesis.

Most of the colon cancers originate from a polyp. Nonneoplastic variety, which includes hyperplastic, mucosal, inflammatory, and hamartomatous polyps, is probably not associated with an increased risk of cancer. Adenomatous polyps are seen in 30% of the population over 50 years and these increases with advancing age. 60% of these lesions are situated beyond splenic flexure of the colon. The transformation of polyps from adenoma to carcinoma involves several genetic alterations:

- chromosomal instability
- epigenetic changes
- microsatellite instability.

Colorectal cancer is the final result of many stepwise mutations that causes the progression of normal bowel mucosa into cancerous. Various genes involved are *APC*, *P53*, *DCC*, and *SMAD4*. Other proposed mechanisms are the defective DNA repair process and microsatellite instability. Various familial cancer syndromes are described related to theses gene mutations including familial adenomatous polyposis (FAP), Lynch syndrome also known as hereditary nonpolyposis colorectal cancer (HNPCC), Peutz–Jeghers syndrome, etc. [3].

5.4 WHEN TO SUSPECT?

Symptoms of CRC include blood in stools, further leading to anemia, altered bowel habits, that is, constipation and increased frequency of bowel movements, abdominal pain, weakness, abdominal distension, etc. Most of the symptoms are often neglected by young people due to the misconception that cancer is the disease of elderly. When a relative is diagnosed with CRC at a young age or if more than one relative in a family are affected by CRC, the risk for developing cancer is 2–6 times higher than the general population. Blood in stools and constipation are symptoms of hemorrhoids but can be the earliest manifestation of CRC. Most of the right-sided colon cancers are presented with altered bowel habits, abdominal pain, and abdominal lump; whereas, left-sided lesion is presented with intestinal obstruction and change in bowel habits. Locally advanced tumors may present with other symptoms, such as with pneumaturia, if a colovesical fistula is present, with hydronephrosis, if the growth obstructs the ureter or with other symptoms, depending on the tumor location.

Unless promptly examined and diagnosed by a medical practitioner, CRC will remain unrecognized and progress into the terminal stage. Studies have shown that CRC in young adults presents late and is aggressive in nature. Around 10% of people present with a mass in the abdomen, which can be detected in a clinical examination.

5.5 SCREENING FOR COLORECTAL CANCER

Certain tests help in the early detection of CRC and are recommended by American Society of Colon and Rectal Surgeons. It also helps in evaluating suspicious growth in the large bowel.

Thus, if a person does not have any risk factors or symptoms or no history of CRC among family members, screening by flexible sigmoidoscopy and fecal occult blood test is advised at the age of 50 years (Figure 5.2). This is reduced to 45 years recently due to an increase in the incidence of CRC in young adults. In people who have a strong family history of colorectal or any cancer in the abovementioned syndromes, they should undergo screening at a very young age, preferably by 12–14 years of age and be continued every 1–2 yearly [3].

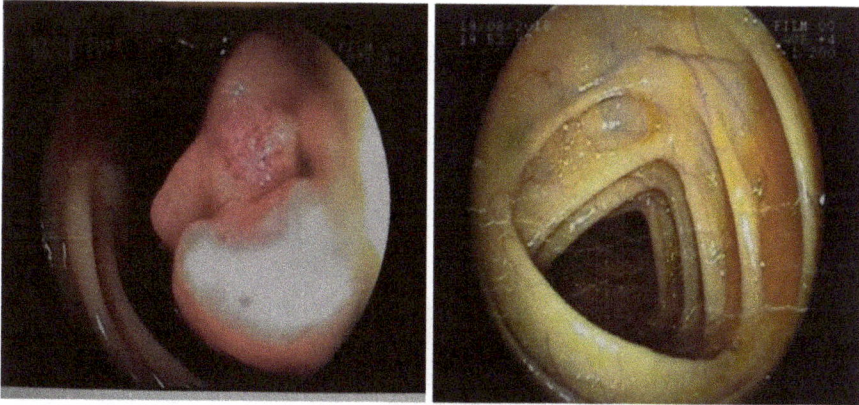

FIGURE 5.2 Colonoscopy images showing an ulceroproliferative lesion in the sigmoid colon 20 cm from the anal verge with normal transverse and ascending colon.

And, suspicious growth or change in the bowel wall can be biopsied by a sigmoidoscope and can be further evaluated. Usually, young adults who avoid medical examinations for the symptoms of CRC due to misconception or negligence, it results in progression to advanced disease at the time of presentation or they present with complications such as obstruction, profuse bleeding, or perforation of the bowel.

5.6 TREATMENT MODALITIES

Diagnosis of CRC is made by various tests including colonoscopy and biopsy, blood tests for tumor markers, and imaging studies such as CT and MRI scans. Once the diagnosis is confirmed, staging of cancer is done to decide further management. The treatment of CRC is multimodal management including chemotherapy, radiotherapy, and surgery.

In an elective setting, CRC is treated by chemotherapy before and after surgery depending on the stage of cancer and surgical removal of tumor followed by radiation (Figure 5.3).

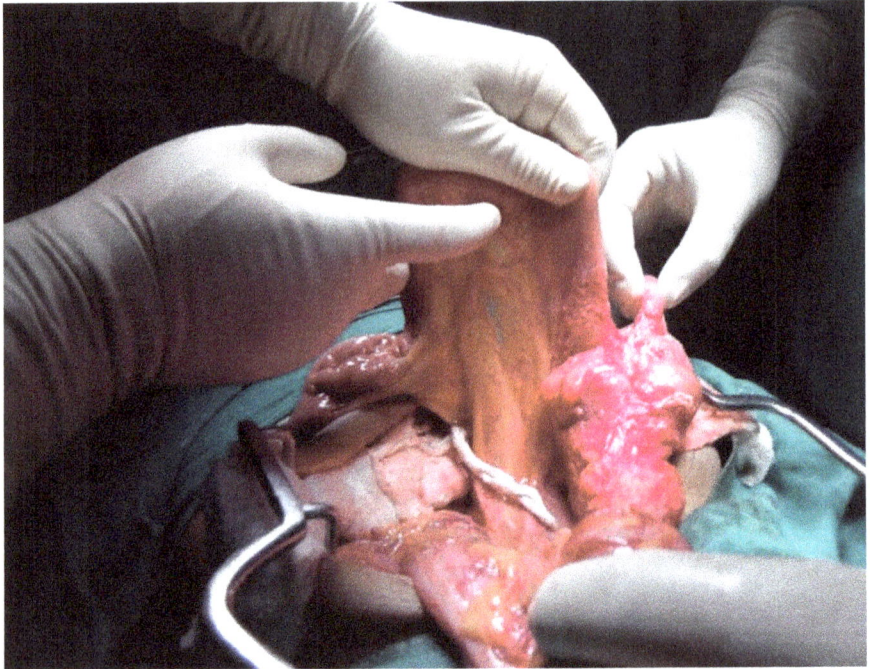

FIGURE 5.3   Intraoperative picture of colon carcinoma.

If the patient presents to the emergency department due to later stage or complicated disease, prompt resuscitation and emergency surgery is the preferable way of management, which usually includes two-staged procedures such as diversion ileostomy or colostomy followed by definitive surgery in a later setting.

5.7   HOW TO PREVENT?

Lifestyle modifications play an important role in preventing CRCs. This includes:

- diet control
- physical activity
- weight reduction
- avoidance of smoking and alcohol
- reduced consumption of red meat and processed food
- high-fiber diet

- vitamin D and calcium supplementation
- chemoprevention by celecoxib in FAP
- timely screening and medical check-ups.

Colorectal cancers are preventable, treatable, and beatable, if promptly diagnosed. Delay in diagnosis or seeking treatment results in complications and increased mortality. Let us be a little concerned. Not all cancers are *PINK*. Let's beat Colon cancer..!!

Footnote: All images included in the chapter belong to the author's compilation of various cases encountered during clinical practice. Consent was taken from patients to include the photographs for academic purposes.

KEYWORDS

- **colorectal cancer**
- **large bowel malignancy**
- **young adults**

REFERENCES

1. Benson AL. Epidemiology, disease progression, and economic burden of colorectal cancer. *J Manag Care Pharm*. 2007;13:5–18.
2. Howlader N, Noone AM, Krapcho M, Miller D, Bishop K, Altekruse SF, et al. SEER Cancer Statistics Review, 1975–2013, National Cancer Institute. Bethesda, MD.
3. Patel SG, Ahnen DJ. Familial colon cancer syndromes: an update of a rapidly evolving field. *Curr Gastroenterol Rep*. 2012;14(5):428–438.
4. Cohan J, Varma MG. *Large Intestine: Current Diagnosis and Treatment Surgery*, 14th edition. McGraw Hill Education: 2015, pp. 695–709.
5. Winawer SJ, Zauber AG, Ho MN, O'brien MJ, Gottlieb LS, Sternberg SS, et al. Prevention of colorectal cancer by colonoscopic polypectomy. *N Engl J Med* 1993; 329 (27):1977–1981.
6. Sirica AE. Classification of neoplasms. In: Sirica AE, Alphonse (ed). *The Pathobiology of Neoplasia*. Boston: Springer; 1989, pp. 25–38.
7. Kumari P, Sharma N, Khatri PK, Narayan S, Kumari S, Harsh KK, et al. Age wise distribution of colorectal cancer: An institutional observational study. *IOSR J Dental Med Sci*. 2017;16(1):11–12.
8. American Cancer Society. Colorectal Cancer Facts & Figures 2017-2019. Atlanta: American Cancer Society; 2017.

9. Arnold M, Sierra MS, Laversanne M, Soerjomataram I, Jemal A, Bray F. Global patterns and trends in colorectal cancer incidence and mortality. *Gut.* 2017;66(1):683–691.

10. Risio M. The natural history of adenomas. *Best Pract Res Clin Gastroenterol.* 2010; 24 (3):271–280.

11. Lau PC, Sung JJ. Flat adenoma in colon: two decades of debate. *J Digest Dis.* 2010; 11 (4):201–207.

12. Toribara NW, Sleisenger MH. Screening for colorectal cancer. *N Engl J Med.* 1995; 332 (13):861–867.

CHAPTER 6

Nanotechnology: An Emerging Technology for Therapeutics

JESIYA SUSAN GEORGE¹, K. P. JIBIN², V. PRAJITHA², V. R. REMYA¹, and SABU THOMAS¹*

¹International and Inter University Centre for Nanoscience and Nanotechnology, Athirampuzha, India

²School of Chemical Sciences, Mahatma Gandhi University, Kottayam, India

*Corresponding author. E-mail: sabuthomas@mgu.ac.in.

ABSTRACT

Nanotechnology is an emerging technology, which has tremendous scope in the field of therapeutics in the current and future era. Nanotechnology is science, engineering, and technology in which the materials are manipulated on a nanoscopic scale. In this chapter, we summarize the recent developments and advances of nanotechnology in the field of medicine/ chemotherapy. A clear understanding of the various nanosystems in drug delivery system (DDS) has been discussed. Nanoemulsions can be formulated for drug delivery systems to achieve better drug loading, drug solubility and controlled release. Similarly, solid lipid nanoparticles (SLNPs) attracting the worldwide attention of drug formulators. They consist of solid lipid particles in the nanosize, along with a solid hydrophobic core with a phospholipid coating. The solid core contains the dispersed drug in the fat matrix. Drug delivery systems based on magnetic nanoparticles and dendrimers have been discussed.

6.1 INTRODUCTION

Ayurveda is the universally accepted world's oldest holistic healing system, originated in India 500 years ago with a basic of Indian Vedic culture [1]. It consists of drugs obtained from different renewable sources, such as herbs, animals, marine, etc. Herbal drugs have a complex structure with many active constituents such as Tannins, Flavonoids, Terpenoids, etc. The presence of all these active ingredients provides a synergistic effect and also enhances the therapeutic effect too. Herbal drugs such as Strychnos nux-vomic, Gloriosa superba, and Rauwolfia serpentine show excellent medicinal strength toward various diseases, Figure 6.1 shows the typical image of the Gloriosa superba flowers. But all these plants were included in the Red List (verge of extinction) created by International Union for Natural resources [2, 3].

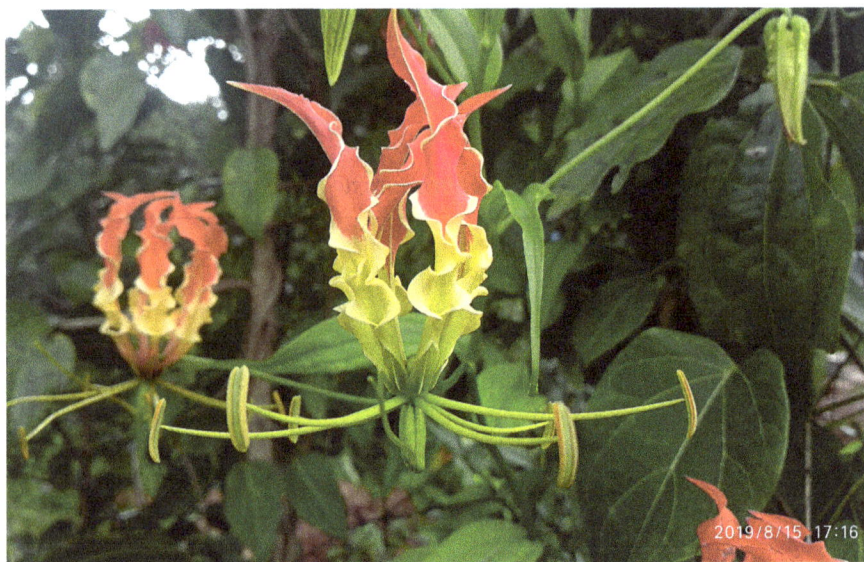

FIGURE 6.1 Image of *Gloriosa superba* flower (Photo by Vijayanrajapuram. https://commons.wikimedia.org/wiki/File:Gloriosa_superba_at_Madikai_Ambalathukara_in_Kasaragod.jpg via https://creativecommons.org/licenses/by-sa/4.0/)

Nanotechnology is the technology of materials that deal with very small dimension materials, usually in the range 1–100 nm in any dimension. Outstanding properties of nanomaterials help to find applications in almost every area. Nanotechnology has a lot of importance in healthcare and medicine, Figure 6.2 summarizes the main application of nanomaterials. However, the use of harmful nanoparticles in therapeutics creates side effects in patients. The nanodrug carriers can be effectively applied in Ayurveda, which will help to reduce the dosage of medicine, which is usually not achievable in normal Ayurvedic treatment [4].

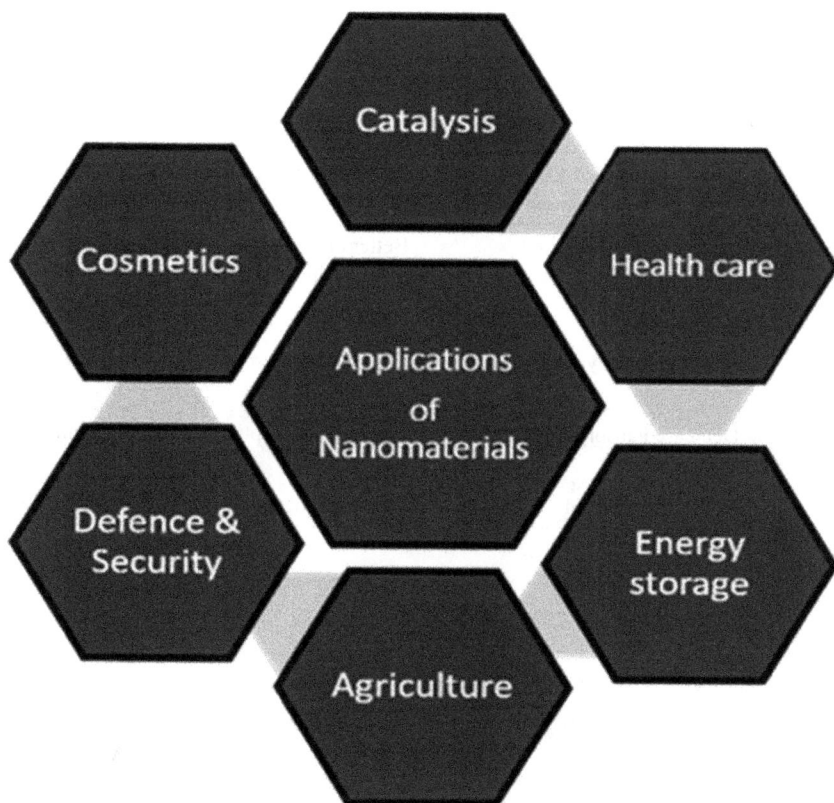

FIGURE 6.2 Applications of nanomaterials.

Traditional drug formulation in Ayurveda shows good efficiency but the drug delivery device lacks standardization and scientific justification. Conventional drug delivery systems (DDS) employed in Ayurveda has many disadvantages over the novel DDS, Table 6.1 list outs the main advantages of novel DDS over the conventionals.

6.1.1 DRUG DELIVERY SYSTEM USING NANOCARRIERS

Nanocarriers are considered as a transport medium for drugs commonly used nanocarriers include dendrimers, polymeric nanoparticles, nanoemulsions, magnetic nanoparticles, solid lipids nanoparticles, liposomes, etc. These systems have the ability to encapsulate various biologically active molecules and drugs in them. Figure 6.3 gives an idea about the widely used nano-DDS.

TABLE 6.1 Advantages of Novel Drug Delivery System

Numbers	Disadvantages of Conventional Drug Delivery System	Advantages of Novel Drug Delivery System
1	Bulk dosage is required	Better efficiency at lower dosage with a reduced and repeat dose administration
2	Lower stability	High stability
3	Lower solubility	Enhanced pharmacological activity and solubility
4	Decreased absorption rate and bioavailability	Increased absorption rate and bioavailability
5	Not target oriented	Target oriented with controlled drug release

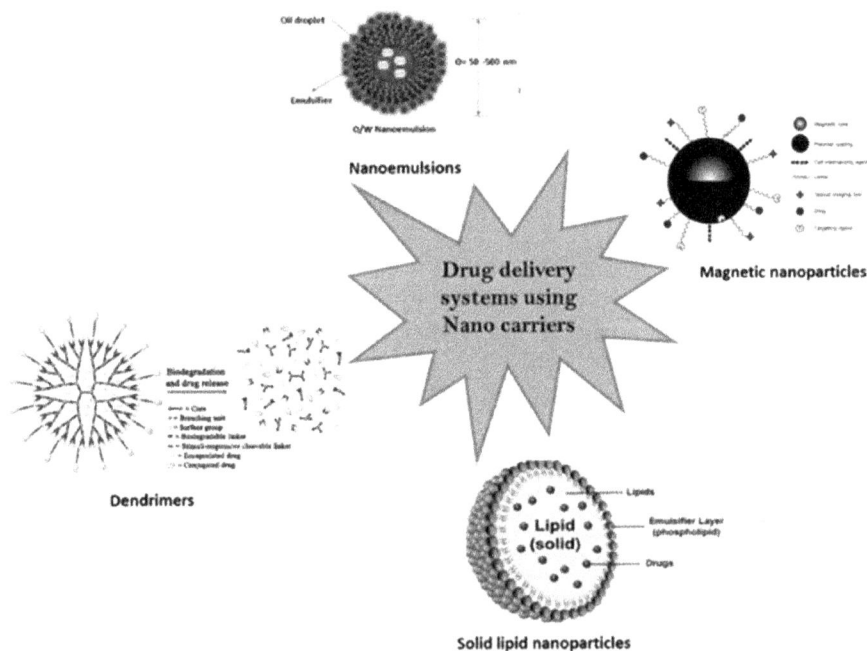

FIGURE 6.3 Drug delivery systems using nanocarriers.

6.2 LIPOSOMES

Liposomes are small artificial vesicles with a spherical shape, constructed from cholesterol, and other natural nontoxic phospholipids. They are biocompatible, biodegradable, nontoxic, and nonimmunogenic in nature. Figure 6.4 shows the typical structure of liposomes, it has a hydrophobic tail directed toward the outside and a hydrophilic tail directed toward the inside, hence hydrophobic drugs can be easily encapsulated. The size, as well as hydrophobic and hydrophilic nature, is responsible for the efficient drug delivery. The preparation method employed, surface charge on the liposome, and lipid composition are the main factors that determine the final property of liposomes. However, the fluidity and rigidity of liposomes vary with bilayer composition and charge on them. Lower solubility, oxidation of lipid bilayer, and higher production cost are the main disadvantages of liposomes [5, 6]

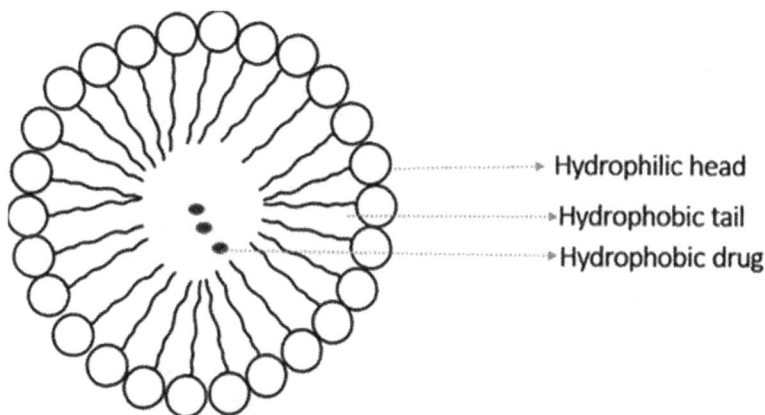

FIGURE 6.4 Typical structure of liposomes.

6.3 NANOEMULSION

Nanoemulsions are defined as isotropic dispersion of two immiscible liquids, normally consist of an organic system dispersed in an aqueous system or aqueous system dispersed in the organic system. An emulsion is thermodynamically unstable system, which can be stabilized by adding emulsifying agents/ surfactant (emulsifier). Emulsifier stabilizes the nanoemulsion via steric hindrance and repulsive electrostatic interactions. Two important destabilization mechanisms found in nanoemulsions are Ostwald ripening and creaming. These nanoemulsions exhibit higher loading efficiency of active ingredients than microemulsions and incorporation of magnetic nanoparticles and other nanoparticles into the nanoemulsion system enhances the site-specificity also. Generally, nanoemulsions are prepared by microfluidization, high-pressure homogenization, spontaneous emulsion, and phase inversion temperature. There are three types of nanoemulsions [7, 8]:

1. Oil in water nanoemulsion.
2. Water in oil nanoemulsion.
3. Bicontinuous nanoemulsion.

Nanoemulsion consists of oil, aqueous phase, and emulsifying agents. Linseed oil, castor oil, olive oil, peanut oil, etc., are the widely used oils in the emulsion. Emulsifying agent is a substance that acts as a stabilizer in emulsions. Essential features of a good emulsifying agents involve nontoxicity, compatability, and lower surface tension (less than 10 dynes/cm).

6.3.1   NANOEMULSIONS IN DRUG DELIVERY

The unique and excellent combination of properties of the nanoemulsions made it a promising candidate in drug delivery, such as excellent stability against droplets, enhanced drug loading, solubility, and better bioavailability. A DDS is defined as a medium or carrier for administrating a pharmaceutical product to a patient. There are various DDSs including transdermal, intranasal, oral, and ocular As shown in Figure 6.5, the small size of the nanoemulsion significantly reduces the gravity as well as Brownian movement and thereby prevents the sedimentation and creaming that occurs during storage, in addition these small droplets prevent the coalescence and surface fluctuations. The small size of the nanoemulsion significantly reduces the gravity as well as Brownian movement and thereby prevents the sedimentation and creaming that occurs during storage, in addition these small droplets prevent the coalescence and surface fluctuations. Wetting, spreading, and penetration of the drugs are very easy in nanoemulsion DDSs as a result of their lower surface tension and interfacial tension of the whole system. Oral drug delivery is the most convenient, cost-effective, and easiest way for the administration of drugs, in order to dominate the current pharmaceutical market, drugs with lower solubility create serious problems in the gastrointestinal tract. One of the important drawbacks for nanoemulsion is that it requires highly sophisticated instruments such as homogenizers, microfluidizers, ultrasonics for the preparation [9].

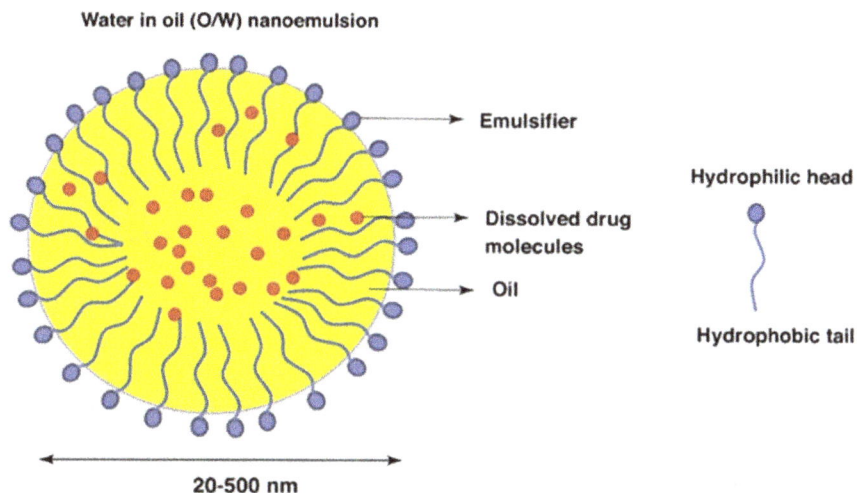

FIGURE 6.5 Nanoemulsions in drug delivery reused with permission from Elsevier.
Source: Reprinted with permission from Ref. [9]. © 2019 Elsevier.

6.4 NANOPARTICLES

Nanoparticles are those in which at least one dimension should be in nanorange, for example, graphene, graphene oxide, metal oxide, etc., which can be either crystalline or amorphous form and has the ability to encapsulate or adsorb the drug and thereby protecting it against chemical and enzymatic degradation. As per the surface chemistry, pristine graphene is inherently hydrophobic in nature hence it has poor water dispersibility, whereas GO consists of some reactive functional groups in its surface and gives a hydrophilic nature. In order to use Graphene for biological applications either some functionality should be introduced into it or requires surfactants. In general, nanoparticle which is to be used in the biological field must have biocompatibility which is essential, before preclinical, and clinical studies can be undertaken. The designing of the system for the controlled release of drug with optimized dosage at a specific site requires for successful therapy [10].

6.4.1 MAGNETIC NANOPARTICLES

In recent years, both nano- and micro-magnetic particles are extensively used for biomedical applications, they were used from 1970 onwards as therapeutic drug carriers. Magnetic targeting has some exceptional advantages in drug delivery over conventional systems. They have the ability to target a specific site and thereby enhancing the uptake at the target site at a lower dosage resulting in enhanced therapeutic effect. A promising site-directed application in the field of nanomedicine is drug targeting using magnetic nanoparticles directed at the target tissue by means of an external magnetic field. In the current scenario, metal/metal oxide nanoparticles are most widely used in magnetic DDS, which are often coated with some organic materials, such as fatty acids, polysaccharides, or some polymers to improve the colloidal stability as well as to prevent the separation into particles and carrier. Commonly used magnetic nanoparticles for drug delivery includes superparamagnetic iron oxide nanoparticles, colloidal magnetic iron oxide, etc. Figure 6.6 shows an image delivery of magnetic nanoparticles loaded with the drug into the tumor site under the influence of an external magnetic field. However, in this system, magnetic nanoparticles will behave magnetically only under the influence of an external magnetic field and they became inactive once the field is removed. Magnetic particles with a size less than 10 nm generally shows the above-explained phenomenon, due to their single domain state [11, 12].

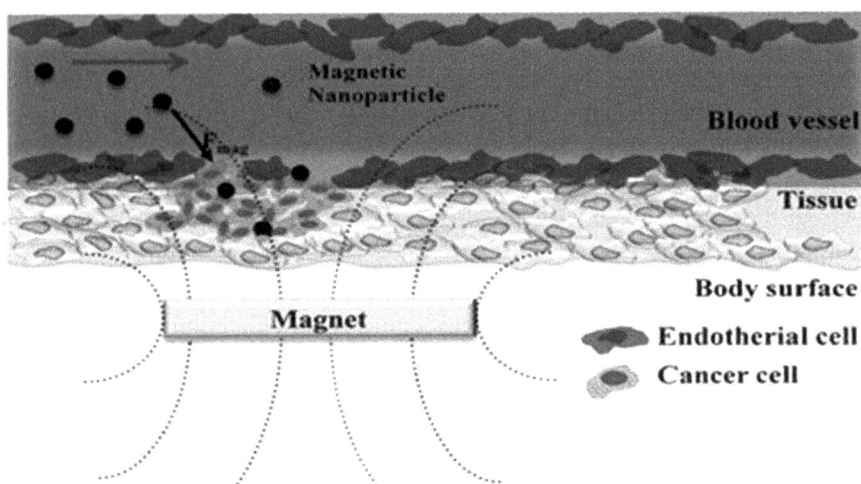

FIGURE 6.6   Drug delivery assisted with magnetic nanoparticles.

Source: Reprinted with permission from Ref. [21]. © 2019 Elsevier.

6.5   DENDRIMERS

Dendrimers are highly branched macromolecular chains with a three-dimensional structure in nanometer dimensions. Dendrimers are synthesized by two different approaches, they are divergent and convergent approach. Figure 6.7 shows the schematic representation of the two synthesis strategies. In the divergent method, dendrimer is formed by the assembly of multifunctional core. It consists of several steps, in each step resulting product is extended outward by the series of reactions [13–15].

A. Divergent synthesis

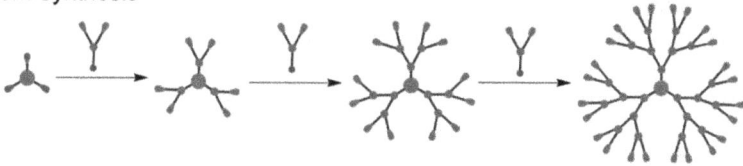

B. Convergent synthesis

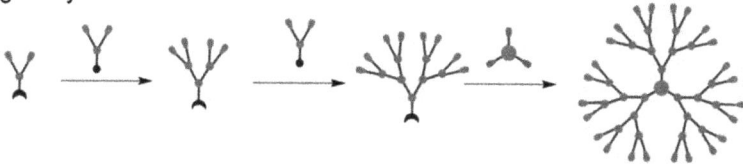

C. Combined divergent/converngent synthesis

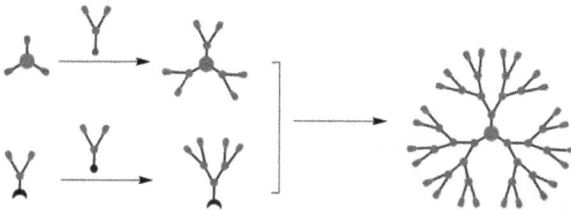

FIGURE 6.7 Schematic representation of dendrimeric nanoparticles synthesis.
Source: Reprinted with permission from Ref. [16]. © 2019 Elsevier.

Controlled surface functionality, monodispersity, and other extraordinary properties of dendrimer make it a good candidate for drug delivery applications. For dendrimer-aided drug delivery applications, either drug can be physically entrapped inside the dendrimer system or drug can be chemically bonded to the surface dendrimer. The physical entrapping of the drug make into possible by the efficient utilization of the internal cavity of a dendrimer. However, in the second method, guest drug molecules can be anchored on the surface of dendrimers via noncovalent chemical linkages such as hydrogen bonding.

6.6　SOLID LIPID NANOPARTICLES

These are the novel materials for the controlled release of drugs. They are in the submicron size range (50–1000 nm) that consists of biocompatible and biodegradable materials capable of incorporating lyophilic and lyophobic drugs. For the formulation of solid lipid nanoparticles (SLNs), lipids are the matrix materials emulsifiers, and water. Charge modifiers, that improve long circulation time and targeting ability, are also used to meet the requirements of stability and targeting aspects [17].

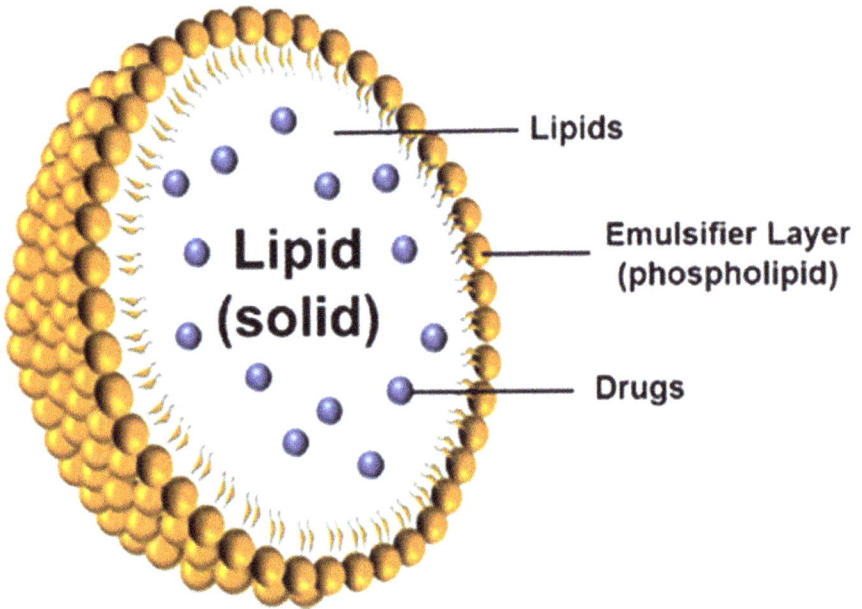

FIGURE 6.8　Solid lipid nanoparticles.

Source: Reprinted with permission from Ref. [18]. © 2019 Elsevier.

The main advantage of sSolid lipid Nnanoparticles (SLNPs) is that they are solid at both temperature and at body temperature. They will offer a synergistic effect of liposomes, polymers, and emulsions and thereby lowering the disadvantages of individual particles. Figure 6.8 represents the typical structure of SLNP. It has a hydrophobic solid core covered by a phospholipid coating, the hydrophobic tails of the emulsifiers phospholipid are embedded in the hydrophobic core solid matrix. Hence SLNPs have strong entrapment tendency toward the hydrophobic drugs than the conventional liposome.

Generally, the drug loading capacity of SLNP is limited to 25% with respect to the lipid matrix, which depends on the drug solubility, structure, and polymorphic state of lipid. Generally, drug incorporated SLNP is prepared by high-pressure homogenization technique with a drug level lower than the saturation solubility of the matrix lipid. The drug is partitioned into the aqueous lipid phase during production and it precipitates later on cooling. Simultaneously the drug again partitioned into aqueous lipid matrix, finally the concentration of the outer shell increases which purely consist of lipid molecules [19,20].

6.7 CONCLUSION

The benefits of nanomedicines are indubitable and unstoppable; in this review chapter, we extensively discussed the use of nanotechnology in Ayurveda, especially in DDSs. The understanding of the use of these nanoparticles in the therapeutic field is very important because the field of nanotechnology has high demand due to its unconditional offers. Drug delivery systems based on magnetic nanoparticles, solid lipid nanoparticles, dendrimers, nanoemulsions, liposomes, and nanoparticles were extensively discussed.

KEYWORDS

- **nanocarriers**
- **Ayurveda**
- **drug delivery**
- **nanotechnology**
- **theraputics**

REFERENCES

1. Seema, A. (2014). Recent development of herbal formulation—a novel drug delivery system. *International Ayurvedic Medical Journal*, 2(6), 952–958.
2. Kaur, H., Yadav, P., Prajapati, P., Khatik, G. L., Haque, A., Vyas, M., & Verma, S. (2020). Application of nanotechnology for ayurvedic drugs and formulations. *Drug Invention Today*, 10, 811–817.

3. Ankanna, S., Suhrulatha, D., & Savithramma, N. (2012). Chemotaxonomical studies of some important monocotyledons. *Botany Research International*, 5(4), 90–96.

4. Chakrapany, S., & Chandan, S. (2014). Nano carriers of novel drug delivery system for 'ayurveda herbal remedies' need of hour—a bird's eye view. *American Journal of PharmTech Research*, 4(2), 60–69.

5. Rathod, S., & Deshpande, S. G. (2010). Design and evaluation of liposomal formulation of pilocarpine nitrate. *Indian Journal of Pharmaceutical Sciences*, 72(2), 155.

6. Vahedi, A., & Kouhi, M. (2020). Correction to: liquid crystal-based surface plasmon resonance biosensor. Plasmonics, 15(1), 73–73.

7. Jaiswal, A. K., Kaur, R., Eappen, K., Dua, K., & Bali, V. (2014). Multidisciplinary approach in the treatment of pathologic migration of lower anterior teeth: a case report. *Baba Farid University Dental Journal*, 5(1), 123–127.

8. Tomiotto-Pellissier, F., Miranda-Sapla, M. M., Machado, L. F., da Silva Bortoleti, B. T., Sahd, C. S., Chagas, A. F., et al. (2017). Nanotechnology as a potential therapeutic alternative for schistosomiasis. *Acta Tropica*, 174, 64–71.

9. Karami, Z., Zanjani, M. R. S., & Hamidi, M. (2019). Nanoemulsions in CNS drug delivery: recent developments, impacts and challenges. *Drug Discovery Today*, 24(5), 1104–1115.

10. Liu, J., Cui, L., & Losic, D. (2013). Graphene and graphene oxide as new nanocarriers for drug delivery applications. *Acta Biomaterialia*, 9(12), 9243–9257.

11. Dobson, J. (2006). Magnetic nanoparticles for drug delivery. *Drug Development Research*, 67(1), 55–60.

12. Mody, V. V., Cox, A., Shah, S., Singh, A., Bevins, W., & Parihar, H. (2014). Magnetic nanoparticle drug delivery systems for targeting tumor. *Applied Nanoscience*, 4(4), 385–392.

13. Liu, M., & Fréchet, J. M. (1999). Designing dendrimers for drug delivery. *Pharmaceutical Science & Technology Today*, 2(10), 393–401.

14. Patri, A. K., Majoros, I. J., & Baker Jr, J. R. (2002). Dendritic polymer macromolecular carriers for drug delivery. *Current Opinion in Chemical Biology*, 6(4), 466–471.

15. Naylor, A. M., Goddard III, W. A., Kiefer, G. E., & Tomalia, D. A. (1989). Starburst dendrimers. 5. Molecular shape control. *Journal of the American Chemical Society*, 111(6), 2339–2341.

16. Lyu, Z., Ding, L., Huang, A. T., Kao, C. L., & Peng, L. (2019). Poly (amidoamine) dendrimers: covalent and supramolecular synthesis. *Materials Today Chemistry*, 13, 34–48.

17. Manjunath, K., Reddy, J. S., & Venkateswarlu, V. (2005). Solid lipid nanoparticles as drug delivery systems. *Methods and Findings in Experimental and Clinical Pharmacology*, 27(2), 127–144.

18. Lin, C. H., Chen, C. H., Lin, Z. C., & Fang, J. Y. (2017). Recent advances in oral delivery of drugs and bioactive natural products using solid lipid nanoparticles as the carriers. *Journal of Food and Drug Analysis*, 25(2), 219–234.

19. Pardeshi, C., Rajput, P., Belgamwar, V., Tekade, A., Patil, G., Chaudhary, K., & Sonje, A. (2012). Solid lipid based nanocarriers: an overview. *Acta Pharmaceutica*, 62(4), 433–472.

20. Wissing, S. A., Kayser, O., & Müller, R. H. (2004). Solid lipid nanoparticles for parenteral drug delivery. *Advanced Drug Delivery Reviews*, 56(9), 1257–1272.

21. Park J.H., Saravanakumar G., Kim K., Kwon I.C. (2010) Targeted delivery of low molecular drugs using chitosan and its derivatives. Adv Drug Deliv Rev 62:28–41.

CHAPTER 7

Polyionenes as Antimicrobial Agents

K. S. JOSHY[1], STEFAN JACKSON[2], AISWARYA SATIAN[3], and HONG CHI[1*]

[1]*Shandong Provincial Key Laboratory of Molecular Engineering, School of Chemistry and Pharmaceutical Engineering, Qilu University of Technology (Shandong Academy of Sciences), Jinan 250353, China*

[2]*Amity Institute of Nanotechnology, Amity University, Noida, Uttar Pradesh, India*

[3]*Mount Carmel College, Palace Road, Bangalore, India*

Corresponding author. E-mail: stefaj619@gmail.com

ABSTRACT

Antimicrobial drug resistance is increasing at an alarming rate and has resulted in causing threat to the public health sector. Due to inefficiency of drugs and as a result of the advent of new resistance mechanisms, the microbial agents have developed multidrug resistance, thereby enhancing the morbidity and mortality rates, and earning the title "super bugs." In addition to this improper sanitary facilities and inappropriate dietary habits have further peaked the multidrug resistance (MDR) spread. MDR has affected human health in ways beyond human comprehension such as prolonged illness, immense risk of death as well as high expenditures in hospital and medical bills. This ever-increasing crisis has led to new avenues such as antimicrobial polymers that possesses zero toxicity to cells. Inherent antimicrobial capacity along with various antimicrobial modes, biocompatibility, stability, structure, functionalities, low cost synthesis, and eco-friendly nature are few among the most promising features of the antimicrobial polymers. Quaternary ammonium salts (QAS) and quaternary phosphonium salts (QPS) are the most common types of antimicrobial polymers, but in-order to effectively combat the microbes there was a need of membrane active cationic polymers. Thus emerged "Polyionenes." The additional dimension and the commercial availability of numerous building blocks are the key features that render the MDR pathogens ineffective. Polyionenes along with its key features ease of synthesis and scale-up have thus made its place in being the one of the most important family in anti-microbial polymers.

7.1   INTRODUCTION

The ever increasing ineffectiveness of conventional antibiotics has become problematic in the field of microbial infections, particularly those caused by resistant bacteria [1]. The slow pace of new antibiotics is being discovered along with increased use of antibiotics in the field of medicine and agriculture, leading to the emergence of new antibiotics that pose a threat. The excessive usage of antibiotics in areas including societal enhancement and food habits have resulted in the emergence of resilient bacterial strains that complicate our well-being [2]. Thereby, the interest in exploring new avenues to comprehend the problems associated with resistant bacteria has increased especially by the scientific community, thus leading to the consideration of bacterial membrane anionic lipids as alluring targets to design novel antibacterial agents. When all is said and done, antimicrobial polymers are hydrophilic cationic macromolecules that can explicitly destroy microorganisms, for example, bacteria, fungi, or protozoans with practically zero cytotoxicity to cells. Most of the antimicrobial polymers possess quaternary ammonium centers as the cations, while others have cations, for example, phosphonium, sulfonium, or metal centers [3]. Effective antimicrobial agents are critical weapons in our perpetual battle against transmiTable diseases, hospital acquired, and surgical site multidrug-resistant infections. By the usage of highly effective, skin compatible, and inexpensive water-soluble macromolecular antimicrobials, polyionenes are developed by employing a catalyst-free polyaddition polymerization. In this research, develop a methodology for the improvement and development of highly soluble macromolecule polybenzenes in the highly efficient and highly frigid, highly polluted waters, with polymerization without catalysts with monomers that are available to eat. A progression of antimicrobial polyionenes is prepared through a basic polyaddition reaction in which both the polymer-forming reaction and charge installation occur simultaneously. The composition and structure of polymers have been adapted to study their effects on antimicrobial activity against a broad spectrum of pathogenic microorganism. Polymers with optimized and improved compositions have potential antimicrobial activity; the polymers show high antimicrobial efficacy against various clinically secluded multidrug-resistant microorganisms, yet demonstrate limitlessly superior skin biocompatibility.

Ganewatta et al. synthesized various antimicrobial macromolecules utilizing pine tree-derived natural resin acids (or rosins), which are having relatively good antimicrobial activities [4]. Pendent groups implemented from polymer backbones were cationic charges. Due to a local balance of amphiphilicity, antimicrobial agents such as antimicrobial peptides and anti-microbial polymers with facially amphiphilic orientation show even more great antimicrobial properties.

7.2 ANTIMICROBIAL POLYMERS

Due to the low propensity to cause drug-resistant microorganisms, antimicrobial polymers have been attracting more interest these days. A fusion of small antimicrobial agents or with inherent antimicrobial activity is the constituents of polymeric macromolecular antimicrobial agents. The functionalization of small antimicrobial agents is usually processed via releasing small molecular antibiotics. The inherent antimicrobial capacity of antimicrobial polymers with different antimicrobial modes stops the development of drug-resistant microorganism strains. In addition, due to the polymeric structures, antimicrobial polymers might impart a higher antimicrobial effectiveness. In the form of dispersion, antimicrobial polymers can be dispersed in solution as antibiotics and preservatives and can be deposited onto the substrate surfaces by physically for disinfection or fixed via covalent bonds. In comparison to the constrained mobility of those being covalently fixed on surfaces, antimicrobial polymers dispersed in solution, attack pathogens with free mobility are much larger than its counterpart. The limited or free mobility of antimicrobial polymers, deposited physically on the substrate surfaces, can be fixed onto or be released from the surfaces to attack pathogens accordingly.

In many major aspects of modern medicine, antimicrobial chemotherapy has revolutionized it and has reduced the effects of infectious diseases such as death and ailments. Most classes of antibiotics, which are being used today, were discovered in the golden era of antibiotics during the 1940s to 1960s. To design antimicrobial agents, molecular targets of pathogens, which are absent or significantly different from human cells such as cell wall, 60S ribosomes, cell membranes, genetic materials, and biosynthetic pathways, are utilized. The rapid emergence of resistant pathogenic populations of microorganisms has been observed due to environmental pressure caused by the action of antibiotics combined with short life cycles and lateral gene transfer mechanisms. For example, the introduction of antibiotics—β-lactam, penicillin, and methicillin, generalized outbreaks of penicillin-resistant *Staphylococcus aureus* and methicillin-resistant *S. aureus* occurred after a few years. Efflux pumps, chemical modifications such as phosphorylation, acetylation, or hydrolysis, altering target, and reprogramming biosynthesis are few among the many various resistance mechanisms, most of which are against small molecule antimicrobials. The expeditious growth of acquired resistance in bacteria that cause major healthcare crisis is the most prominent issue. For example, the number of unique lactamase enzymes has grown from zero to over 1000, since the introduction of the first-lactam antibiotics. Along with a 40-year lull in the pipeline of novel antimicrobial agents and decades of use and misuse of antibiotics have led to consequences of a global superbug threat that could lead human civilization to a preantibiotic era. As a result of the catastrophic nature of the increasing resistance to existing antibiotics, it is a worldwide concern at high priority. Antibiotic resistance appears to be unavoidable. Subsequently, it is fundamental to ceaselessly create antimicrobial agents with novel methods of activity to confront the advancing resistance. Being is fueled by the combined knowledge on antimicrobial peptides (AMPs) and polymer disinfectants that have emerged as two distinct fields since the 1980s, antimicrobial polymers are a class of novel antimicrobial agents. There are a few books such as an assortment of reviews and features on antimicrobial polymers distributed in the course of recent years that give more extensive and different perspectives. Rapid expansion of novel antimicrobial polymers and related research has been witnessed in the last decade. It is progressively perceived that microbial membranes provide an effective target for the development of de novo designed antimicrobial agents. Ongoing comprehension of the innate immunity intervened by macromolecules features the significance of short amphiphilic peptides that modulate host defenses against microbial pathogens. AMP molecules are almost produced by all forms of life. AMPs are potent, wide-range antimicrobials that act as the first line of defense against a wide range of attacking pathogens encompassed of yeast, bacteria, protozoa, fungi, and viruses by rapid and direct killing as well as several other means of regulating host immune systems. More than 2000 AMPs with diverse sequences of amino acids and a range of structures have been revealed as per the decades of studies. However, all AMPs demonstrate a typical trademark: the presence of an amphiphilic structure (in some literature, amphipathic is often utilized). The optimal amphiphilicity, which comes from hydrophobic residues (e.g., isoleucine, valine) and cationic amino acids (e.g., lysine, arginine), empowers AMPs to fold into cationic and facially amphiphilic secondary structures. This feature allows AMPs to interact strongly with biological membranes. Strikingly, receptor-mediated antimicrobial activity is naturally not present in AMPs. For instance, it was shown that all-D synthetic enantiomer homologous of cecropins and magainins has similar potency to all-L natural peptides. This nonspecific property has appeared to be a class of promising anti-infective agents that are expected to concede long-term resistance development compared to small molecule antibiotics.

Basically, a wide range of living cells contains a cytoplasmic membrane made of lipid bilayers that fill in as a defensive boundary to isolate and shield the cell from its encompassing environment. What is more than being a "semipenetrable film," it goes about as a gateway directing the transport of substances to and from the intracellular space. Thereby, the cytoplasmic membrane has a crucial role in the survival of the cell. Most generally acknowledged mechanism of antimicrobial activity of AMPs is immediate microbial killing by the disruption, reorganization, or pore development of cell membranes, bringing about the leakage of cellular contents and inevitable cell death. Albeit still under discussion, a few models, for example, "barrel stave," "toroidal pore," and "carpet model," have been proposed to clarify the membrane damaging interaction of AMPs with lipid bilayers. The crucial method of microbicidal activity of synthetic antimicrobial polycationic agents is additionally observed to be like that of AMPs. It is translated in terms of basic sequential processes: (1) It starts by the adsorption on microbial cell surface. This most imperative step is likewise the basis of selectivity toward microorganisms; (2) Then, the polycations diffuse through the cell wall as well as (3) interact with the membrane of cytoplasm; (4) This association may irreversibly harm the integrity of the cell membrane; (5) In this manner, it results in the release of cytoplasmic parts including K^+ ions, DNA/RNA; and (6) at last, it leads to cell death. Notwithstanding the membrane interruption by the integration of cationic polymers with lipid membranes, they may likewise destabilize the membrane surface by dislodging divalent cations, for example, Ca^{2+} associated with the layer phospholipids. The foundation of selectivity of AMPs or polymer mimics toward bacterial or fungal cell membranes that originate from the critical distinction between the cellular membrane lipid composition and surface components. Typically, in terms of charge, the cytoplasmic membrane leaflets of mammalian cells are asymmetric. For instance, the external leaflet of human erythrocyte membrane is made out of neutral (zwitterion) lipids, for example, phosphatidylcholine, sphingomyelin, and phosphatidylethanolamine, while the inward leaflet contains negative charge originating from phosphatidylserine. Conversely, the presence of phosphatidylglycerol, phosphatidylserine, or cardiolipin in microbial cell membrane external leaflets make the external surface appealing to cationic atoms, for example, AMPs. Likewise, bacterial and parasitic cells have extra cell envelope segments, basically, the cell wall that gives adequate mechanical strength to withstand changes in osmotic pressure forced upon by the environment. In Gram-positive bacteria, teichoic acids that are connected to either the peptidoglycan cell wall or to the cell membrane confer net negative charges in light of the presence of phosphate moieties in their structure. Gram-negative microscopic bacterial organisms have an extra external membrane possessing phospholipids and lipopolysaccharides. The lipopolysaccharides confer a firmly negative charge to cell surface. Glycoproteins and polysaccharides are present in fungal cell walls, for the most part glucan and chitin that are broadly interconnected together to shape a complex network. The phosphodiester linkages result in extra negative charges in fungal cell surface. Generally, the overall shot of organisms to create resistance toward an agent relies upon the target specificity of the antimicrobial mechanism of action. This is the conspicuous actuality for the fast resistance improvement against antimicrobial agent, since they are very particular to assault a particular microbial target. Conversely, polycations are generally nonspecific in their activity on microorganisms. In any case, it is doubtful to expect that microbial pathogens are unfit to create resistance against these macromolecules. It needs to be noticed that there are few reports demonstrating bacterial resistance development toward AMPs and synthetic polymers. Nevertheless, widespread and quick resistance improvement toward membrane active, cell lysing antimicrobial macromolecules might be far-fetched contrasted with small molecule antimicrobials interceded with specific receptor sites. It has been visible that there is a lot of more prominent number of passes required to provoke resistance in microorganisms against AMPs or synthetic mimics of AMPs under in-vitro experiments. Then again, it is equivocal in in-vivo conditions, where a huge number of defense agents and mechanism are available in the host and may characterize the microbial adjustments against cationic macromolecules.

These highlights might be the reason AMPs have been effectively present in biological frameworks as viable defensive macromolecules in numerous forms of life for a million years. Synthetic mimics of AMPs are quickly growing demonstrating that AMPs have shaped a superior stage to build-up a class of cutting-edge antimicrobial therapeutics. A few kinds characteristic of AMPs and mimics of AMPs, for example, manufactured AMPs, 93 peptides, 94, 95 peptides, 96 and AA peptides 97 have been created with practically identical or stunningly better activities than the regular adaptations. Be that as it may much of the time expensive manufactured methodologies, quick proteolytic corruption, low bioavailability, or toxicity limits their across the board clinical applicability. The capacity to tweak the basic highlights into different architecture and functionalities, low cost synthesis, powerful biological activity, and steadiness make engineered antimicrobial polymers favorable over different analogs of AMPs compared with circulatory time and reduced residual toxicity to the environment. The general term "antimicrobial polymers" incorporate a few classes of materials, for example, cationic polymers, biocide-discharging polymers, and antimicrobial conjugated polymers. Engineered polymer disinfectants, with cationic functionalities that rose simultaneously with AMPs, show solid biocidal activities. These macromolecules normally have cationic functionality, for example, quaternary ammonium groups and hydrophobic alkyl moieties have been for the most part derived from poly(styrene)s, poly(vinylpyridine)s, poly(methacrylate)s, etc. However, earlier variants of polycationic biocides indicated big lethality to human cells. This property could be just in accordance with their targeted application, which is in the solid state as intense disinfectants or biocidal coatings. In this manner, the improvement of both antimicrobial and biocompatible polymers is basic to empower far-reaching foundational or topical clinical utilization of these macromolecules [5, 6].

7.2.1 CONVENTIONAL ANTIMICROBIAL POLYMERS

Due to biocidal diffusion, the prepared conventional antimicrobial agents, which are based totally on natural or low-molecular-weight compounds, are easily touchy to resistance and might result in environmental contamination and toxicity to the human body. By promoting antimicrobial efficacy and decreasing residual toxicity, antimicrobial polymeric materials offer a valid approach addressing these problems. Added to the abovementioned facts, chemical stability, nonvolatility, and long-term activity are the main characteristics of antimicrobial polymers. Polymers containing covalently bonded antimicrobial moieties avoid the problem of the permeation of low-molecular-weight biocides from the polymer matrices compared to the antimicrobial polymeric materials, which are achieved by physically entrapping or coating organic and/or inorganic active agents to the materials during or after processing. Long-term durability in an eco-friendly manner is one of the promising features of such antimicrobial polymers. Among them, the maximum extensively used and studied antimicrobial polymers are the ones antimicrobial polymeric materials containing quaternary ammonium salt (QAS) and/or quaternary phosphonium salt (QPS). Generations of QAS possessing various systems have been explored as disinfectants since Domagk found the antimicrobial assets of benzalkonium chlorides in 1935. QAS has been found as the most popular antimicrobial polymeric material as per a survey on approximately 500 United States Environmental Protection Agency that registered disinfectant products for households have been applied in 57.8% of the formulations. As in keeping with the reports, it has been stated that the yearly global-wide consumption of QAS changed into zero, 5 million heaps in 2004, and is predicted to exceed to around 0.7 million tons. QPS has been developed for supplying new progress in cationic biocides as it has systems and antimicrobial activities just like QAS. Due to the intrinsic property of the corresponding QAS/QPS, polymeric QAS/QPS ought to acquire broad-spectrum antimicrobial activities through both direct polymerizations of monomers containing QAS/QPS corporations or covalently incorporating QAS/QPS moieties inside everyday synthetic or herbal polymers. In the meantime, antibiotic resistance may be conquered by polymeric QAS/QPS as capability drivers. Preparation of polymerizable QAS/QPS monomers that are ultimately polymerized or copolymerized with other monomers is one method of synthesizing polymers with pendant QAS/QPS. Quaternization of polymers containing either tertiary ammonium/phosphonium groups or alkyl halides is another approach. Monomeric stability can be a limiting factor within the direct polymerization process. While the quaternization degree is limited by the impact of neighboring groups and steric hindrance, the potential limitations of monomeric stability are screened by postquaternization. Properties of the as-prepared polymers may range in terms of the quaternization degree, since it is difficult to achieve complete functionalization by postquaternization of polymeric tertiary ammonium/phosphonium salts. The most common methods for determination of the antimicrobial ability of water-soluble QAS/QPS polymers are measurements of the minimum inhibitory concentration and minimum bactericidal concentration of polymers. For the estimation of antimicrobial performance of water-insoluble polymers, the shaking flask test and inhibition zone measurement are two general approaches in which the inhibition zone measurement is normally applied to detect the diffusion of biocidals.

To form a fast-swelling, antimicrobial superabsorber synthesis of a hemocompatible, antimicrobial 3,4-en-ionene (PBI) derived by polyaddition of trans-1,4-dibromo-2-butene and $N,N,N',$N'-tetramethyl-1,3-propanediamine was carried out by cross-linking via its bromine end groups using tris(2-aminoethyl)amine according to a very recent study by Arne Strassburg et al. By forming a hydrogel, the granulated material is taking on 96-fold of its weight and the superabsorber is taking over the 30-fold of its weight in 60 s. The production of the bacterium *S. aureus* is fully prevented. To form an interpenetrating hydrogel (IPH) with varying PBI content material within the range of 2.0–7.8 wt%, the PBI network was swollen with 2-hydroxyethyl acrylate and glycerol dimethacrylate followed by photopolymerization. Atomic force microscopy and transmission electron microscopy were used to confirm the nanophasic structure of the IPH. Even at the minimum PBI concentration, the bacterial cells of the nosocomial strains such as *S. aureus*, *Escherichia coli*, and *Pseudomonas aeruginosa* are killed at the IPH. Even after washing the hydrogels for as much as 4 weeks, the antimicrobial activity becomes retained. By the usage of a new quantitative test for PBI detection in solution, the IPHs show minor leaching of PBI far under its antimicrobial active concentration. Formation of the inhibition zone and the termination of bacterial cells in the medium of the IPH cannot be obtained as the leaching was exposed to be insufficient. The successful fast swelling superabsorber, as a result of the end-group cross-linking of the PBI, takes up water within less than a minute to a multifold of its own weight. The hydrogels formation via polybenzimidazole granulates are also fast swelling in water. The limitations of the inefficiency of not being able to hold back liquids under pressure can be overcome by the use of this material, thus finding applications as a promising additive for wound bandages. Addition of intrinsic antimicrobial properties in this way further allows no bacterial growth in its surroundings. A clear stable material with 1.4–7.8 wt% PBI can be obtained after the rendering of such a material into an IPH. Long-term antimicrobial activity is shown by the IPHs against several nosocomial bacterial strains. Antimicrobial activity is allowed post 4 weeks of washing by the minor leaching of the PBI. Wound dressing, for example, for burns or infected wounds are few fields of applications where IPH is a promising material [7, 8].

Figure 7.1 generally describes the action mode of polymers, represented by AMPs, against pathogens via electrostatic interactions. First antimicrobial polymers approach cell membranes of pathogens; by formation of pores, it disrupts the cytoplasmic membranes, probably in various mechanisms, for example, carpet barrel-stave and toroidal pore; further due to increase in diffusion of water and ions, leading to further damage of integrity and structural organizations of the cell membranes due to osmotic imbalances in cellular systems and finally leading to leakage of cytoplasmic contents and cell lysis [3, 6]. The less negatively charged and the more stable form than those of bacteria, the cell membranes of mammalian cells, which are rich in phosphatidylcholine, phosphatidylserine, and cholesterol, are rich in phosphatidylethanolamine and phosphatidylglycerol without cholesterol, thus thereby leading to the facilitation of antimicrobial polymers to differentiate between pathogens and mammalian cells. However, polyhexamethylene biguanide and synthetic AMPs could kill bacteria and *Mycobacterium* by targeting DNA as indicated in the recent works. In the case of poly(norbornene) containing guanidine units and other AMPs, similar antimicrobial mode was previously suggested.

Thereby, we have come to point where its vital task to fine-tune the chemistry, topology, and morphology of polymers to attack the cell membranes or/and genetic substances of pathogens effectively rather than mammalian cells based on the knowledge, to develop safe and effective antimicrobial polymers. At present, due to electrostatic interaction with the negatively charged cell membranes, majority of antimicrobial polymers target pathogens as shown in Figure 7.1. The integrated forms of various units, for example, amine (primary, secondary, tertiary), quaternary ammonium, guanidinium/biguanide salt, quaternary pyridinium, quaternary imidazolium, 20 quaternized 1,3-thiazole and 1,2,3-triazole, 21 phosphonium and sulfonium are being utilized as antimicrobial polymers in different styles.

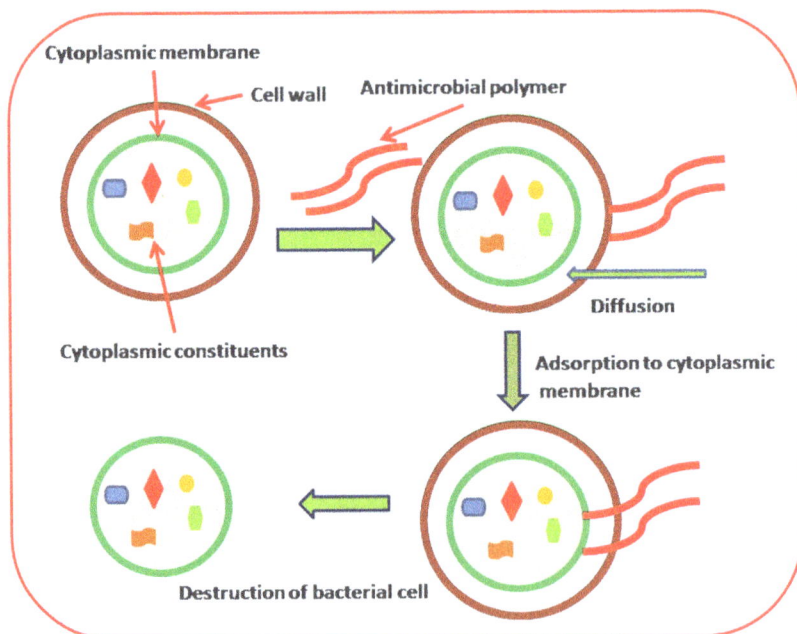

FIGURE 7.1   Schematic representation of the mode of action of antimicrobial polymers on pathogens.

The investigation of the effects of the amine types on antimicrobial activity has been studied similarly. It has been mentioned that more antimicrobial effectiveness and much less hemolytic properties were observed in the case of protonated primary amines and protonated tertiary amines of polyacrylates than quaternary amines and comparable results were observed for poly(methacrylamide). Strong antimicrobial activity was shown in the case of protonated primary amines in aminohexyl polyacrylates. Added to such a fact, it was observed that primary amines of polyacrylates possessing low molecular weight showed antimicrobial activity, but the corresponding quaternary amines lost the activity probably as a result of loss of hydrophobicity required to disrupt the cell membranes of pathogens. Also, high antimicrobial activity was shown by protonated secondary amines in poly(diallyl ammonium chloride) than quaternary ammonium. Therefore, via hydrogen bonding together with electrostatic interactions, protonated primary and secondary amines might be able to interact with the cell membranes of pathogens to improve antimicrobial activity. On the other hand, higher antimicrobial activity was displayed by protonated tertiary amines incorporated with polystyrene than the quaternary ammonium; whatsoever, quaternization of tertiary amines of polyacrylates could improve antimicrobial response. Via the introduction of hydrophobic units, the hydrophobicity of polymers can be achieved from hydrophobic backbones. From recent work, it has been studied that high antimicrobial activity can be achieved via the incorporation of hydrophobic valine units with lysine to form star-shaped polypeptide. Hydrophobicity can be introduced by the application of alkylation. For different polymers, the optimal length of alkyl units is different in order to attain a potent antimicrobial activity. Incorporation of antimicrobial polymers into bulk of substrates can be done to improve the durability. Integration of antimicrobial triazole units into the backbones of polymers could be casted in melt into films with antimicrobial activity. Better understanding of the biological properties of both pathogens and mammalian cells, such as cell membrane compositions, pH and redox status, and genetics, is very essential to incorporate further developments in antimicrobial polymers with high efficiency and safety. In the meanwhile, on the premise of the current knowledge, new potent antimicrobial species are still desirable. To explore the different distribution of negative charges on the cell membranes of pathogens and human cells, it should be meaningful to establish the development of polymers with optimal spatial distribution of antimicrobial units such as amines, peptides, and other potent species. An optimal matching between the positively charged units of polymers and the negatively charged units on the cell membranes of the pathogens should significantly improve the efficacy of antimicrobial polymers. However, without side effects on mammalian cells, even though it was indicated that the charge density of polymers on the surfaces needs to be higher than a threshold value and is a key factor to achieve antimicrobial potency. However, exploration for the antimicrobial applications can be established via the large pool of polymers for gene delivery, majority of which are polyamines [5].

7.2.2   *BILE ACIDS FOR THE SYNTHESIS OF ANTIMICROBIAL POLYMERS*

For the preparation of antimicrobial polymers, it was noted that bile acids are potential candidates. Amphiphilic steroidal acids such as bile of mammals and other vertebrates are rich in bile acids. Conjugated formation of bile salts with taurine or glycine in the liver serves as surfactants in the solubilization of dietary lipids and fats via the formation of micelles that allow digestion of food. Applications of bile acids have found its place in the areas of gene delivery, drug delivery, sensing, polymeric gels, antimicrobial agents as well as other biological applications. The 5b framework of bile acids or the cis A-B ring junction having two faces with dramatically different properties imparts a curvature to the ring system. Facial amphiphilicity is created by the hydroxyl groups of bile acid molecules being positioned in a-face while their methyl groups being positioned in the b-face [4]. Hydrophobic cores that are provided by the steroidal nucleus possessing four fused rings can preferentially embedded into cell membranes. The hydrophilic chemical functionalization that is needed to achieve robust molecular designs and architectures to investigate key determinants of its surface activity and the ability to selectively interact with membrane lipids are offered by the presence of hydroxyl and carboxylic acid groups. A variety of structures having bile acids as repeating units in the polymer backbone, as pendant groups along the polymer chain in block or statistical polymers and chain end-functional polymers are few among the various recent advances of bile acid in macromolecular research. Zhu and coworkers have carried out notable advances on bile acid polymers. Atomic transfer radical polymerization, reversible addition-fragmentation chain transfer,, and ring-opening metathesis polymerization are few among the many controlled polymerization methods that have been used to make side chain bile acid-containing polymers. Step-growth polymerization via incorporating a variety of linkers such as esters, anhydrides, triazoles, β-amino esters, and sulfides are used in the preparation of polymers containing bile acids in the main chain. Highly efficacious and inexpensive antimicrobial polymers for numerous applications are prepared using polycondensation method. Ammonium polyionenes, a unique class of polyelectrolytes, can be prepared by growth polymerizations to obtain cations in the backbone at regular and specific sites. The general method of preparation consists of a reaction between ditertiary amines and dihalides via a Menshutkin reaction. Strong- and fast-acting antimicrobial activities are well presented by these polymers. Whatsoever, the fact that only little knowledge is available on the regard of the preparation of hydrophobic polyionenes that incorporate natural product-derived chemicals targeted for antimicrobial applications persists. The possibility to develop dihalides monomers from bile acids such as lithocholic acid can be used to prepare quaternary ammonium polyionenes. Development of water-soluble cationic polymers with degradable ester linkages via usage of lithocholic acids in the main chain has become formulated with ease. The development of difunctional monomers from lithocholic acid and the usage of them to make cationic polymers that contain quaternary ammonium groups along the polymer backbone play a crucial role in the formation of micelles in water that acts as excellent antimicrobial polymers [4].

7.3   POLYIONENES AS ANTIMICROBIAL AGENTS

In order to effectively combat microbes, several classes of membrane-active cationic polymers have emerged as antimicrobial materials. Polyionenes being a promising candidate in the class of antimicrobial compounds among numerous classes of antimicrobial compounds have emerged in this field due to ease of synthesis and scale-up. The cationic charge density and hydrophobicity of these polymers can be tailored by the careful selection of building blocks and the cationic charge resides along the backbone in polyionenes (Figure 7.2). Polyionenes are rendered to be alluring materials to combat multidrug resistant (MDR) pathogens as a result of this additional dimension to tailor the polymer structure properties along with numerous commercially available building blocks. It has been discovered in recent research that these membrane-active polymers are effective against numerous MDR species including *Acinetobacter baumannii*, *E. coli*, *Klebsiella pneumoniae*, methicillin-resistant *S. aureus*, *Candida albicans*, and many others. Commercially available aromatic bis-halides and bis-dimethylamine-containing monomers were used in the synthesis of these polymers through addition polymerization. The potentiality of polyionenes with broad spectrum of antimicrobial function, excellent killing kinetics, and in-vivo skin biocompatibility can be observed. Another important factor was that these polymers were active against clinically isolated pathogens. This leads to the conclusion that polyionenes are an important family of antimicrobial polymers [5].

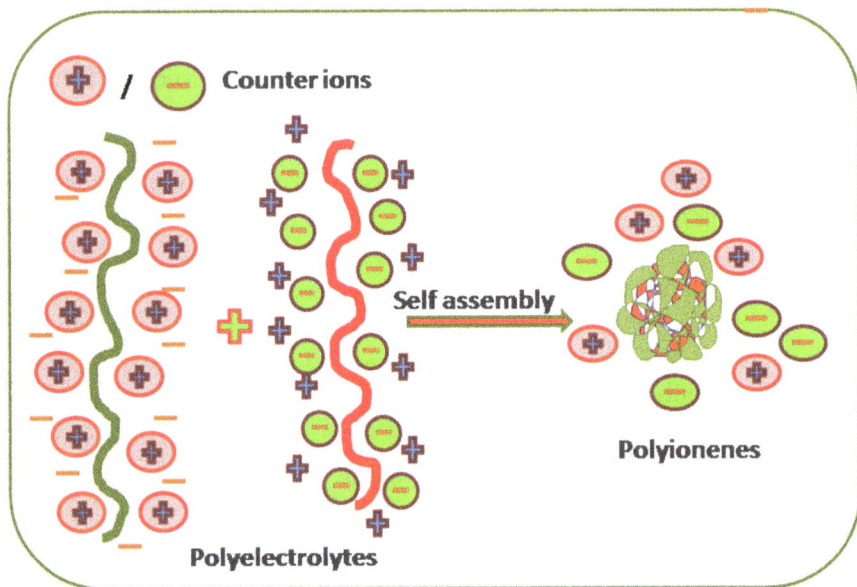

FIGURE 7.2   Schematic representation of polyionenes.

The quaternized nitrogen is placed in the polymer backbone in polyionenes in which the distal charges are pendent to the backbone, possess high charge density and highly efficient processability, demonstrating high antimicrobial activity. By choosing appropriate commercially available monomers, charge density and hydrophobicity of polyionenes can be readily tuned in comparison to polycarbonates and polyacrylates. Studies have been conducted on polyionenes as antimicrobials. For example, alkyloxyethylammonium ionenes with varying pendent groups and alky spacers in the main chain as biocides have been done by Agarwal and coworkers using polyaddition reaction of *N,N,N',N'*-tetramethylmethanediamines and a,u-dibromoalkanes. It was also found that such polyionenes have excellent antimicrobial activity and were not hemolytic toward red blood cells by Tiller's group. On a general perspective, the chain rigidity and alkyl groups of varying length are two major factors that determine the antimicrobial efficacy of polyionenes, which were used to modulate hydrophobicity [6].

Reports have stated that quaternary ammonium PEI (QPEI) has been endowed with excellent antibacterial activities. The approximate ratio of primary, secondary, and tertiary amine groups of branched water-soluble polyethylenemine is equal to 1:2:1. The higher density of quaternary ammonium groups along its backbone causes the QPEI to be effectively antibacterial. QPEI has a stronger antibacterial effectiveness in comparison to the small-molecular-weight QASs because of the macromolecular effect of concentrating antibacterial groups. The action mechanism of antibacterial quaternary ammonium compounds is assumed to be a set of events starting with cationic binding and electrostatic interaction between the microorganism cell wall components and the QPEI, causing a strong adsorption that later disrupts the membrane function, resulting in leakage of constituents such as K1 ions, DNA, and RNA and eventually causing cell death. According to that, quaternary ammonium affects lysis of bacterial cells and demonstrates high bactericidal effect. Thus, sterilizing process is the antibacterial mechanism of QPEI. A 100% antibacterial ratio against *E. coli* cells following contact time of 4 min can be observed in the case of QPEI. Determination of *N*-alkylated poly(ethyleneimine) against a variety of Gram-positive and Gram-negative bacteria was studied by Lin et al. The dependency of antibacterial activity on molecular weight of the conjugate can found easily. There are results that prove, for example, *N*-alkylated PEI of 2 and 0.8 kDa had low bactericidal activity. To add more, a structure–activity relationship analysis has shown that in order to create antibacterial surfaces immobilized long polymeric chains have to be positively charges as well as hydrophobic (but not excessively so). This particular design methodology has been validated with macroscopic surfaces as well as with nanoparticles. Reports have been formulated showing a study against oral pathogens and QPEI-based nanoparticles. The few among the many oral pathogens include *Enterococcus faecalis*, *Streptococcus mutans*, *Actinomyces viscosus*, *Lactobacillus casei*, and whole saliva. The nanoparticles demonstrated enduring microbial protection against all these pathogens.

Quaternary amine-containing antimicrobial poly(bile acid)s that contain a hydrophobic core of lithocholic acid in the main chain were developed by Mitra et al. in a recent study. Core-shell micelles can be formed by these cationic polymers. Furthermore, biocidal activity against both Gram-positive and Gram-negative bacterial species was demonstrated by these polymers. The fact that the micelles can deliver hydrophobic antibiotics that functionally have dual antimicrobial activities were also well exhibited. Dosage-dependent toxicity for polymers with longer linkers was displayed by the cytotoxicity assays against HeLa cells. Micelles formation in aqueous media with a cationic surface and a hydrophobic core were evident from these novel polyionenes. Added to such a fact, prominent broad-spectrum antimicrobial activities were exhibited by these polyionenes. As a result of the negative charge on the bacterial cell surface, polymers possessing cations or comprising positive charges on their surfaces may have a contact disinfectant effect. Development of a number of polymers that demonstrate antibacterial properties were toward this purpose, including soluble and insoluble pyridinium-type polymers and water-soluble pyridinium-type polycations having bactericidal properties. Furthermore, through either water or air, poly(vinyl-*N*-hexylpyridinium) surface coating has proven to kill 90%–99% of Gram-negative and Gram-positive bacteria. Compounds, bearing quaternary ammonium groups, usually act primarily by its interaction with the cell wall and then the disruption of negatively charged bacterial cell membrane. As per structure–activity relationship analysis, it has been revealed to us that in order to create antibacterial surfaces, immobilized long polymeric chains need to be water resistant (but not excessively so) and positively charged [6].

Using a polymerization of noncatalytic polymeric acids with monomers found in the market, macromolecular polyolene in water-soluble polyols in high-efficiency and skin-compatible water has been developed by Shaoqiong Liu et al. Preparation of a series of antimicrobial agents is carried out with a simple polyamination reaction with the training of polymers and the installation of the device intervening simultaneously. To study the effects of antimicrobial activity on a broad spectrum of pathogenic microbes, the polymorphic components and structures are modulated. Polymers with optimized compositions have a powerful antimicrobial activator with minimal inhibitory concentrations. These polymers demonstrate a high antimicrobial efficacy against several clinically isolated microdegree microbes and show a biocompatibility of the skin much higher compared to the other clinical surgical scrubs used (chlorhexidine and betadine). The microbicide activity of the polymer is mediated smooth through the membrane as demonstrated by confocal microscopy. Unlike molecular antibiotic smallpox, the repeated use of the drug does not induce resistance to drugs. Even more important, the polymers show an optimal bactericidal activity in a pattern of blood glucose by *P. aeruginosa*. The powerful and profitable antimicrobial polymers have been successfully synthesized by simple polymerization in most of the available material available on the merchandise programs.

Polymers prove to show low but effective dose with high-therapeutic index in an MDR *Klebsiella pneumoniae* 8637-caused pneumonia mouse model. Polymers are also more dependent on survival and a faster relocation of bacteria from the main organs and the blood of impairment from the treatment of polymers. Even more important, the treatment of polymers does not cause toxicity to the function of kidneys and rods nor interferes with the balance of blood electrolytes at the therapeutic dose. The policy is a promising candidate to cure pneumonia caused by MDR *K. pneumoniae* due to its in-vivo efficacy and insignificant toxicity.

Antimicrobial polymers are used as therapy for the cure of MDR *K. pneumoniae* pulmonary infections. Md Anisur Rahman designed a class of antimicrobial cationic polymers that grouped the local facial amplitude of the replicate unit to improve interactions with the bacterial membrane without requiring a global conformal arrangement associated with intracellular loss. The macromolecular architecture of macromolecular economy demonstration can be observed with a series of polymers based on its multicultural natural products. We have demonstrated that the selectivity of derivatives of copolymeric acid with three groups of the critical texts is more powerful than the lithocholic and deoxycholic acid, particularly against Gram-negative bacteria. True face amphiphilic training is attributed to this with ion-group hydrophobic-oriented, multifaceted hydrocarbon faces and structures on the opposite faces. When there is contact with bacterial membrane, such as local amphiphilicity facile, it adds via a flexible backbone macromolecular in a concerted manner.

The antimicrobial polymers described by ShrinivasVenkataraman have high selectivity and a spectrum versus pathogenic (versus mammalian cell) that gives a way to combat infections with only a severe possibility of resistance. Antimicrobial fungal biodegradability materials that are usually derived from inexpensive renewable resources yield polysaccharides as a liver uptake for broader applications. Here, we bring a friendly approach to one's vacuum to access powerful antimicrobial polymers from solubility, a matter based on renewable plants and other readily accessible reagents. It demonstrated an excellent antibacterial activity in the solution site using these polymers with an optimal composition, but can only have limited anti-fungal effects. The smooth transformation of these polymers in antimicrobial hydrogels and reactions with photo-mediated thiol reactions can be activated by using reactive alloys installed on the polymeric platform. Through more pathogenic agents (100% by *S. aureus*, *E. coli*, and *P. aeruginosa*), it can be the hydrogel or the hydrogel thickeners and they have very high efficiencies.

The rapid development of formulations and prototypes in various shapes such as gels and surface varnish, minimizing, or completely eliminating the need to optimize polymers to satisfy diverse applications is due to the installation of reactive groups onto antimicrobial platforms. The demonstration of the potential usefulness of biodegradable polymers based on catalyzing properties can be addressed as applications such as antimicrobial materials and reversals for the prevention of infections.

7.4 CONCLUSION AND FUTURE PERSPECTIVES

Many researchers have been targeted on the development of new antimicrobial polymeric materials and exploration of their biocidal activities and action modes. Polymers possess wide spectrum of antimicrobial activity with excipients of low-molecular weight, covalently bonded moieties, and long-term biocidal efficacy with no leaching of active moieties and their applications can expanded by designing and employing different polymeric structures. However, there is still a high requirement for developing antimicrobial materials aspired at multispecies pathogenic microbes including bacteria, fungi, protozoa, prions, viruses, etc. In particular, the nonenveloped viruses, which do not possess lipid bilayer envelope surrounding the capsid, those are very stable and virulent, and it is difficult to control and/or destroy by conventional antimicrobial materials. There are so many studies that are currently going onto investigating structure–bioactivity relationship to achieve an optimal balance between antimicrobial activity and cytotoxicity. In the case of polyionenes, polymeric structures under mild conditions each bond-forming event creates a positive charge. This enabled an initial survey of a new class of antimicrobial polyionenes.

KEYWORDS

- **antimicrobial polymers**
- **multidrug resistance**
- **polyionenes**
- **membrane active cationic polymers**
- **quaternary ammonium salts**

REFERENCES

1. Luepke, K. H., Suda, K. J., Boucher, H., Russo, R. L., Bonney, M. W., Hunt, T. D. and Mohr, J. F. Past, present, and future of antibacterial economics: increasing bacterial resistance, limited antibiotic pipeline, and societal implications. *Pharmacotherapy* 37(1) (2017): 71–84.
2. Arora, G., Andaleeb, S. and Vipin, C. K. (Eds). Drug resistance in bacteria, fungi, malaria and cancer. Philadelphia: Springer, 2017.
3. Muñoz-Bonilla, A. and Fernández-García, M. Polymeric materials with antimicrobial activity. *Progress in Polymer Science* 37(2) (2012): 281–339.
4. Ganewatta, M. S., Rahman, M. A., Mercado, L., Shokfai, T., Decho, A. W., Reineke, T. M. and Tang, C. Facial amphiphilic polyionene biocidal polymers derived from lithocholic acid. *Bioactive Materials* 3(2) (2018): 186–193.
5. Ren, W., Cheng, W., Wang, G. and Liu, Y. Developments in antimicrobial polymers. *Journal of Polymer Science Part A: Polymer Chemistry* 55(4) (2017): 632–639.
6. Lou, W., Venkataraman, S., Zhong, G., Ding, B., Tan, J. P. K., Xu, L., Fan, W. and Yang, Y. Y. Antimicrobial polymers as therapeutics for treatment of multidrug-resistant Klebsiella pneumoniae lung infection. *Acta Biomaterialia* 78 (2018): 78–88.
7. Liu, S., Ono, R. J., Wu, H., Teo, J. Y., Liang, Z. C., Xu, K., Zhang, M., Zhong, G., Tan, J. P. K., Ng, M., Yang, C., Chan, J., Ji, Z., Bao, C., Kumar, K., Gao, S., Lee, A., Fevre, M., Dong, H., Ying, J. Y., Li, L., Fan, W., Hedrick, J. L. and Yang, Y. Y. Highly potent antimicrobial polyionenes with rapid killing kinetics, skin biocompatibility and in vivo bactericidal activity. *Biomaterials* 127 (2017): 36–48.
8. Beyond, N., Subramani, K. and Ahmed, W. Antimicrobial nanoparticles in restoration composites: emerging nanotechnologies in dentistry. Philadelphia: William Andrew Publishing, 2017. 41–58.

CHAPTER 8

Antirheumatic Potential of *Justicia gendarussa* Root Extract on Chronic Arthritic Models

S. K. KAVITHA[1*] and A. HELEN[2]

[1]National Institute of Malaria Research Field Unit, ICMR, Bangalore, India

[2]Department of Biochemistry, University of Kerala, Thiruvananthapuram, Kerala, India

*Corresponding author. E-mail: kavitha.skumar@gmail.com

ABSTRACT

Inflammation triggers a varied assortment of physiological and pathological progressions. More recent evidence suggests that a much broader range of diseases have divulging markers for inflammation. Rheumatoid arthritis (RA) is an inflammatory arthritis that distresses nearly 1% of the world's adults. The drugs frequently in use for the treatment of RA include nonsteroidal anti-inflammatory drugs, disease-modifying antirheumatic drugs, corticosteroids, and biologic response modifiers. These managements exert anti-inflammatory actions with severe adverse effects. As a consequence, alternative treatments based on medicinal plants and natural plant products are becoming increasingly popular in India, US, and other countries. In the light of this remark, *Justicia gendarussa*, a medicinal plant, which is widely used for the treatment of inflammation and rheumatic diseases in folk medicine, was selected for this study to investigate its antirheumatic potential. This chapter converses about the antirheumatic efficacy of *Justicia gendarussa* on chronic arthritic models. Through this work, the beneficial potential of *Justicia gendarussa* was explored and this may provide a novel approach in anti-inflammatory research. This chapter is a result of me and my PhD guide's interest in inflammation and anti-inflammatory agents. This book may provide additional knowledge about the design and development of new drug delivery systems potentially useful in the treatment of chronic inflammatory-based diseases.

8.1　INTRODUCTION

Immune system is dynamic to persist, since an overactive immune coordination may cause lethal illness owing to overwhelming sensitized reaction leading to sequences of derangements, loss of standard capacity to differentiate self from nonself, resultant in immune reactions against one's own tissues and cells called autoimmune diseases [27]. Arthritis is an inflammation of synovial joint due to immune-facilitated reaction. The pathophysiological portent of arthritis comprises dysregulation of proinflammatory cytokines and proinflammatory enzymes, which fallouts in high level of prostaglandins, leukotrienes, and nitric oxide; in addition, there is also manifestation of an adhesion molecule, matrix metalloproteinase and hyperspread of synovial fibroblasts [56]. Regulation of all these factors is preserved through transcription factor called nuclear factor kB [58]. Rheumatoid arthritis (RA) is a relatively common type of arthritis and its serious forms can cause severe disability [2]. It is a chronic advanced illness, emerging over months or years, and linking basically the synovial joints of the body [2]. RA has 19th century origins and 20th century pedigree [87].

　　Free-radical mechanisms have been implicated in the pathology of numerous human ailments, including RA [10, 18]. Throughout phagocytosis, monocytes, neutrophils, and macrophages produce superoxide radicals, hydrogen peroxide, and the exceedingly reactive hydroxyl radicals [72]. These cytotoxic reactive oxygen species may cause oxidative impairment in the cells [32, 57]. Stimulated oxygen intermediates together with highly reactive radicals, such as the hydroxyl radicals, are able to terminate membrane lipids, proteins, deoxyribonucleic acid, hyaluronic acid, and cartilage [15]. Enzymatic mechanisms comprise superoxide dismutase (SOD), catalase, and glutathione peroxidase (GPX) [32]. Vitamins A, C, E and glutathione are some of the main nonenzymatic antioxidants in the body [26].

　　More than a few lines of indication recommend that oxidative stress has a role in the pathology of RA [4]. The inadequacy of antioxidant defense systems and the hastening of the oxidative reactions can be the outcomes of the pro-oxidant/antioxidant disparity in RA [4]. Furthermore, it was also bring into being that individuals with innately low levels of protecting antioxidants in their plasma, such as vitamins A and E, carotene, and selenium, are also at greater risk of developing RA [4, 28].

Lysosomes are produced from the endosomal membrane system through a complex mechanism involving membrane and protein sorting and trafficking. It is now generally conceded that lysosomal instability in tissues of the rheumatoid joint plays some part in the rheumatoid process either directly [90]. Lysosomal enzymes and their release into the cytoplasm stimulate the formation of inflammatory mediators [70]. These enzymes play a major role in the destruction of structural macromolecules in connective tissue and cartilage proteoglycans [20]. They are also capable of destroying extracellular activities by increased extracellular activities of lysosomal enzymes [52]. They are also skillful in destroying extracellular structures and may contribute in mediating tissue damage in rheumatic ailments [52].

A number of experimental arthritis models have been used to impressionist human RA, ranging from immunization with cartilage components to infection with joint tropic organisms [86, 92]. These have added to the basic understanding of joint disease and to the development of effective antiarthritic agents. The preferred models of the joint pathology that occur in human RA are rat adjuvant-induced arthritis (AIA) and collagen-induced arthritis (CIA).

India is identified as the "Emporium of Medicinal plants" due to handiness of quite a lot of medicinal plants in the diverse bioclimatic zones. Concentration in medicinal plants as a re-emerging well-being aid has been drove by the growing costs of prescription drugs in the preservation of personal health and well-being and the bioprospecting of new plant-derived medicines [44]. Many pharmacological class of medications obtainable in the market are derived from natural products prototype including atropine from *Atropa belladonna* (Solanaceae), reserpine from *Rauwolfia serpentina* (Apocyanaceae), digoxin from *Digitalis purpurea* (Scrophulariaceae), and quinine from *Cinchona officinalis* (Rubiacea).

The practice of natural remedies for the treatment of inflammatory and painful conditions has a long history, beginning with Ayurvedic treatment and extending to the European and other systems of old-style medicines [37, 84]. Many hundreds of plants comprise well-known anti-inflammatory agents [55]. There are characteristic anti-inflammatory herbs in almost each family in the plant kingdom [55]. For some plants, intrinsic anti-inflammatory activity is inferred from other identified pharmacological activities related to modulation of the complex inflammatory response. For some, the anti-inflammatory activity has been widely studied while preliminary evidence has been recognized for others.

The plant particular for our study is *Justicia gendarussa* (JRM) Burm. F. [61]. JRM has many characteristic features such as it is a shade loving plant that grows quickly and it is an evergreen shrub that can be seen throughout India and also in all Asian countries such as Malaysia, Indonesia, Sri Lanka, and Bangladesh [50, 69]. It is a rare medicinal plant that belongs to the family Acanthaceae. JRM is erect and branched that measures up to 0.6–1.2 m in height. The leaves of this plant are simple, opposite, lanceolate or linear lanceolate, acute at base, tapering into rounded apex, and glabrous and shining leaves (8–12.5 cm long and 1.2–2 cm broad) with prominent purple veins beneath [33]. The stem of JRM is quadrangular, thickened at and above the nodes, and internodes measure 2–7 cm long. The flowers of this plant are in terminal or axillary spikes and are irregular, bisexual, sessile, and white with pink or purple spots inside and red in the throat and lip [69].

Commonly, JRM is also known as willow-leaved *justicia* (Figure 8.1). The plant possesses wide-ranging spectrum of activities due to the manifestation of active constituents such as alkaloids, flavonoids, phenolic compounds, steroids, carbohydrate, carotenoids, and terpenoids [33]. In a study that studied the quantitative estimation of 40 phytoconstituents of leaves of JRM, it shows the presence of alkaloids ($1.62 \pm 0.081\%$ w/w), flavonoids ($2.03 \pm 0.105\%$ w/w), triterpenoids ($0.199 \pm 0.009\%$ w/w), carotenoids ($7.88 \pm 0.394\%$ w/w), phenolic compounds ($2.21 \pm 0.11\%$ w/w), sugar ($8.74 \pm 0.435\%$ w/w), and starch ($5.85 \pm 0.292\%$ w/w) [33, 60]. Reports show the presence of beta-sitosterol, lupeol, an alkaloid, friedelin, and aromatic amines in leaves of JRM [33]. In traditional medical system, different parts of JRM have been mentioned to be useful in a variety of diseases [30]. The fresh leaves of JRM are pounded into a paste, warmed and rubbed or applied onto the affected area, which is then bandaged to ease muscle pains, broken/fractured bone, muscle sprains, and cuts [97]. In Vietnamese folk medicine as a poultice to treat rheumatism and arthritis, the leaves of JRM are being used [3]. The leaves of JRM are used as an analgesic to treat hemiplegia, rheumatism, arthritis, headache, and earache in Sri Lankan traditional medicine [69]. It is also used in India for the treatment of chronic rheumatism, cephalalgia, cough, and bronchitis [9]. A decoction prepared by boiling JRM roots in milk is used for the treatment of chronic rheumatic disorders, dysuria, fever, carbuncles, and diarrhea [38] and a paste made from leaves is used in fracture, itches, and wound in Bangladeshi folk medicine [47].

The contemporary study was commenced to study the effect of methanolic extract of JRM roots in lessening inflammation, oxidative stress, and lysosomal instability during experimentally-induced arthritis. The model systems used were AIA and type II CIA in rats. Indomethacin, which is a nonsteroidal anti-inflammatory drug and cyclooxygenase inhibitor, is used as a reference drug to study the process of inflammation. The findings of these investigations are presented and discussed in this chapter.

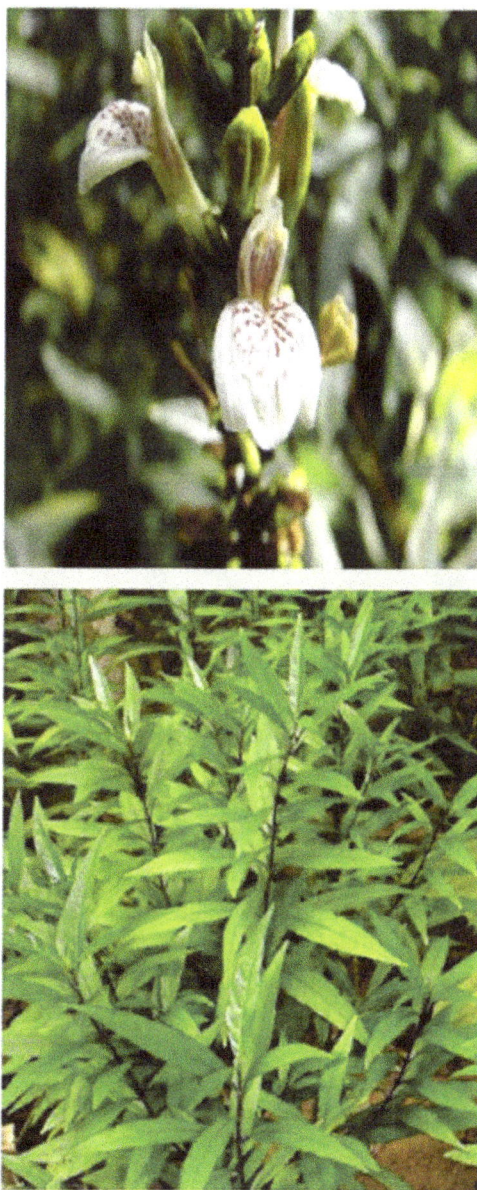

FIGURE 8.1 *Justicia gendarussa* plant.

8.2   MATERIALS AND METHODS

8.2.1   EXPERIMENTAL ANIMALS

Male Wistar rats weighing (150–200 g) were used in this experimental study. The animals in the study were breed and reared in the department animal house in polypropylene cages and kept in an environment with controlled temperature (24–26 °C), humidity (55%–60%), and photoperiod (12:12) light-dark cycle. The rats were given a commercially well-adjusted diet (Amrut laboratory animal feeds, Maharashtra, India) and tap water was provided ad libitum. The trial protocol was sanctioned by the Institutional Animal Ethics Committee [39] and the precaution of laboratory animals was taken as per the guidance of committee [93] for the perseverance of the Committee for the Purpose of Control and Supervision of Experiments on Animals, Registration No. 218/CPCSEA, under project number IAEC-KU-7/2006-2007 BC AH (7).

8.2.2   PLANT MATERIAL

JRM was collected from the medicinal garden of Poojappura Research Institute, Trivandrum, Kerala, India [40]. The plant was recognized and authenticated by Dr G Valsala Devi, Curator, Department of Botany, University of Kerala, Kariavattom [34]. A receipt specimen was deposited at Department of Botany, University of Kerala, Kariavattom (Voucher No. 5797) [34].

8.2.3   PREPARATION OF METHANOLIC EXTRACT OF JRM ROOTS

JRM roots were isolated, cleaned, dried, and weighed (50 g) [34]. It was defatted with petroleum ether (boiling point 60–80 °C) and extracted thrice with methanol. This was concentrated in SpeedVac at 50 °C and used as JRM (yield is 3.68 g with respect to plant material).

8.2.4   ADJUVANT-INDUCED ARTHRITIS

The antiarthritic effect of JRM was studied in AIA [89]. For AIA immunizations, 0.1 mL of complete Freund's adjuvant containing heat-killed mycobacteria in paraffin oil was injected to the right hind paw of animals. Drugs were administered from 5th day. The edema of right hind paw was evaluated from day 7–21 postinjection of adjuvant using plethysmometer [19]. Period of experiment was 21 days. Rats were then sacrificed after overnight fasting by euthanasia. Various tissues such as joint cartilage, liver, spleen, and gastric mucosa were isolated for evaluation of biochemical parameters.

8.2.4.1 EXPERIMENTAL DESIGN

Group I: Control

Group II: Adjuvant-induced arthritic control rats

Group III: Adjuvant-induced arthritic rats supplemented with JRM (100 mg/ kg body weight)

Group IV: Adjuvant-induced arthritic rats supplemented with indomethacin (INDO 3 mg/kg body weight)

8.2.5 TYPE II CIA IN RATS

For immunizations, bovine collagen type II (CII) was liquefied in 0.1 M acetic acid at a concentration of 4 mg/mL and blended in an equal volume of incomplete Freund's adjuvant [25]. Each rat was given intradermal doses of 100 µL at two sites on the back on day 0 and then received booster injections at two sites (100 µL in divided doses) on day 7. Inflammation peaked on day 14. Rats that showed severe arthritis were excluded from the study. Normal nonimmune rats were used as negative controls. Drugs were administered from 14th day. Polyarthritic index was checked on 14th day, 21st day, 28th day, 45th day, and 60th day. To quantitatively calculate the polyarthritic index, a clinical scoring system was used that correlates the arthritis sternness with joint size. Inflammation was graded as follows: Grade 0: paws with no swelling and focal redness, Grade 1: paws with swelling of finger joints, Grade 2: paws with mild swelling of ankle or wrist joints, Grade 3: paws with severe inflammation of entire paws, and Grade 4: paws with deformity or ankylosis [77].

8.2.5.1 EXPERIMENTAL DESIGN

Collagen-induced arthritis was induced in rats by injecting CII in complete Freund's adjuvant [18] into the base of rat tail of male adult Wistar rats [1].

Group I: Control

Group II: Rats with type II CIA

Group III: CIA supplemented with methanolic extract of JRM roots (100 mg/kg/day orally by gastric intubation)

Group IV: CIA supplemented with indomethacin (3 mg/kg/day orally by gastric intubation).

Each paw was graded and scores were totaled, so that the possible maximal score per rat was 12 [77]. Duration of experiment was 60 days. Rats were then sacrificed after overnight fasting by euthanasia. Various tissues such as joint cartilage, liver, spleen, and gastric mucosa were isolated for evaluation of biochemical parameters.

8.2.6 ASSAY OF TOTAL CYCLOOXYGENASE (COX) ACTIVITY (EC 1.14.99.1)

8.2.6.1 REAGENTS

- Tris–HCl buffer (100 mM, pH 8)
- 5 mM glutathione
- 5 mM hemoglobin
- 200 μM arachidonic acid
- 10% TCA in 1 N HCl
- 1% thiobarbiturate.

8.2.6.2 PROCEDURE

The examination of COX was done by TBA method [76]. The assay mixture encloses 1 mL Tris–HCl buffer, 50 μL hemoglobin, and 50 μL enzyme. The reaction was started by the addition of 100 μL arachidonic acid and incubated at 37°C for 20 min. The reaction was terminated by the addition of 10% TCA in HCl, mixed well and 200 μL thiobarbituric acid was added and condensed, heated in a boiling water bath for 20 min, cooled, and centrifuged at 1000 rpm for 3 min. The supernatant was measured at 530 nm for COX activity.

8.2.7   ASSAY OF COX-2 INHIBITION

8.2.7.1   REAGENTS

- 0.1 M Tris–HCl buffer (pH 7.8)
- 1 mM EDTA.

8.2.7.2   PROCEDURE

Cells/tissues were spun at 1000–2000 g for 10 min at 4 °C and sonicated in cold 0.1 M Tris–HCl buffer (pH 7.8) containing 1 mM EDTA and once again spun at 10,000 g for 15 min at 4 °C. COX-1 or COX-2 inhibition was checked using a colorimetric assay kit purchased from Cayman Chemicals, USA. The employed SC 560 is used as specific COX-1 inhibitor, so that only COX-2 activity will be expressed. The results were expressed as % COX-2 inhibition [96].

8.2.8   ASSAY OF LIPOXYGENASE (LOX) (EC 1.13.11.12)

8.2.8.1   REAGENTS

- 50 mM Tris–HCl buffer (pH 7.4)
- Sodium phosphate buffer (pH 6.5)
- 10 mM sodium linoleate.

8.2.8.2   PROCEDURE

The assay of LOX was measured by Axelrod [11]. 70 mg of linoleic acid and equivalent weight of Tween 20 were dissolved in 4 mL oxygen-free water, mixed back and forth with a pipette avoiding air bubbles. Sufficient amount of 0.5 N NaOH was added to yield a clear solution (0.55 mL) and made up to 25 mL using oxygen-free water. This was divided into 0.5 mL portion and flushed with nitrogen gas before closing and it is kept frozen until needed.

8.2.8.3   ASSAY OF 5-LIPOXYGENASE (5-LOX)

The assay mixture contains 2.75 mL Tris–HCl buffer (pH 7.4), 0.1 mL sodium linoleate, and 50 μL of the enzyme. The increase in OD was measured at 234 nm.

8.2.8.4   ASSAY OF 15-LIPOXYGENASE (15-LOX)

The assay mixture contains 2.75 mL sodium phosphate buffer (pH 6.1), 0.1 mL sodium linoleate, and 50 μL of the enzyme. The increase in OD was measured at 280 nm.

8.2.9   ASSAY OF SOD (E.C.1.15.1.1)

8.2.9.1   REAGENTS

- 0.25 M sucrose buffer
- 10% ammonium sulfate
- 0.05 M sodium pyrophosphate buffer
- 186 μM phenazine methosulfate
- 300 μM nitroblue tetrazolium
- 780 μM NADH
- Glacial acetic acid
- *n*-butanol.

8.2.9.2   PROCEDURE

Activity of SOD was measured by the method of Kakkar et al. [31]. Tissues were homogenized in 0.25 M sucrose and differentially centrifuged under cold conditions to get the cytosol fraction. Before estimation of SOD, precipitate the protein from the supernatant with 90% ammonium sulfate. The precipitated proteins were removed by centrifugation. The SOD in the supernatant fraction was dialyzed overnight in Tris–HCl buffer (0.0025 M, pH 7.4) and freed from $(NH4)_2SO_4$. The supernatant was used as the enzyme source. Assay concoction contained 1.2 mL sodium pyrophosphate buffer, 0.1 mL of 1.2 µM phenazine methosulfate, 0.3 mL of nitroblue tetrazolium, 0.2 mL NADH and nearly diluted enzyme preparations and water in a overall volume of 3 mL. Reaction was started by the addition of NADH. After incubation at 30 °C for 90 s, the reaction was stopped by the addition of 1 mL glacial acetic acid [23]. Reaction mixture was stirred robustly and shaken with 4 mL of *n*-butanol [23]. The mixture was allowed to stand for 10 min, centrifuged, and butanol layer was taken out. Color intensity of the chromogen in the butanol fraction was measured at 560 nm against butanol [23]. A system devoid of the enzyme served as control. One unit of the enzyme activity is defined as the enzyme concentration required inhibiting the chromogen production by 50% in 1 min under the assay condition [23]. The specific activity is expressed in units/mg protein.

8.2.10   ASSAY OF CATALASE (EC.1.11.1.6)

8.2.10.1   REAGENTS

- 1.5 M phosphate buffer (pH 7.00)
- H_2O_2 phosphate buffer [1.5 M phosphate buffer ($1.25 \times 10 - 2\ H_2O_2$) (pH 7.0)]

Diluted 0.16 mL H_2O_2 (30% w/v) to 100 mL with buffer. The OD of the solution was about 0.5 at 240 nm with 1 cm light path.

8.2.10.2   PROCEDURE

The enzyme activity was assayed by the method used by Maehly and Chance [46]. The enzyme extract was prepared by homogenizing the tissue in phosphate buffer and centrifugation at 5000 rpm. The reaction mixture contained phosphate buffer, 2 mM H_2O_2, and the enzyme extract. The decrease in the absorbance at 230 nm was measured spectrophotometrically. Specific activity was expressed in terms of units per mg protein.

8.2.11 ESTIMATION OF GLUTATHIONE (GSH) CONTENT

8.2.11.1 REAGENTS

- Precipitating solution: 1.67 g glacial metaphosphoric acid, 0.2 g disodium EDTA, and 30 g sodium chloride were dissolved in 100 mL distilled water.
- Phosphate solution: 42.5 g disodium hydrogen phosphate was dissolved in 1 L distilled water.
- DTNB reagent: 40 g dithionitrobenzoic acid or Ellman's reagent was dissolved in 100 mL 1% sodium citrate solution. This solution is stable for 13 weeks.
- GSH standard: 50 mg/dL was prepared.

8.2.11.2 PROCEDURE

The method of Benke et al., [14] was used for estimating the GSH content. Tissues were homogenized in precipitating solution containing glacial metaphosphoric acid and EDTA at 4 °C. The homogenate was filtered and to 0.2 mL filtrate, 1 mL of 10 mM dithiobisnitrobenzoic acid in 0.1% sodium citrate was added and the absorbance was read at 412 nm. The values of unknown samples were drawn from standard curve plotted by assaying different known concentrations of GSH [18]. The amount of GSH was expressed as mg/100 g tissue [18].

8.2.12 ASSAY OF MYELOPEROXIDASE (MPO) (EC 1.11.1.7)

8.2.12.1 REAGENTS

- 50 mM potassium phosphate buffer (pH 7)
- 0.5% hexadecyltrimethylammonium bromide in phosphate buffer
- o-dianisidine dihydrochloride (0.167 mg/mL)
- 0.0005% hydrogen peroxide.

8.2.12.2 PROCEDURE

MPO was determined by the method of Bradley et al. [16]. MPO activity was evaluated as an index of neutrophil infiltration. Tissues were first homogenized in a solution containing 50 mM potassium phosphate buffer, pH 7.0 containing 0.5% hexadecyltrimethylammonium bromide. This was freeze, warm up thrice, and then centrifuged at 20,000 g for 30 min at 4 °C. An aliquot of the supernatant was tolerable to react with a solution of o-dianisidine dihydrochloride (0.167 mg/mL) and 0.0005% hydrogen peroxide. MPO activity has been defined as the concentration of enzyme degrading 1 μmol of peroxide/min at 37 °C and was expressed as units/mg of protein.

8.2.13 ASSAY OF NITRIC OXIDE SYNTHASE (NOS) (EC 1.14.13.39)

8.2.13.1 REAGENTS

- HEPES solution (36 mg/100 mL)
- L-arginine (350 mg/100 mL)
- $MnCl_2$ (20 mg/10 mL)
- Dithiothreitol (30 μg/mL)
- NADPH (84 μg/mL)
- Tetrahydrobiopterin (63 μg/mL)
- 2 μM oxygenated hemoglobin in HEPES buffer (prewarm at 37 °C).

8.2.13.2 PROCEDURE

We used the method described for the determination of NOS. The tissues/freeze ruptured cells were used as the enzyme source. Tissues were homogenized in HEPES buffer prewarmed to 37 °C. The reaction mixture contained substrate L-arginine, $MnCl_2$, dithiothreitol, NADPH, tetrahydrobiopterin, enzyme source, and 2 μM oxygenated hemoglobin in a total volume of 1 mL. The increase in absorbance was read at 401 nm.

8.2.14 ASSAY OF MALONDIALDEHYDE (MDA)

8.2.14.1 REAGENTS

- 1.5% potassium chloride
- 8.1% SDS
- 20% acetic acid (pH 3.5)

- 0.8% thiobarbituric acid
- Butanol:pyridine mixture (15:1).

8.2.14.2   PROCEDURE

Determination of MDA in the tissues was performed to estimate the amount of lipid peroxidation in the damaged tissues [18]. The test was done according to the method by Okhawa et al. [53]. A standard curve was prepared using 1,1,3,3-tetraethoxypropane. Tissues were homogenized in 10 volumes of buffer and centrifuged at 4000 rpm/min to obtain the supernatant. The reaction mixture containing supernatant, thiobarbituric acid, and acetic acid buffer was heated at 100 °C for 1 h. The samples were then centrifuged and the absorbance of the supernatant was measured at 532 nm. The results were expressed as mmol/100 g wet tissue.

8.2.15   ASSAY OF B-GLUCURONIDASE (EC 3.2.1.31)

8.2.15.1   REAGENTS

- 0.1 M citrate buffer (pH 4.6)
- *p*-nitrophenyl-*N*-acetyl-β-D-glucuronide
- Stop reagent: 0.4 M glycine-NaOH (pH 10.5).

8.2.15.2   PROCEDURE

Estimation of β-glucuronidase was done by the method developed by Kawai et al. [32, 36]. The reaction concoction contained 0.1 M citrate buffer (pH 4.6) containing *p*-nitrophenyl-*N*-acetyl-β-D-glucuronide as substrate and enzyme source. After incubation at 37 °C for 1 h, the reaction was stopped by addition of discontinuing reagent. The absorbance was measured at 405 nm [24].

8.2.16   ASSAY OF B-HEXOSAMINIDASE (EC 3.2.1.30)

8.2.16.1   REAGENTS

- 0.1 M citrate buffer (pH 4.6)

- p-nitrophenyl-*N*-acetyl-β-D-glucosaminide
- Stop reagent: 0.4 M glycine-NaOH (pH 10.5).

8.2.16.2   PROCEDURE

The level of β-hexosaminidase was estimated by the method developed by Rubin et al., [73]. The reaction mixture contained 0.1 M citrate buffer (pH 4.6) containing *p*-nitrophenyl-*N*-acetyl-β-D-glucosaminide as substrate and enzyme source. After incubation at 37 °C for 4 h, the reaction was stopped by addition of stopping reagent [0.4 M glycine-NaOH (pH 10.5)]. The absorbance was measured at 405 nm [24].

8.2.17   STATISTICAL ANALYSIS

Statistical analysis was prepared by following method described by Steel et al. [83]. Results were evaluated using statistical program SPSS version 11.5 (SPSS Inc., Chicago, IL, USA). Comparisons between the groups were performed by one-way analysis of variance (ANOVA) followed by Duncan's post-hoc multiple comparison tests [6]. The results were presented as mean value ± standard error mean for six samples. Significance was defined at $p < 0.05$.

8.3   RESULTS

8.3.1   OUTCOME OF JRM ON PAW VOLUME IN AIA RATS [19]

The emblematic period path of the development and progression of disease [18] (as assessed by paw volume) is shown in Figure 8.2. Inflammation and redness developed over a 24-hour time period in rat paw induced with adjuvant. The right and the left hind paw volumes were recorded just before the first treatment at 0, 7th 11th, and 21st days after daily oral treatment with JRM and indomethacin. By 20 days, all animals showed evidence of disease, predominantly in the hind paw [18]. JRM (100 mg/kg) exhibited a significant inhibition of paw volume during 7th, 11th, and 21st days compared with arthritic control.

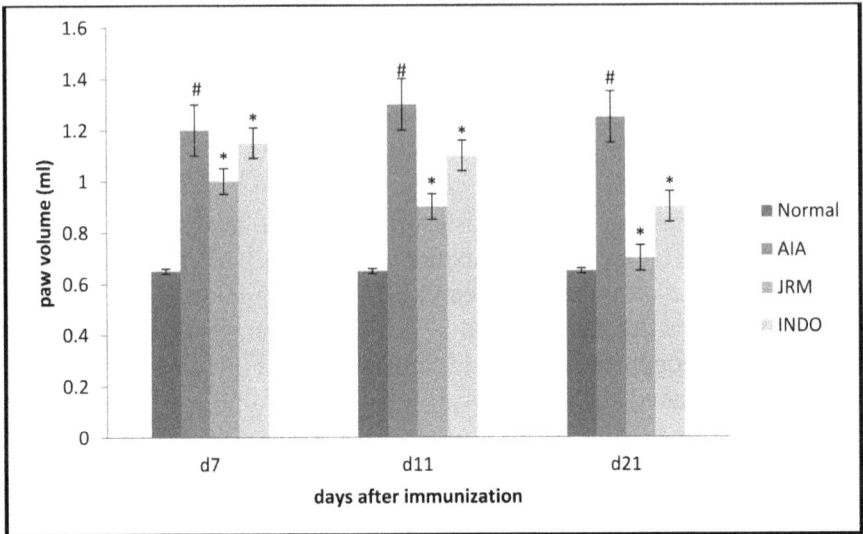

FIGURE 8.2   Effect of JRM on paw volume. Rats were immunized in the paw with CFA and treated with JRM (100 mg/kg) or INDO (3 mg/kg) for 21 days. Normal: nonimmunized normal rats, AIA: rats immunized with CFA, JRM: immunized rats given JRM (100 mg/kg), and INDO: immunized rats given indomethacin (3 mg/kg). Results are expressed as mean ± SEM (n = 6). #Significantly different from normal ($p < 0.05$). *Significantly different from AIA control ($p < 0.05$).

8.3.2   STUDY ON BODY WEIGHT CHANGES IN AIA RATS

Figure 8.3 shows the changes in body weight of normal and experimental rats. All the rats in the different experimental groups were weighed at the start of the experiment [54]. This was taken to be the initial weight. Weekly weight measurements were taken in all the groups [54]. The final weight measurement was conducted on the last day of the experiment. For naive rats, the weight increased with animal's growth; although in arthritic control rats, a decrease in body weight was observed. JRM inhibits the loss of body weight on adjuvant-induced arthritic animal. The loss of body weight is predominant in indomethacin-treated group. Improvement in weight was observed from the third week onward. At the end of 21 days, the body weight of JRM-treated rats resembled that of normal rats.

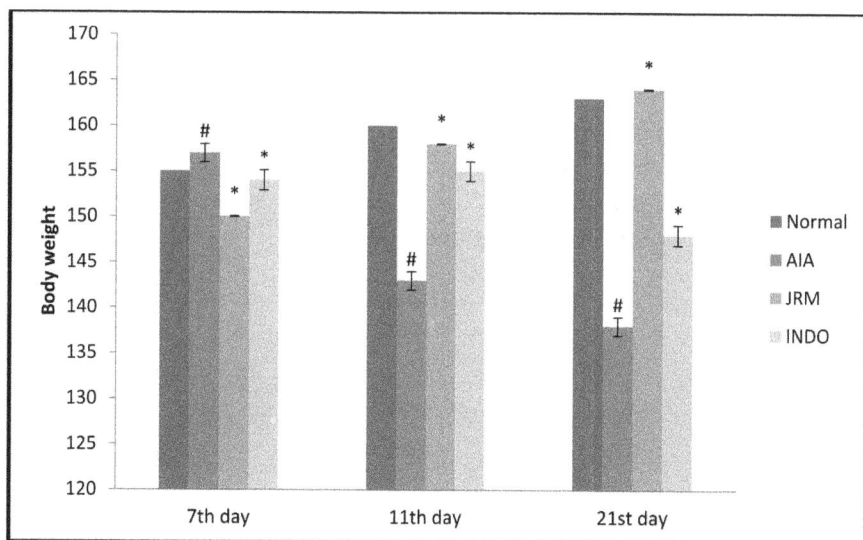

FIGURE 8.3 Effect of JRM on body weight changes in AIA rats. Rats were immunized in the paw with CFA and treated with JRM (100 mg/kg) or INDO (3 mg/kg) for 21 days. Normal: nonimmunized normal rats, AIA: rats immunized with CFA, JRM: immunized rats given JRM (100 mg/kg), and INDO: immunized rats given indomethacin (3 mg/kg). Results are expressed as mean ± SEM (n = 6). #Significantly different from normal ($p < 0.05$). *Significantly different from AIA control ($p < 0.05$).

8.3.3 EFFECT OF JRM ON THE INFLAMMATORY MEDIATOR COX IN MONONUCLEAR CELLS OF AIA RATS

To estimate the activity of COX, rat mononuclear cells were isolated. Normal rats disclosed very less activity of COX in mononuclear cells. Treatment with JRM significantly declined COX activity in rat monocytes compared to arthritic control (Figure 8.4).

8.3.4 EFFECT OF TREATMENT WITH JRM ON 5-LOX AND 15-LOX ACTIVITIES IN MONONUCLEAR CELLS OF AIA RATS [67]

The inhibitory effects of JRM on 5-LOX and 15-LOX activities were tested in vivo using lysed mononuclear cells isolated from rat blood. Induction of arthritis increased 5-LOX and 15-LOX activities in rat mononuclear cells. Treatment with JRM significantly decreased 5-LOX activities in rat mononuclear cells compared to arthritic control (Figure 8.5A and B). The positive control indomethacin group also brought about decrease in both the enzyme activities and the effect was more or less same compared to JRM. This in vivo study showed that JRM has the potential to significantly decrease both 5-LOX and 15-LOX activities in mononuclear cells.

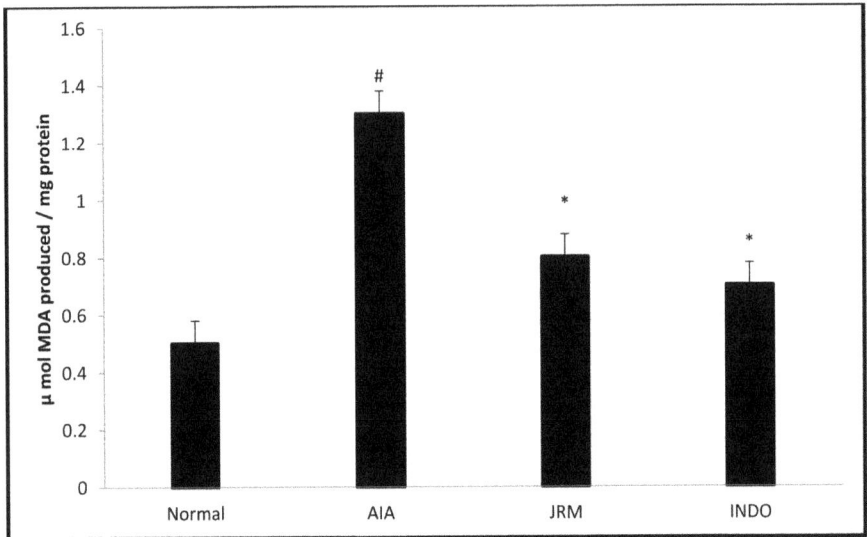

FIGURE 8.4 Effect of JRM on COX activity in mononuclear cells of AIA rats. Rats were immunized in the paw with CFA and treated with JRM (100 mg/kg) or INDO (3 mg/kg) for 21 days. Normal: nonimmunized normal rats, AIA: rats immunized with CFA, JRM: immunized rats given JRM (100 mg/kg), and INDO: immunized rats given indomethacin (3 mg/kg). Results are expressed as mean ± SEM (n = 6). #Significantly different from normal ($p < 0.05$). *Significantly different from AIA control ($p < 0.05$).

8.3.5 EFFECT OF JRM ON MPO ACTIVITY IN GASTRIC MUCOSA, CARTILAGE, AND LIVER OF AIA RATS

To demonstrate the effect of JRM on neutrophil infiltration, gastric mucosa, cartilage, and liver were isolated. MPO activity was found significantly increased in the tissues in the arthritic group. This effect was significantly reduced in rats treated with JRM (Figure 8.6).

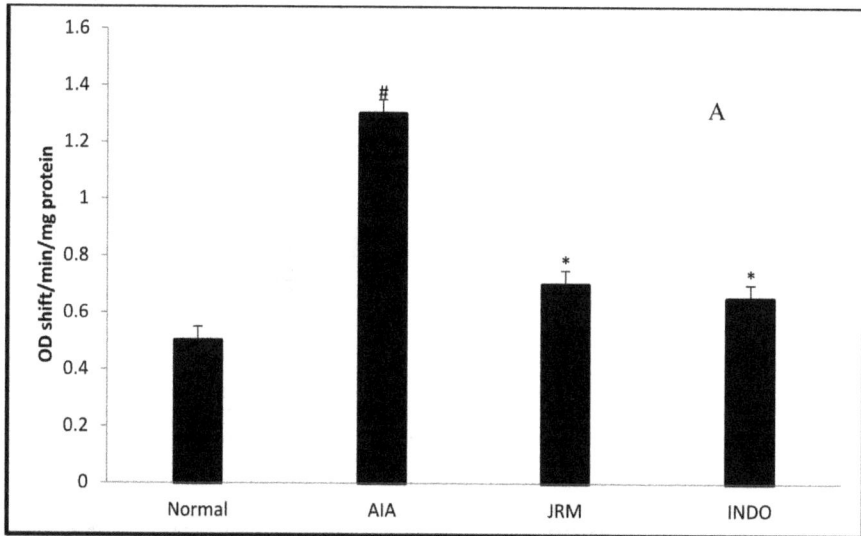

(A)

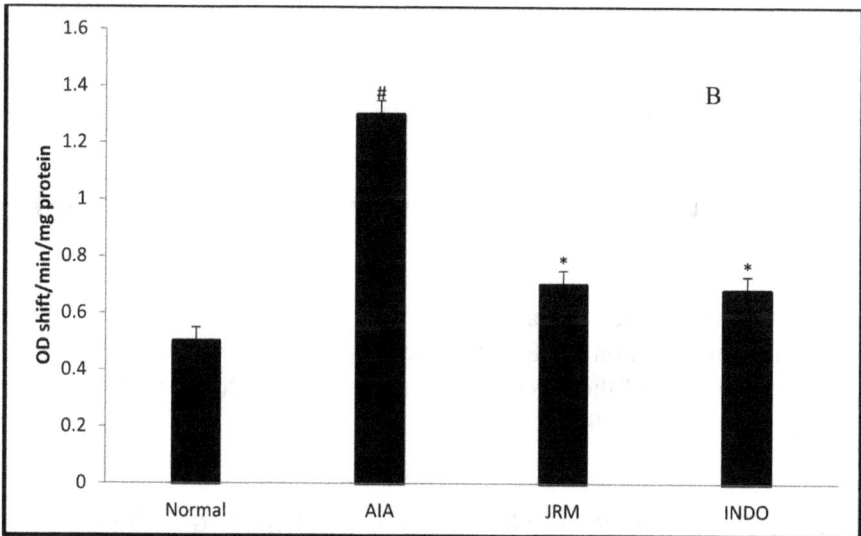

(B)

FIGURE 8.5 (A) Effect of JRM on 5-LOX activity in rat mononuclear cells and (B) Effect of JRM on 15-LOX activity in rat mononuclear cells. Rats were immunized in the paw with CFA and treated with JRM (100 mg/kg) or INDO (3 mg/kg) for 21 days. Normal: nonimmunized normal rats, AIA: rats immunized with CFA, JRM: immunized rats given JRM (100 mg/kg), and INDO: immunized rats given indomethacin (3 mg/kg). Results are expressed as mean ± SEM (n = 6). #Significantly different from normal ($p < 0.05$). *Significantly different from AIA control ($p < 0.05$).

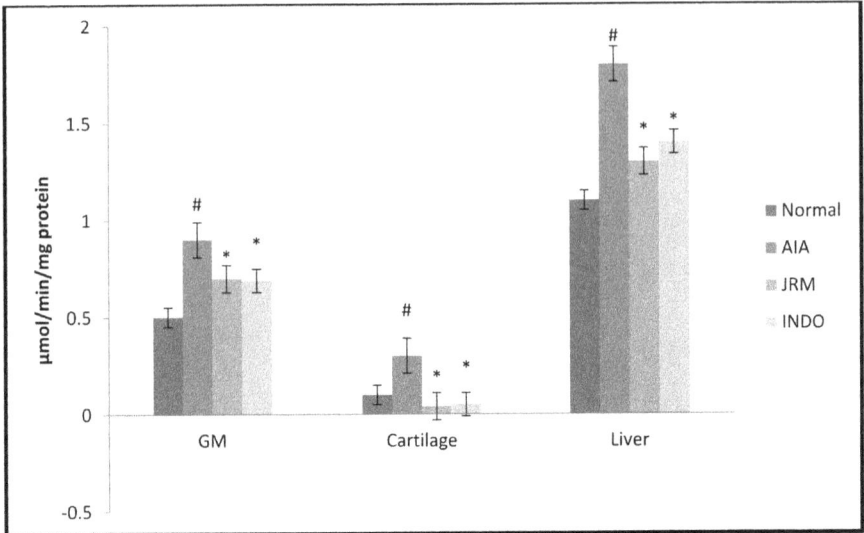

FIGURE 8.6 Effect of JRM on MPO activity in gastric mucosa (GM), cartilage, and liver of AIA rats. Rats were immunized in the paw with CFA and treated with JRM (100 mg/kg) or INDO (3 mg/kg) for 21 days. Normal: nonimmunized normal rats, AIA: rats immunized with CFA, JRM: immunized rats given JRM (100 mg/kg), and INDO: immunized rats given indomethacin (3 mg/kg). Results are expressed as mean ± SEM (n = 6). #Significantly different from normal ($p < 0.05$). *Significantly different from AIA control ($p < 0.05$).

8.3.6   EFFECT OF JRM ON NOS ACTIVITY IN CARTILAGE AND LIVER OF AIA RATS

The NOS was significantly raised in the AIA rats as compared to the control rats [1]. Administration of JRM significantly reduced the NOS level in the cartilage and liver of the inoculated rats. Treatment with indomethacin also generated similar results (Figure 8.7).

8.3.7   EFFECT OF LIPID PEROXIDATION IN CARTILAGE, LIVER, AND SPLEEN OF AIA RATS AS AN INDICATIVE OF OXIDATIVE STRESS [12]

The effect of JRM on lipid peroxidation in arthritic rats was studied by assaying MDA levels in cartilage, liver, and spleen. All groups tested, except for the group receiving oral JRM showed an increase in MDA concentration when compared to the control. Indomethacin administration also showed similar effect (Figure 8.8).

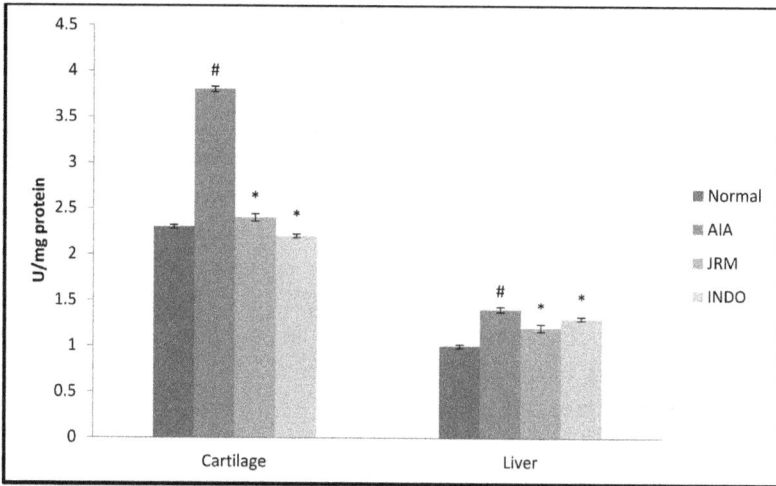

FIGURE 8.7 Effect of JRM on NOS activity in cartilage and liver of AIA rats. Rats were immunized in the paw with CFA and treated with JRM (100 mg/kg) or INDO (3 mg/kg) for 21 days. Units:picomol citrulline released per minute. NC: nonimmunized normal rats, AIA: rats immunized with CFA, JRM: immunized rats given JRM (100 mg/kg), and INDO: immunized rats given indomethacin (3 mg/kg). Results are expressed as mean ± SEM (n = 6). #Significantly different from normal ($p < 0.05$). *Significantly different from AIA control ($p < 0.05$).

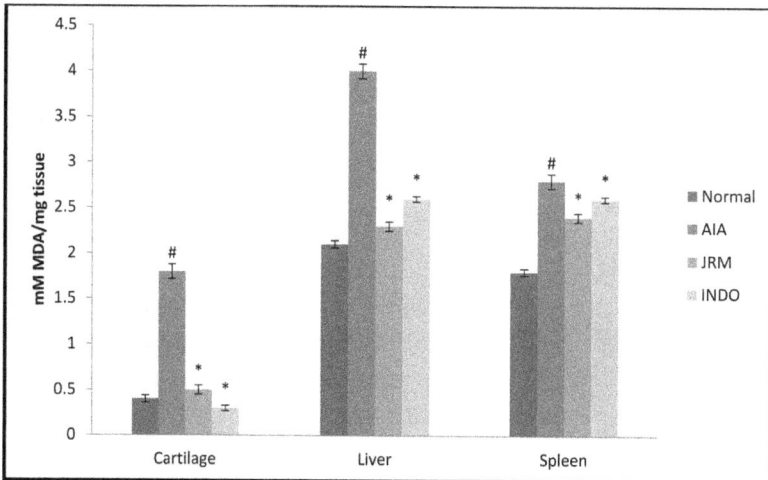

FIGURE 8.8 Effect of JRM on lipid peroxidation in cartilage, liver, and spleen of AIA rats. Rats were immunized in the paw with CFA and treated with JRM (100 mg/kg) or INDO (3 mg/kg) for 21 days. Normal: non immunized normal rats, AIA: rats immunized with CFA, JRM: immunized rats given JRM (100 mg/kg), and INDO: immunized rats given indomethacin (3 mg/kg). Results are expressed as mean ± SEM (n = 6). #Significantly different from normal ($p < 0.05$). *Significantly different from AIA control ($p < 0.05$).

8.3.8   ANTIOXIDANT STATUS IN CARTILAGE, LIVER, AND SPLEEN OF AIA RATS WITH THE TREATMENT OF JRM [17]

The effect of JRM on antioxidant status in arthritic rats was measured by assaying the activities of SOD, catalase, and level of reduced GSH [4]. Figure 8.9(A)–(C) elucidates the significant decrease in the level of tissue SOD [81], catalase, and increased levels of GSH content in AIA rats (group II) when compared to control rats (group I) [1]. In the present study, administration of JRM to arthritic rats caused a significant increase in elevated SOD level, a significant increase in catalase, and reduced GSH. The drug treatment has significantly increased these antioxidant levels when compared with the AIA control.

8.3.9   EFFECT OF JRM ON β-GLUCURONIDASE AND β-HEXOSAMINIDASE ACTIVITIES IN SERUM, CARTILAGE, LIVER, AND SPLEEN OF AIA RATS

Tables 8.1 and 8.2 show the effect of JRM on the activities of β-glucuronidase and β-hexosaminidase in serum, cartilage, liver, and spleen of AIA rats. In AIA-induced rats, the activities of these enzymes were significantly increased when compared to control rats [82]. Administration of JRM to AIA rats significantly decreased the activities of these enzymes with respect to AIA control.

8.3.10   EFFECT OF JRM ON ARTHRITIC INDEX IN CIA RATS

Time course of the inflammatory symptoms is given in Table 8.3. The first signs of CIA developed between 11 and 13 days as seen by increase in paw volume and clinical score. Treatment with JRM wielded a substantial attenuation in the incidence of CIA [18]. The mean arthritis severity score, viz., swelling in the digits and the alteration in hind paw diameter was found decreased with respect to CIA group.

8.3.11   EFFECT OF JRM ON PROGRESSION OF CIA

Mild periarticular erythema and swelling of paws and ankles started within 12–14 days after the first injection of collagen. Hind paws of the experimental rats showed significant swelling after a period of 21 days (Figure 8.10).

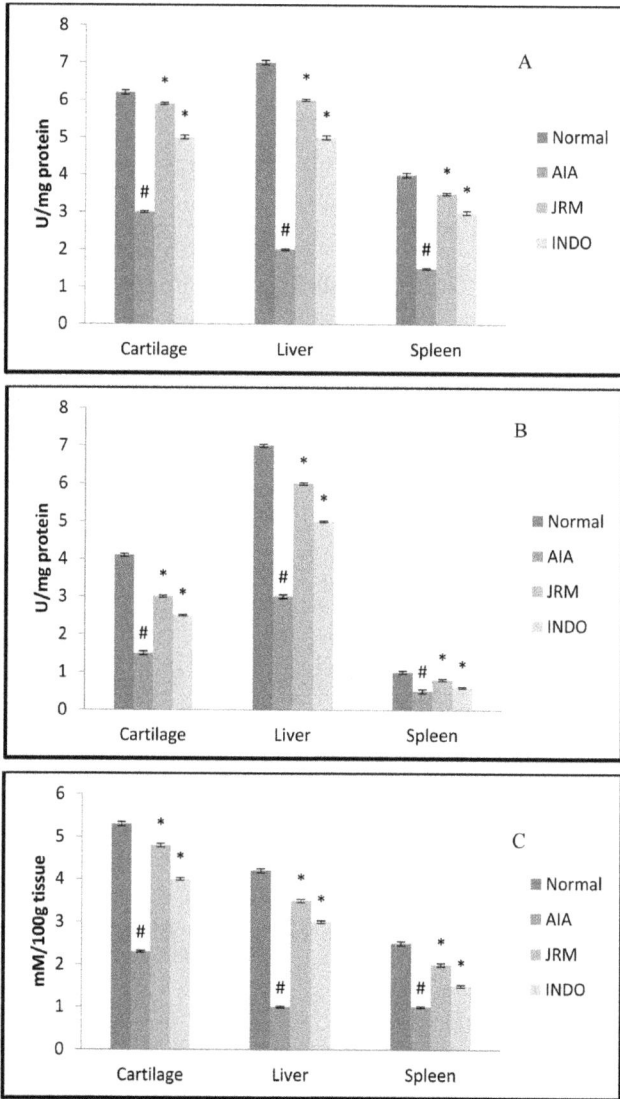

FIGURE 8.9 (A) Effect of JRM on SOD activity in AIA rats. (B) Effect of JRM on catalase activity in AIA rats. (C) Effect of JRM on glutathione levels in AIA rats. Rats were immunized in the paw with CFA and treated with JRM (100 mg/kg) or INDO (3 mg/kg) for 21 days. Units—SOD: enzyme concentration required to inhibit chromogen by 50%, catalase: μmol H_2O_2 decomposed/min/mg protein, catalase: units/mg protein, and glutathione: mM/100 g tissue. Normal: nonimmunized normal rats, AIA: rats immunized with CFA, JRM: immunized rats given JRM (100 mg/kg), and INDO: immunized rats given indomethacin (3 mg/kg). Results are expressed as mean ± SEM (n = 6). #Significantly different from normal ($p < 0.05$). *Significantly different from AIA control ($p < 0.05$).

Maximum paw volume occurred around day 21 in CIA rats. The paw volume in each CIA rat exposed a time-dependent increase in hind paw volume (Figure 8.10).

TABLE 8.1   Activity of β-hexosaminidase (μM PNP Liberated/min/mg Protein)

Groups	Serum	Cartilage	Liver	Spleen
Normal	0.025 ± 0.001	0.082 ± 0.006	28.33 ± 6.6	18.33 ± 6.6
AIA	0.095 ± 0.001[#]	0.14 ± 0.007[#]	49.50 ± 7.5[#]	27.16 ± 5.6[#]
JRM	0.024 ± 0.001[#]	0.073 ± 0.007[#]	27.66 ± 2.6[#]	17.53 ± 5.9[#]
INDO	0.022 ± 0.001[*]	0.07 ± 0.007[*]	26.50 ± 3.7[*]	18.03 ± 4.6[*]

Rats were immunized in the paw with CFA and treated with JRM (100 mg/kg) or indomethacin (3 mg/kg) for 21 days. Normal: nonimmunized normal rats, AIA: rats immunized with CFA, JRM: immunized rats given JRM (100 mg/kg), and indomethacin: immunized rats given indomethacin (3 mg/kg). Results are expressed as mean ± SEM (n = 6).
[#]*Significantly different from normal (p < 0.05).*
[*]*Significantly different from AIA control (p < 0.05).*

TABLE 8.2   Activity of β-glucuronidase (μM PNP Liberated/min/mg Protein)

Groups	Serum	Cartilage	Liver	Spleen
Normal	0.025 ± 0.001	0.028 ± 0.007	29.83 ± 4.7	14.15 ± 2.5
AIA	0.091 ± 0.007[#]	0.094 ± 0.007[#]	41.50 ± 7.6[#]	30.65 ± 3.5 [#]
JRM	0.040 ± 0.006[#]	0.045 ± 0.007[#]	33.83 ± 2.4[#]	17.53 ± 4.6[#]
INDO	0.034 ± 0.007[*]	0.037 ± 0.007[*]	31.83 ± 2.7[*]	18.03 ± 2.7[*]

Rats were immunized in the paw with CFA and treated with JRM (100 mg/kg) or indomethacin (3 mg/kg) for 21 days. Normal: nonimmunized normal rats, AIA: rats immunized with CFA, JRM: immunized rats given JRM (100 mg/kg), and Indomethacin: immunized rats given indomethacin (3 mg/kg). Results are expressed as mean ± SEM (n = 6).
[#]*Significantly different from normal (p < 0.05).*
[*]*Significantly different from AIA control (p < 0.05).*

TABLE 8.3   Effect of JRM on Arthritic Index in CIA Rats

	Day 14	Day 21	Day 28	Day 45	Day 60
CIA	5.8 ± 1.8	10 ± 1.7	10.8 ± 1.2	11 ± 1.2	11.5 ± 0.9
JRM	5.9 ± 1.7	9.1 ± 0.8	8.5 ± 0.9[*]	7.8 ± 1.6[*]	6.5 ± 1.3[*]
INDO	6.2 ± 1.2	8.5 ± 1.9	8.0 ± 1.4[*]	7.3 ± 0.9[*]	7.0 ± 0.9[*]

CIA was induced by intradermal injection of type II collagen in CFA into the base of rat tails. JRM (100 mg/kg) was given orally from day 14 to day 60 after booster immunization. Polyarthritic index was evaluated at day 14, day 21, day 28, day 45, and day 60. Results are expressed as mean ± SEM (n = 6). [*]Significantly different from CIA control (p < 0.05)

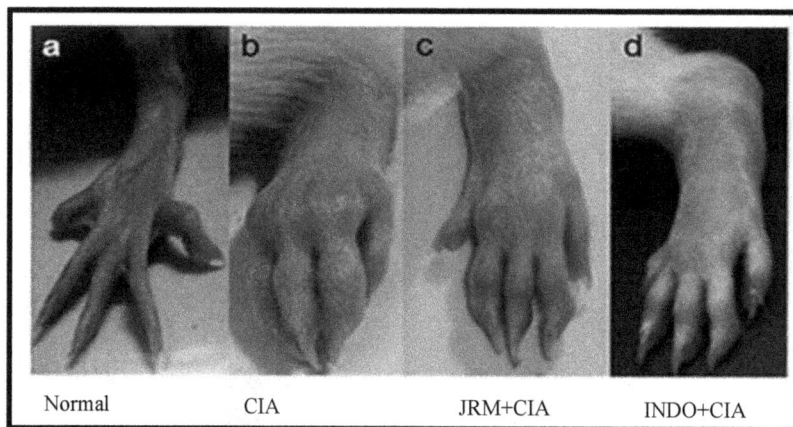

FIGURE 8.10 Effect of JRM and indomethacin on progression of CIA. CIA was induced by intradermal injection of type II collagen in CFA into the base of rat tails. JRM (100 mg/kg) was given orally from day 14 to day 60 after booster immunization. Normal: non immunized normal rats, CIA: rats immunized with type II collagen in CFA, JRM: immunized rats given JRM (100 mg/kg), and INDO: immunized rats given indomethacin (3 mg/kg).

8.3.12 EFFECT OF JRM ON BODY WEIGHT CHANGES IN CIA RATS

Body weight was measured on 14th, 28th, 42nd, and 56th days. Animals immunized with collagen disclosed symptoms of CIA such as inflammation in joints within 12–16 days. Collagen-induced disease with very high arthritic score was evident from joint inflammation, reduced weight-bearing capacity, and loss of body weight (Figure 8.11).

8.3.13 EFFECT OF JRM ON COX ACTIVITY IN MONONUCLEAR CELLS OF CIA RATS AND COX-2-SPECIFIC INHIBITION IN PAW TISSUES OF CIA RATS

To evaluate the activity of COX, mononuclear cells were isolated. Normal rats showed very less activity of COX in mononuclear cells. Increased total COX activity was found in the mononuclear cells of CIA rats compared with the normal control. Treatment with JRM and indomethacin significantly decreased the activity of overall COX in mononuclear cells with respect to CIA control (Figure 8.12). Our following objective was to better understand the ability of JRM root. Methanolic extract to inhibit COX-2 was determined using colorimetric COX inhibitor screening assay kit employing SC-560 as

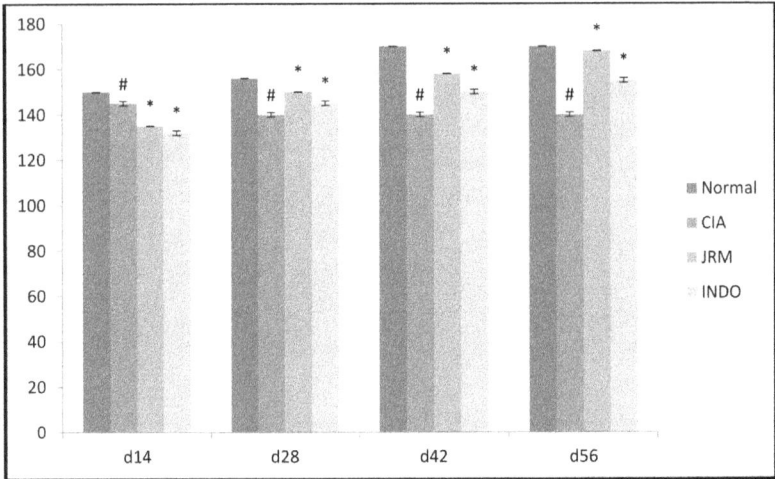

FIGURE 8.11 Effect of JRM on body weight changes in CIA rats. CIA was induced by intradermal injection of type II collagen in CFA into the base of rat tails. JRM (100 mg/kg) was given orally from day 14 to day 60 after booster immunization. Normal: nonimmunized normal rats, CIA: rats immunized with type II collagen in CFA, JRM: immunized rats given JRM (100 mg/kg), and INDO: immunized rats given indomethacin (3 mg/kg). [#]Significantly different from normal ($p < 0.05$). [*]Significantly different from CIA control ($p < 0.05$).

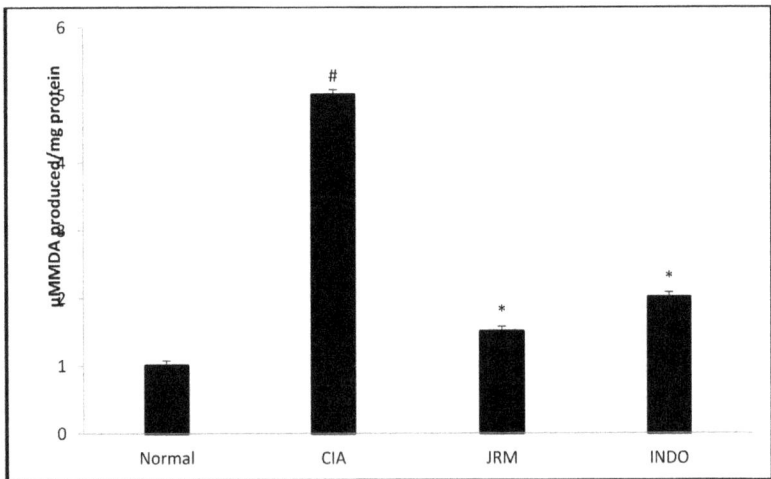

FIGURE 8.12 Effect of JRM on cyclooxygenase activity in CIA rats. CIA was induced by intradermal injection of type II collagen in CFA into the base of rat tails. JRM (100 mg/kg) was given orally from day 14 to day 60 after booster immunization. Normal: nonimmunized normal rats, CIA: rats immunized with type II collagen in CFA, JRM: immunized rats given JRM (100 mg/kg), and INDO: immunized rats given indomethacin (3 mg/kg). [#]Significantly different from normal ($p < 0.05$). [*]Significantly different from CIA control ($p < 0.05$).

COX-2 inhibitor. COX-2 was highly induced in CII-induced rat paw. COX-2 inhibition percentage is shown in Figure 8.13. Paw tissues taken from the JRM-treated group showed 60% COX-2 inhibition [96]. Indomethacin-treated group exhibited 11% COX-2 inhibition.

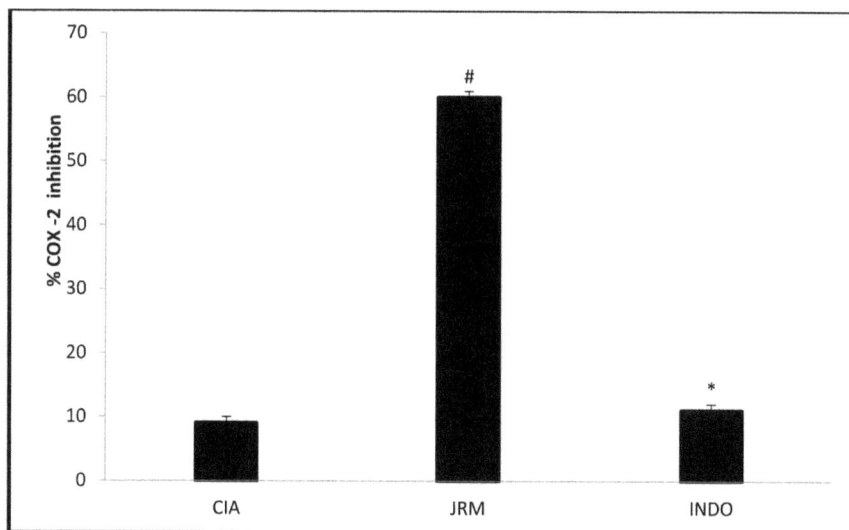

FIGURE 8.13 Effect of JRM on COX-2 inhibition. CIA was induced by intradermal injection of type II collagen in CFA into the base of rat tails. JRM (100 mg/kg) was given orally from day 14 to day 60 after booster immunization. CIA: rats immunized with type II collagen in CFA, JRM: immunized rats given JRM (100 mg/kg), and INDO: immunized rats given indomethacin (3 mg/kg). #Significantly different from CIA ($p < 0.05$). *Significantly different from JRM ($p < 0.05$).

8.3.14 EFFECT OF JRM ON THE LEVELS OF INFLAMMATORY MEDIATOR 5-LOX IN MONONUCLEAR CELLS OF CIA RATS

Blood from the retro-orbital vein of CIA rats on day 60 was collected and the consequence of JRM on 5-LOX activity in mononuclear cells was studied [67]. The cells were isolated from rat blood by density-gradient centrifugation using histopaque and lysed by freeze-thaw cycles. Normal rats showed very low activity of 5-LOX in rat blood mononuclear cells compared to cells isolated from normal rats. Induction of arthritis using CII significantly increased the activity of 5-LOX in rat blood mononuclear cells compared to cells isolated from normal rats [79]. Treatment with JRM significantly decreased the activity of 5-LOX in mononuclear cells (Figure 8.14) with respect to CIA control [67]. Treatment with indomethacin also showed significant change in 5-LOX activity with respect to arthritic rats.

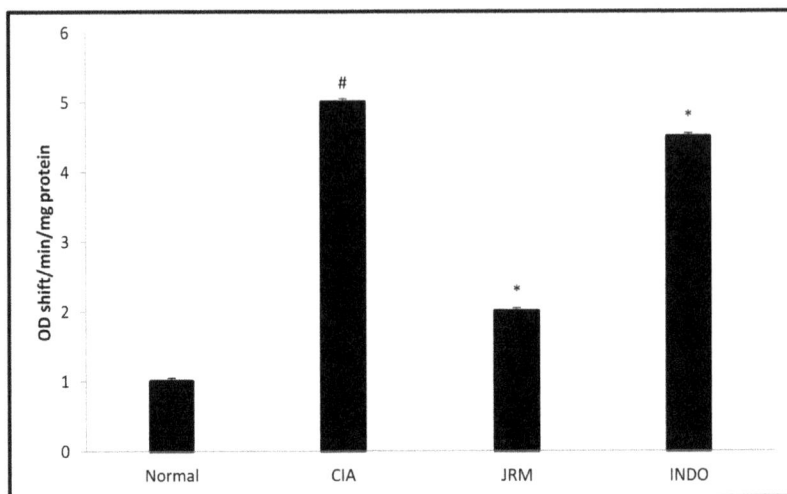

FIGURE 8.14   Effect of JRM on 5-LOX activity in CIA rats. CIA was induced by intradermal injection of type II collagen in CFA into the base of rat tails. JRM (100 mg/kg) was given orally from day 14 to day 60 after booster immunization. Normal: nonimmunized normal rats, CIA: rats immunized with type II collagen in CFA, JRM: immunized rats given JRM (100 mg/ kg), and INDO: immunized rats given indomethacin (3 mg/kg). #Significantly different from normal ($p < 0.05$). *Significantly different from CIA control ($p < 0.05$).

8.3.15   EFFECT OF JRM ON MPO ACTIVITY IN CIA RATS

The effect of JRM on MPO activity was studied in gastric mucosa, cartilage, and liver of arthritic rats. Arthritis induction significantly increased the activity of MPO in the gastric mucosa, cartilage, and liver (Figure 8.15). Treatment of CIA rats with JRM significantly ($p < 0.05$) decreased the activity of MPO with respect to the CIA control rats.

8.3.16   EFFECT OF JRM ON NOS ACTIVITY IN CARTILAGE AND LIVER OF CIA RATS

As shown in Figure 8.16, the NOS level in the collagen-induced arthritic rats was significantly raised when compared with the normal group. There is a significant decreasing effect in the NOS activity in the JRM-treated and indomethacin-treated group compared with the CIA group.

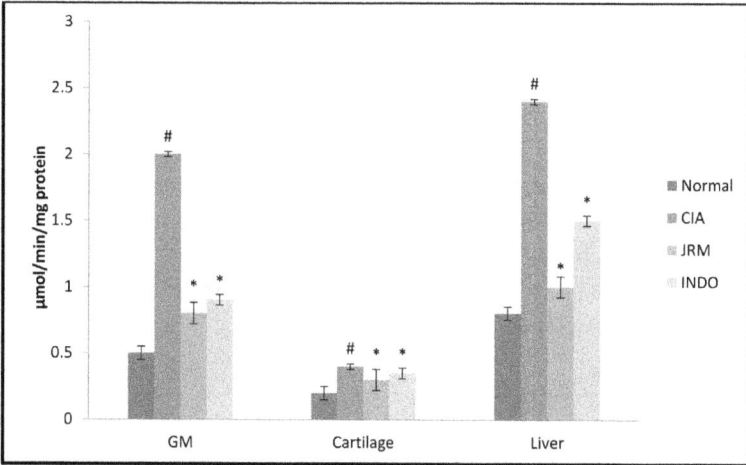

FIGURE 8.15 Effect of JRM on myeloperoxidase activity in CIA rats. CIA was induced by intradermal injection of type II collagen in CFA into the base of rat tails. JRM (100 mg/kg) was given orally from day 14 to day 60 after booster immunization. Normal: nonimmunized normal rats, CIA: rats immunized with type II collagen in CFA, JRM: immunized rats given JRM (100 mg/kg), and INDO: immunized rats given indomethacin (3 mg/kg). #Significantly different from normal ($p < 0.05$). *Significantly different from CIA control ($p < 0.05$).

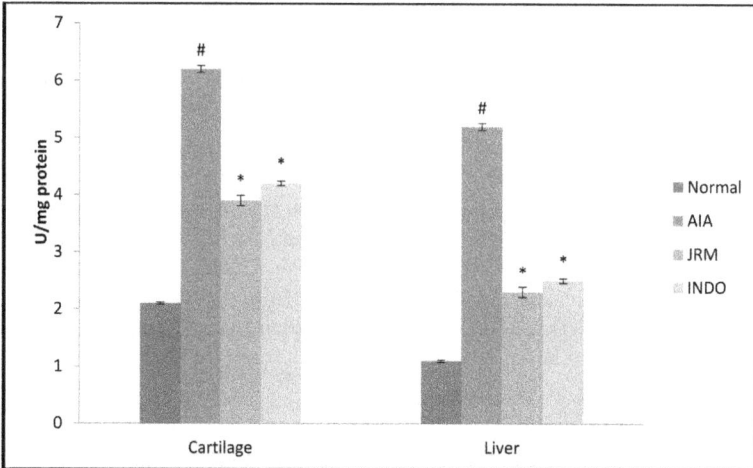

FIGURE 8.16 Effect of JRM on nitric oxide synthase activity in CIA rats. CIA was induced by intradermal injection of type II collagen in CFA into the base of rat tails. JRM (100 mg/kg) was given orally from day 14 to day 60 after booster immunization. Units: picomol citrulline released per minute. Normal: non immunized normal rats, CIA: rats immunized with type II collagen in CFA, JRM: immunized rats given JRM (100 mg/kg), and INDO: immunized rats given indomethacin (3 mg/kg). #Significantly different from normal ($p < 0.05$). *Significantly different from CIA control ($p < 0.05$).

8.3.17   EFFECT OF JRM ON LIPID PEROXIDATION IN CARTILAGE, LIVER, AND SPLEEN OF CIA RATS [52]

Figure 8.17 depicts the effect of JRM on lipid peroxidation status in cartilage, liver, and spleen of control and investigational rats. The levels of lipid peroxidation (MDA) were found to be significantly increased in the arthritic rats compared to the normal rats [59]. Administration of JRM to arthritic rats altered the above changes by modifying the lipid peroxide levels closely to that of normal rats [12]. Indomethacin-treated group also displayed related results as that of JRM-treated group.

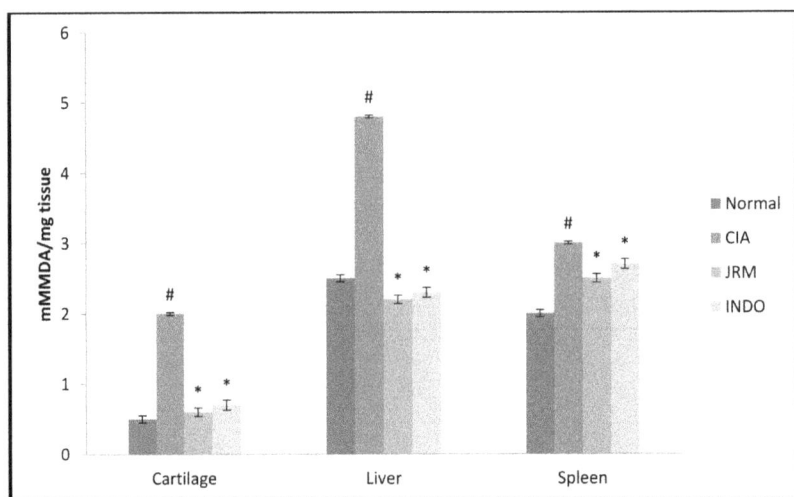

FIGURE 8.17   Effect of JRM on lipid peroxidation in CIA rats. CIA was induced by intradermal injection of type II collagen in CFA into the base of rat tails. JRM (100 mg/kg) was given orally from day 14 to day 60 after booster immunization. Normal: non immunized normal rats, CIA: rats immunized with type II collagen in CFA, JRM: immunized rats given JRM (100 mg/kg), and INDO: immunized rats given indomethacin (3 mg/kg). [#]Significantly different from normal ($p < 0.05$). [*]Significantly different from CIA control ($p < 0.05$).

8.3.18   EFFECT OF JRM ON ANTIOXIDANT ACTIVITIES IN CARTILAGE, LIVER, AND SPLEEN OF CIA RATS

The effect of JRM on antioxidant prominence in collagen-induced arthritic rats was measured by assessing the activity of SOD, catalase, and reduced GSH [17]. Figure 18(A)–(C) elucidates the noteworthy decrease in the activities of tissue SOD and catalase and levels of GSH content in collagen-induced

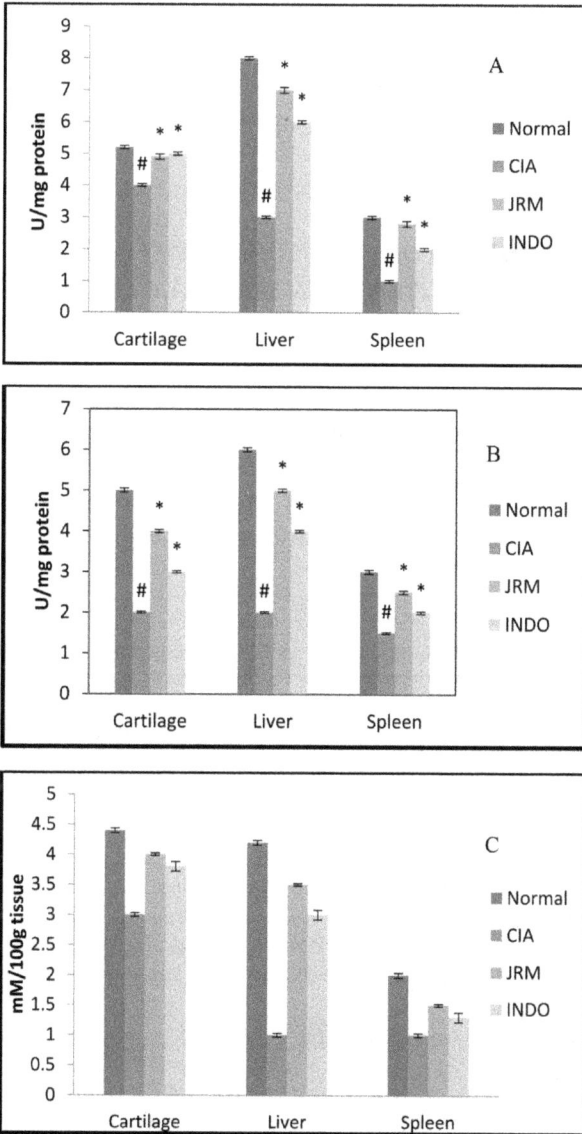

FIGURE 8.18 (A) Effect of JRM on SOD activity in CIA rats. (B) Effect of JRM on catalase activity on CIA rats. (C) Effect of JRM on glutathione levels in CIA rats. Units— SOD: enzyme concentration required to inhibit chromogen by 50%, Catalase: μmol H_2O_2 decomposed/min/mg protein, catalase: units/mg protein, and glutathione: mM/100 g tissue. Normal: nonimmunized normal rats, CIA: rats immunized with CFA, JRM: immunized rats given JRM (100 mg/kg), and INDO: immunized rats given indomethacin (3 mg/kg). Results are expressed as mean ± SEM (n = 6). #Significantly different from normal ($p < 0.05$). *Significantly different from CIA control ($p < 0.05$).

rats (group II) when compared to normal rats (group I). In the present study, administration of JRM to CIA rats caused a substantial increase in elevated SOD level, a major increase in catalase, and reduced GSH. The drug action has significantly increased these antioxidant levels when compared with the CIA control.

8.3.19 EFFECT OF JRM ON β-GLUCURONIDASE AND β-HEXOSAMINIDASE ACTIVITIES IN SERUM AND CARTILAGE OF CIA RATS

Tables 8.4 and 8.5 show the effect of JRM on the activities of β-glucuronidase and β-hexosaminidase in serum and cartilage of CIA rats. In CIA-induced rats, the activities of these enzymes were suggestively augmented when compared to control rats [22]. Administration of JRM to CIA rats pointedly decreased the activities of these enzymes with respect to CIA control.

TABLE 8.4   Activity of β-hexosaminidase (μM PNP Liberated/min/mg Protein)

Groups	Serum	Cartilage
Normal	0.025 ± 0.007	0.082 ± 0.006
ARTH	$0.120 \pm 0.001^{\#}$	$0.197 \pm 0.001^{\#}$
JRM	$0.037 \pm 0.001^{\#}$	$0.058 \pm 0.002^{\#}$
INDO	$0.080 \pm 0.002^{*}$	$0.097 \pm 0.004^{*}$

Rats were immunized in the paw with type II collagen and treated with JRM (100 mg/kg) or indomethacin (3 mg/kg) for 21 days. Normal: nonimmunized normal rats, CIA: rats immunized with type II Collagen in CFA, JRM: immunized rats given JRM (100 mg/kg), and Indomethacin: immunized rats given indomethacin (3 mg/kg). Results are expressed as mean ± SEM (n = 6).

$^{\#}$*Significantly different from normal (p < 0.05).*

**Significantly different from CIA control (p < 0.05).*

8.4   DISCUSSION

This chapter appraises the antiarthritic potential of JRM using two experimental model systems—adjuvant induced and type II CIA [82]. Freund's adjuvant and type II CIA in rats are a well-established experimental model for the study of the pathophysiology of many types of human arthritis, especially RA [13]. JRM root methanolic extract at a dosage of 100 mg/kg [6, 35, 95] displayed significant antiarthritic effect and the activity was analogous with that of indomethacin [64, 65].

TABLE 8.5 Activity of β-glucuronidase (μM PNP Liberated/min/mg Protein)

Groups	Serum	Cartilage
Normal	0.025 ± 0.009	0.031 ± 0.006
CIA	0.015 ± 0.008[#]	0.194 ± 0.001[#]
JRM	0.035 ± 0.001[#]	0.047 ± 0.005[#]
INDO	0.047 ± 0.008[*]	0.052 ± 0.005[*]

Rats were immunized in the paw with type II collagen and treated with JRM (100 mg/kg) or indomethacin (3 mg/kg) for 21 days. Normal: nonimmunized normal rats, CIA: rats immunized with type II collagen in CFA, JRM: immunized rats given JRM (100 mg/kg), and Indomethacin: immunized rats given indomethacin (3 mg/kg). Results are expressed as mean ± SEM (n = 6).
[#]*Significantly different from normal (p < 0.05).*
[*]*Significantly different from CIA control (p < 0.05).*

As a result of edema of periarticular tissues, increased paw swelling was observed in the arthritic rats [39, 58]. The swelling got increased in the early phase of inflammation and then remained constant for 2 weeks. An appreciable increase in paw volume was observed in adjuvant-induced group compared to normal rats [94]. A major reduction in paw volume was observed in both JRM- and indomethacin-treated rats compared to the disease-induced arthritic group. This was detected in the starting of the third week of drug treatment. In evaluating the degree of inflammation and therapeutic efficacy of the drugs, the degree of swelling in the paw plays a major role. In JRM-treated groups, the observed reduction in paw swelling from the second week onward may be due to their immunological protection. JRM (100 mg/ kg) formed a reduction in hind paw inflammation after 21 days. Thus, the study discovered that methanolic extract of *JRM* with a concentration of 100 mg/kg body weight produced major inhibition of paw edema compared with adjuvant-induced arthritic rats. Nonsteroidal anti-inflammatory drugs (NSAIDs) hinder pain behaviors induced by inflammation and prevent or reduce the swelling associated with an inflammatory stimulus and the outcome of plant extract is similar to that of NSAIDs. The swelling in the paw was significantly reduced in the JRM-treated rats [20], which designates its interference on COX pathway.

Following AIA induction with CFA and CII, it was found that the rats also showed certain systemic features of inflammation such as uveitis, gastrointestinal tract inflammation, and body weight loss that start 24–48 h before the onset of the arthritis [66]. Changes in the body mass are an advantageous guide to measure the path of the disease and the retort to therapy of anti-inflammatory drugs in hunt [59, 91]. It was observed that there was a change in weight of arthritic rats when we compared it with the normal rats [65]. The loss of body weight observed in arthritic rats may be due to the reduced absorption of glucose and leucine in rat intestine [78]. Diminished weight gain in arthritic rats was significantly recovered by JRM treatment. The increase in body weight during JRM administration tells the rebuilding of absorption ability of the intestine in the arthritic animals [37]. The escalation in absorption capacity could be due to the existence of minerals and antioxidant pigments in the extract. Changes in body weight have been used to calculate the path of illness and the response to therapy of standard. Arthritis is characterized by decrease in weight and is associated with improved production of proinflammatory cytokines such as TNF-α, IL-6, and IL-1 [42]. Treatment with JRM has shown significant increase in body weight when compared to arthritic control.

Prostaglandins are the end products of the COX pathway and PGE2 exclusively is upregulated due to a prominent COX-2 activity in arthritis [71]. From the evidence observed in the animal models of inflammatory arthritis, it powerfully proposes that improved expression of COX-2 is accountable for improved PG production seen in inflamed joint tissues [7, 75]. Cell culture trials utilizing primary cells derived from human synovial tissue or cell types (e.g., monocytes) significant in inflammatory processes have been perilous to an understanding of factors involved in modifying this induction [75]. The role of COX-2 in inflammation has led to drug monitors attempting to identify anti-inflammatory agents selective for COX-2 as well as to the rational design of highly selective COX-2 inhibitors [63]. Our study also provides insight into the proinflammatory activities of COX-2-derived PGs in established arthritis. JRM treatment significantly decreased COX activity and thereby PGE2 production in the paw tissue of JRM-treated rats. COX-1 is constitutively expressed in resident inflammatory cells and there is suggestion for induction of COX-1 during LPS-mediated inflammatory response and cellular differentiation [49]. JRM significantly decreased COX-2 and to a lesser extent COX-1 as well as PGE2 production in paw tissues of arthritic rats. Indomethacin-treated group showed only 11% COX-2 inhibition and remaining is COX-1 inhibition. This may be the reason of indomethacin showing several side effects. Antiarthritic effect exerted by JRM may be due to inhibition of COX-2 and PGE2 production [89].

The main biological functions of leukotrienes are recruitment and initiation of inflammatory cells, chiefly neutrophils, but also macrophages, monocytes, eosinophils, and lymphocytes [5]. Leukotrienes B4 (LTB4) is produced mainly by macrophages and neutrophils, that is, cell sorts that initiative inflammatory processes [5]. Revisions in 5-LOX-activating protein-deficient mice and 5-LOX-deficient mice approve that leukotrienes have a critical role in arthritis. In this study, arthritis induction significantly increased the activity of 5-LOX in blood mononuclear cells. Administration of JRM significantly decreased this arthritis-induced 5-LOX activity. In divergence with COX inhibitors, LTB4 inhibitors had a clear effect on immune complex-induced models and CIA. Preceding studies showed that JRM inhibits 5-LOX and 15-LOX activities in mononuclear cells isolated from carrageenan-induced rat paw edema model. These results hint that *JRM* extract has LOX inhibition activity and gives some recommendation that the extract might be valuable in managing the effects of inflammation.

JRM showed distinct inhibitory effect on the production of leukotrienes by 5-LOX and 15-LOX as well as production of prostaglandin PGE2 by COX-1 and COX-2 enzymes. Together, these results reveal an interesting activity profile with dual inhibition of COX-1 and COX-2 as well as LOX, both major pathways of arachidonic acid metabolism. Such dual inhibitors are reported to have several advantages over the widely used NSAIDs, which preferentially inhibit COX. The inhibitory effects observed in this study complement reported biological activities of the plant in the literature. Among the advantages are a broad range of anti-inflammatory properties as well as reduction of the NSAIDs-associated commonly observed gastrointestinal ulcerogenic activity. From our point of view, the use of dual inhibitor COX/ LOX pathways seems advantageous to the treatment of other inflammatory disorders beyond RA.

The effect of JRM on neutrophil accumulation was appraised in both chronic models by evaluation of MPO. It was observed that a strong reduction in infiltration of polymorphonuclear cells has occurred due to the effect of MPO [18]. The activity of MPO was decreased in JRM-treated rats and increased in adjuvant-induced rats. This increase in MPO activity after CFA and CII challenge was significantly inhibited by treatment with JRM at a dose of 100 mg/kg showing that the extract has the potential to inhibit neutrophil migration into inflamed tissue [88].

NO synthesized by inducible nitric oxide synthase (iNOS) has been associated as a moderator of inflammation in rheumatic and autoimmune diseases [80]. It contributes to the increased permeability of vessels during edema formation. NO, which is an important signaling and effector molecule in inflammation and immunity, combines with superoxides to form peroxynitrite, which, in turn, induces the production of prostaglandin endoperoxide synthase (COX) from monocytes/macrophages resulting in improved synthesis of prostaglandins, which are established mediators of inflammation. As seen from the results, JRM has significantly decreased NOS activity in the tissues thereby modulating NO production and COX activity in monocytes thereby checking prostaglandin production at the inflammatory sites. Our observation that NOS levels in JRM-treated rats was significantly lower as compared to controls and suggests that one of the probable mechanisms for curtailing the progression of AIA and CIA in rats might have been a declined cellular production of NO by inhibiting NOS activity [21, 62].

Weakening of antioxidant defense system can lead to an increase in lipid peroxidation. The degree of lipid peroxidation is measured through MDA level, a pro-oxidant factor that defines the oxidative damage [18]. In the present study, tissue lipid peroxide level was significantly increased in AIAs (group II) when compared to normal group. This phenomenon may be the product of the release of chemical mediators during phagocytosis [41]. A fall of lipid peroxidation activity was observed in standard drug and JRM-treated group. Outcomes of the present study demonstrate that the drug obstructs both inflammation [45] as well as accumulation of lipid peroxides in tissues, which was comparable with indomethacin-treated group. This action can be attributed to the phytochemicals such as flavonoids, alkaloids, tannins, and saponins in the JRM extract [18].

It has been reported that lipid peroxidation and decreased antioxidant status are underlying reasons for the progression of arthritis. MDA levels were found to be significantly ($P < 0.005$) preeminent in the arthritic-treated rats compared to the controls [81]. Increased MDA levels, reflecting the increase in lipid peroxidation, endorse the induction of oxidative stress by adjuvant treatment in the present study. It is well known that lipid peroxidation, leading enhanced oxidative stress, may play an important role in tissue damage. In the present study, MDA coupled to decreased levels of GSH was observed in the arthritic rats. This data is in occurrence with reports by Rasool and Sabina [68], which stated that increased lipid peroxidation and declined antioxidant status in tissues of arthritic rats. Treatment with JRM significantly reduced MDA levels indicative of attenuation of injury in these tissues. GSH, a predominant low molecular weight thiol in the cytoplasm, is requisite for protection of tissues against lipid peroxidation during arthritis [51]. The level of GSH was significantly contracted in arthritic rats indicating greater utilization of this endogenous antioxidant. JRM treatment dampened the depletion of

GSH in the tissues studied probably while shifting the free radicals and this action might have helped to preserve the integrity of cellular membranes in JRM-treated rats.

Our body has a set of endogenous antioxidant enzymes such as SOD, catalase, and GSH. A major systemic event that occurs in the rat following the induction of inflammation is marked alteration in the cellular defense mechanism. The antioxidant enzymes, including SOD, catalase, and GSH, can convert active oxygen molecules into nontoxic compounds. These enzymes thwart the generation of hydroxyl radical and safeguard the cellular constituents from oxidative damage. Induction of arthritis can cause the production of peroxy radical O_2^-, which accompanies with inactivation of catalase, GSH, and SOD enzymes [85].

SOD is an important defense enzyme, which catalyzes the dismutation of superoxide radicals to hydrogen peroxide, thereby reducing the likelihood of superoxide anion interacting with NO to form reactive peroxynitrite. Hydrogen peroxide is successively metabolized into water and nonreactive oxygen species by the activities of catalase and GPX [48]. Catalase is a tetrameric enzyme, which decomposes the hydrogen peroxides into the mild product such as water and molecular oxygen. Catalase is one of the most skilled enzymes, so that it cannot be saturated by hydrogen peroxide at any concentration [43]. The GST catalyzes the conjugation of GSH to a wide range of electrophiles and supports the defending mechanism against CCl_4-mediated oxidative stress. The level of enzymatic antioxidants is found to be conspicuously dropped in the AIA rats and CIA rats. However, rats administered with JRM expressively improved the activities of enzymatic antioxidants. This undoubtedly explains the significant drop in the activities of SOD, catalase, and GSH observed in rats induced with Freund's adjuvant and CII. Administration of JRM caused the intensification of SOD, catalase, and GSH activities, which, in turn, may be liable for its antioxidant properties.

There is increasing evidence that lysosomal enzymes play an important role in the development of acute and chronic inflammation [7, 64]. Alteration in lysosomal integrity and metabolism of connective tissue are the prominent features in adjuvant arthritis [74]. The destruction of cartilage in human RA was reported to be due to the enzymatic degradation of proteoglycans by lysosomal enzymes [29]. Significantly increased activities of lysosomal enzymes are found on the arthritic rats in the extracellular fluid due to decrease in lysosomal stability [90]. The increase in paw edema after adjuvant injection in rats is paralleled by increased extracellular activities of lysosomal enzymes [8]. The preeminent levels of lysosomal enzymes in serum and cartilage of AIA and CIA rats put forward that the leakage or extrusion of these enzymes is a direct consequence of higher endocytotic activity. In the present study, significantly increased activities of lysosomal enzymes are found in arthritic rats than in normal rats. The activities of the enzymes, β-glucuronidase and β-hexosaminidase, were expressively increased as compared to normal rats. Thus, the manifest increase in the activities of lysosomal enzymes in the present study confirms the increased fragility of lysosomal membranes in AIA rats. On the other hand, supplementation of JRM showed significant lessening in the activities of these enzymes in the serum and cartilage. This may perhaps be due to the stabilization of lysosomal membrane.

In conclusion, JRM possesses significant antiarthritic activity. JRM exerts antiarthritic effect by inhibiting 5-LOX and COX-2 activities, increasing lysosomal stability, decreasing neutrophil regulation, decreasing lipid peroxidation, and improving antioxidant status during arthritis.

KEYWORDS

- **inflammation**
- **rheumatoid arthritis**
- **non-steroidal anti-inflammatory drugs**
- **medicinal plants**
- *Justicia gendarussa*

REFERENCES

1. Abdel El-Gaphar, O., Abo-Youssef, A. M., & Abo-Saif, A. A. (2018). Effect of losartan in complete Freund's adjuvant-induced arthritis in rats. *Iranian Journal of Pharmaceutical Research, 17*(4), 1420–1430.
2. Abudoleh, S.M., Disi, A.M., Qunaibi, E.A., & Aburjai, T.A. (2011). Anti-arthritic activity of the methanolic leaf extract of Urtica pilulifera L. on Albino Rats. *American Journal of Pharmacology and Toxicology, 6*, 27–32.
3. Ahmad, F.B., Holdsworth, D.K. (2003). Medicinal plants of Sabah, East Malaysia—Part I. *Pharmaceutical Biology*, 41, 340–346.
4. Alorainy M. (2008). Effect of allopurinol and vitamin e on rat model of rheumatoid arthritis. *International Journal of Health Sciences, 2*(1), 59–67.
5. Alten, R., Gromnica-Ihle, E., Pohl, C., Emmerich, J., Steffgen, J., Roscher, R., Sigmund, R., Schmolke, B., & Steinmann, G. (2004). Inhibition of leukotriene B4-induced CD11B/CD18 (Mac-1) expression by BIIL 284, a new long acting LTB4 receptor antagonist, in

patients with rheumatoid arthritis. *Annals of the Rheumatic Diseases*, *63*(2), 170–176. https://doi.org/10.1136/ard.2002.004499

6. Al Za'abi, M., Al Busaidi, M., Yasin, J., Schupp, N., Nemmar, A., & Ali, B. H. (2015). Development of a new model for the induction of chronic kidney disease via intraperitoneal adenine administration, and the effect of treatment with gum acacia thereon. *American Journal of Translational Research*, *7*(1), 28–38.

7. Anderson, G.D., Hauser, S.D., McGarity, K.L., Bremer, M.E., Isakson, P.C., Gregory, S.A. (1996). Selective inhibition of cyclooxygenase (COX)-2 reverses inflammation and expression of COX-2 and interleukin-6 in rat adjuvant arthritis. *Journal of Clinical Investigation*, 97, 2672–2679.

8. Anderson, A.J (1970). Lysosomal enzyme activity in rats with adjuvant-induced arthritis. *Annals of Rheumatic Diseases*, 29, 307–313.

9. Arokiyaraj, S., Perinbam, K., Agastian, P., Balaraju, K (2007). Immunosuppressive effect of medicinal plants of Kolli hills on mitogen-stimulated proliferation of the human peripheral blood mononuclear cells *in vitro*. *Indian Journal of Pharmacology*, 39(4), 180–183.

10. Aruoma, O.I. (1998). Free radicals, oxidative stress, and antioxidants in human health and disease. *Journal of the American Oil Chemists' Society*, *75*, 199–212.

11. Axelrod, B., Cheesebrough, T.M., Laakso, S (1981). Lipoxygenase from soybeans. *Methods in Enzymology*, 71, 441–453.

12. Ayala, A., Muñoz, M. F., & Argüelles, S. (2014). Lipid peroxidation: production, metabolism, and signaling mechanisms of malondialdehyde and 4-hydroxy-2-nonenal. *Oxidative Medicine and Cellular Longevity*, *2014*, 360438.

13. Bendele, A.M. (2001). Animal models of rheumatoid arthritis. *Journal of Musculoskeletals Neuronal Interactions*, 1, 377–385.

14. Benke, G.M., Cheever, K.L., Mirer, F.E., Murphy, S.D (1974). Comparative toxicity, acetyl choline esterase action and metabolism of methyl parathione (parathione in sun fish). *Toxicology and Applied Pharmacology*, 28; 97–101.

15. Biemond, P., Swaak, A.J., Penders, J.M., Beindorff, C.M., Koster, J.F (1986). Superoxide production by polymorphonuclear leucocytes in rheumatoid arthritis and osteoarthritis: in vivo inhibition by the antirheumatic drug piroxicam due to interference with the activation of the NADPH-oxidase. *Annals of the Rheumatic Diseases*, 45, 249–255.

16. Bradley, P.P., Preibat, D.A., Christensen, R.D., Rothstein, G (1982). Measurement of cutaneous inflammation: estimation of neutrophil content with an enzyme marker. *Journal of Investigative Dermatology*, 78, 206–209.

17. Botezelli, J. D., Cambri, L. T., Ghezzi, A. C., Dalia, R. A., M Scariot, P. P., Ribeiro, C., Voltarelli, F. A., & Mello, M. A. (2011). Different exercise protocols improve metabolic syndrome markers, tissue triglycerides content and antioxidant status in rats. *Diabetology & Metabolic Syndrome*, *3*, 35.

18. Campo, G. M., Avenoso, A., Campo, S., Ferlazzo, A. M., Altavilla, D., & Calatroni, A. (2003). Efficacy of treatment with glycosaminoglycans on experimental collagen-induced arthritis in rats. *Arthritis Research and Therapy*, *5*(3), R122–R131.

19. Cong, H.H., Khaziakhmetova, V.N., Zigashina, L.E. (2015). Rat paw oedema modeling and NSAIDs: Timing of effects. *International Journal of Risk and Safety Medicine*, 27 (1), S76–S77.

20. Dheeba, B., Sampathkumar, P., Kannan, M., Vaishnavi, E., Maragatham. (2012). Therapeutic efficacy of spirulina in the treatment of formaldehyde induced rheumatoid arthritis in Swiss albino mice. *Biosciences Biotechnology Research Asia,* 9 (1), 321–326.

21. Earp, J. C., Dubois, D. C., Almon, R. R., & Jusko, W. J. (2009). Quantitative dynamic models of arthritis progression in the rat. *Pharmaceutical Research, 26*(1), 196–203.
22. Ewan, E. E., & Martin, T. J. (2012). Intracranial self-stimulation of the paraventricular nucleus of the hypothalamus: increased faciliation by morphine compared to cocaine. *Anesthesiology, 116*(5), 1116–1123.
23. Gautam, M. K., Purohit, V., Agarwal, M., Singh, A., & Goel, R. K. (2014). In vivo healing potential of Aegle marmelos in excision, incision, and dead space wound models. *The Scientific World Journal*, 740107.
24. Gregoraszczuk, E. L., Rak-Mardyła, A., Ryś, J., Jakubowicz, J., & Urbański, K. (2015). Effect of chemotherapeutic drugs on caspase-3 activity, as a key biomarker for apoptosis in ovarian tumor cell cultured as monolayer: a pilot study. *Iranian Journal of Pharmaceutical Research, 14*(4), 1153–1161.
25. Guo, W., Yu, D., Wang, X., Luo, C., Chen, Y., Lei, W., Wang, C., Ge, Y., Xue, W., Tian, Q., Gao, X., & Yao, W. (2016). Anti-inflammatory effects of interleukin-23 receptor cytokine-binding homology region rebalance T cell distribution in rodent collagen-induced arthritis. *Oncotarget, 7*(22), 31800–31813.
26. Halliwell, B., Gutteridge, J.M.C., Cross, C.E. (1992). Free-radicals, antioxidants, and human-disease—where are we now. *Journal of Laboratory and Clinical Medicine*, 119, 598–620.
27. Havagiray, R.C., and Nitin, PP. (2009). Antiarthritis Activity of Aristolochia Bracteata Extract in Experimental Animals. *The Open Natural Products Journal*, 2, 6–15.
28. Heliovaara, M., Knekt, P., Aho, K., Aaran, R.K., Alfthan, G., Aromaa, A. (1994). Serum antioxidants and risk of rheumatoid arthritis. *Annals of Rheumatic Diseases*, 53, 51–53.
29. James, S., Clement, B.S., Jonathan, N., Craig, R.S. (1979). A tissue-culture model of cartilage breakdown in rheumatoid arthritis. Quantitative aspects of proteoglycan release. *Biochemical Journal*, 180(2), 403–412.
30. Jothimanivannan, C., Kumar, R.S., Subramanian, N. (2010). Anti-inflammatory and analgesic activities of Aerial parts of *Justicia gendarussa* Burm. *International Journal of Pharmacology*, 1–6.
31. Kakkar, P., Das, B., Viswanathan, P.N. (1984). A modified spectrophotometric assay of superoxide dismutase. *Indian Journal of Biochemistry and Biophysics*, 2, 130–132.
32. Karatas, F., Ozates, I., Canatan, H., Halifeoglu, I., Karatepe, M., Colak, R. (2003). Antioxidant status & lipid peroxidation in patients with rheumatoid arthritis. *The Indian Journal of Medical Research*, 118, 178–181.
33. Kavitha, K., Sridevi Sangeetha, K.S., Sujatha, K., Umamaheshwari, S. (2014). Phytochemical and pharmacological profile of *Justicia gendarussa* Burm f.—review. *Journal of Pharmacy Research*, 8(7), 990–997.
34. Kavitha, S.K., Viji, V., Shobha, B., Kripa, K.V., Helen, A. (2012). Anti-inflammatory potential of an ethyl acetate fraction isolated from *Justicia gendarussa* roots through inhibition of iNOS and COX-2 expression via NF-κB pathway. *Cellular Immunology*, (272), 283–289.
35. Kavitha, S.K., Viji, V., Kripa, K., A, Helen. (2011). Protective effect of *Justicia gendarussa* Burm.f. on carrageenan-induced inflammation. *Journal of Natural Medicine*, **65**, 471–479.
36. Kawai, Y., Anno, K. (1971). Mucopolysaccharides degrading enzymes from the liver of the squid Ommastrephes *solani paciicus*. I. Hyaluronidase. *Biochimica et Biophysica Acta*, 242, 28–436.

37. Kore, K. J., Shete R.V., Desai, V. (2011). Anti-arthritic activity of hydroalcoholic extract of lawsonia innermis. *International Journey of Drug Development and Research*, 3(4), 217–224.

38. Krishna, K.L., Mruthunjaya. K., Patel, J.A. (2009) Antioxidant and hepatoprotective activity of leaf extract of *Justicia gendarussa* burm. *International Journal of Biological and Chemical Sciences*, 3, 99–110.

39. Kumar, R., Singh, S., Saksena, A. K., Pal, R., Jaiswal, R., & Kumar, R. (2019). Effect of Boswellia Serrata Extract on Acute Inflammatory Parameters and Tumor Necrosis Factor-α in Complete Freund's Adjuvant-Induced Animal Model of Rheumatoid Arthritis. *International Journal of Applied and Basic Medical Research*, 9(2), 100–106.

40. Kumar, K.S., Sabu, V., Sindhu. G., Rauf, A.A., Helen. A. (2018). Isolation, identification and characterization of apigenin from *Justicia gendarussa* and its anti-inflammatory activity. *International Immunopharmacology*, 59, 157–167.

41. Langervoort, H.L., Cohn, Z.A., Hirsch, J.G., Humphrey, J.H., Spector, W.G., van Furth, R. (1970). The Nomenclature of mononuclear phagocytic cells, Mononuclear Phagocytes. F.A. Davis Company: Philadelphia.

42. Leela Krishna, V., Chitra, V., Soujanya, R.J. (2011). Anti-arthritic activity of whole plant acalypha indica on type II collagen induced arthritis in Wistar rats. *International Journal of Pharmacy and Pharmaceutical Sciences*, 3(5), 99–102.

43. Lledías, F., Rangel, P., Hansberg, W. (1998). Oxidation of catalase by singlet oxygen. *Journal of Biological Chemistry*, 273, 10630–10637.

44. MacDonald, I. (2013). Science and Technology in the 21st Century: Phytomedicine in Focus. *Research Journal of Recent Sciences*, 2, 1–7.

45. Madhvi, B., Anupam, K., Sandeep, T.; Sandeep K. (2013). Commiphora wightii down regulates HMG CoA reductase in hyperlipidemic rats. *International Journal of Biological & Pharmaceutical Research*, 4(6), 441–447.

46. Maehly, A.C., Chance, B. (1954). The assay of catalases and peroxidases. *Methods of Biochemical Analysis*, 1, 357–359.

47. Mahbubur Rahman, A.H.M., Manik Chandra. B., Rafiul Islam, A.K.M., Zaman, A.T.M.N. (2013). Assessment of traditional medicinal plants used by local people of Monirampur Upazilla under Jessore District of Bangladesh. *Wudpecker Journal of Medicinal Plants*, 2(6), 099–109.

48. Matés, J.M., Sánchez-Jiménez, F. (1999) Antioxidant enzymes and their implications in pathophysiologic processes. *Frontiers in Biosciences*, 4, 339–345.

49. McAdam, B.F., Catella-Lawson, F., Mardini, I.A., Kapoor, S., Lawson, J.A., Fitz Gerald, G.A. (1996). Systemic biosynthesis of prostacyclin by cyclooxygenase (COX)-2: the human pharmacology of a selective inhibitor of COX-2. *Proceedings of the National Academy of Sciences USA*, 96, 272–277.

50. Mohammad, R.U., Suchana, S., Mohammad, A.H., Mohammad, A.K., Mohammad, K.H., Mohammad, A.R. (2011). Chemical and biological investigations of *Justicia gendarussa* (Burm. f). *Dhaka University Journal of Pharma Sciences*, 10(1), 53–57.

51. Naganuma, A., Anerson, M.E., Meister, A. (1990). Cellular glutathione as a determinant of sensitivity to mercuric chlorine toxicity. *Biochemistry and Pharmacology*, 404; 693–697.

52. Narendhirakannan, R.T., Subramanian, M. K. (2007). Anti-inflammatory and lysosomal stability actions of *Cleome gynandra* L. studied in adjuvant induced arthritic rats. *Food and Chemical Toxicology*, 45(6), 1001–1012.

53. Okhawa, H., Oshishi, N., Yagi K. (1979). Assay for lipid peroxides in animal tissues by thiobarbituric acid reaction. *Analytical Biochemistry*, 95(2); 351–358.

54. Okon, U.A., Owo, D.U., Udokang, N.E., Udobang, J.A., Ekpenyong, C.E. (2012). Oral Administration of Aqueous Leaf Extract of Ocimum Gratissimum Ameliorates Polyphagia, Polydipsia and Weight Loss in Streptozotocin-Induced Diabetic Rat. *American Journal of Medicine and Medical Sciences*. 2(3), 45–49.

55. Okoli, C. O., & Akah, P. A. (2004). Mechanisms of the anti-inflammatory activity of the leaf extracts of Culcasia scandens P. Beauv (Araceae). *Pharmacology, Biochemistry, and Behavior*, 79(3), 473–481.

56. Otis, J.S., Niccoli, S., Hawdon, N., Sarvas, J.L., Frye, M.A., Chicco, A.J., et al. (2014). Pro-Inflammatory Mediation of Myoblast Proliferation, *PLoS One*, 9(3): e92363.

57. Parke, D.V., Sapota, A. (1996). Chemical toxicity and reactive oxygen species. *International Journal of Occupational and Environmental Health*, 9, 331–40.

58. Patel, D., Kaur, G., Ghag, S.M., Deshmukh, P. (2013). Herbal medicine—a natural cure to arthritis. *Indian Journal of Natural Products and Resources*, 4, 27–35.

59. Patel, S. S., & Shah, P. V. (2013). Evaluation of anti-inflammatory potential of the multidrug herbomineral formulation in male Wistar rats against rheumatoid arthritis. *Journal of Ayurveda and Integrative Medicine*, 4(2), 86–93.

60. Patel, S., Kapadia, N., Shah, B., Shah, M. (2011). Botanical identification and physicochemical Investigation of leaf of Nili-nirgundi (*Justicia gendarussa*). *International Journal Of Pharmaceutical Sciences Review and Research*, 10(1), 116–121.

61. Paval, J., Kaitheri, S. K., Potu, B. K., Govindan, S., Kumar, R. S., Narayanan, S. N., & Moorkoth, S. (2009). Anti-arthritic potential of the plant Justicia gendarussa Burm F. *Clinics (Sao Paulo, Brazil)*, 64(4), 357–362.

62. Perle, T., Katy, M.G., Clément, P., Daniel, W., Céline, D. (2014). Mechanisms of endothelial dysfunction in rheumatoid arthritis: lessons from animal studies. *Arthritis Research & Therapy*, 16(202), 1–8.

63. Penning, T., Talley, J., Bertenshaw, S., Carter, J., Collins, P., Docter, S., Graneto, M., Lee, L., Malecha, J., Miyashiro, J., Rogers, R., Rogier, D., Yu, S., Andersen, G., Burton, E., Cogburn, J., Gregory, S., Koboldt, C., Perkins, W., Seibert, K., Veenhuizen, A., Zhang, Y., Isakson, P. (1997). Synthesis and biological evaluation of the 1,5-diarylpyrazole class of cyclooxygenase-2 inhibitors: identification of 4-[5-(4-methylphenyl)-3-(trifluoromethyl)-1H-pyrazol-1-yl] benzene sulfonamide (SC-58635, celecoxib). *Journal of Medicinal Chemistry*, 440, 1347–1365.

64. Petchi, R. R., Parasuraman, S., Vijaya, C., Gopala Krishna, S. V., & Kumar, M. K. (2015). Antiarthritic activity of a polyherbal formulation against Freund's complete adjuvant induced arthritis in Female Wistar rats. *Journal of Basic and Clinical Pharmacy*, 6(3), 77–83.

65. Petchi, R. R., Vijaya, C., & Parasuraman, S. (2013). Anti-arthritic activity of ethanolic extract of Tridax procumbens (Linn.) in Sprague Dawley rats. *Pharmacognosy Research*, 5(2), 113–117.

66. Prakken, B.J., Roord. S., Ronaghy, A., Wauben, M., Albani, S., Van Eden, W. (2003). Heat shock protein 60 and adjuvant arthritis: a model for T cell regulation in human arthritis. *Springer Seminars in Immunopathology*, 25, 47–63.

67. Rådmark, O., & Samuelsson, B. (2009). 5-Lipoxygenase: mechanisms of regulation. *Journal of Lipid Research*, 50 Suppl (Suppl), S40–S45.

68. Rasool, M, Sabina, E.P. (2008). Evaluation of the protective potential of Spirulina fusiformis on lipid peroxidation and antioxidant status in adjuvant-induced arthritic mice. *PharmacologyOnline*, 1, 300–310.

69. Ratnasooriya, W.D., Deraniyagala, S.A., Dehigaspitiya, D.C. Antinociceptive activity and toxicological study of aqueous leaf extract of *Justicia gendarussa* Burm. F. in rats. *Pharmacognosy Magazine*. 2007, 3(11), 145–155.

70. Ravichandran, L.V., Puvanakrishna, Joseph, K.T. (1991). Influence of Isoproterenol-induced myocardial infarction on certain glycohydrolases and cathepsin in rats. *Biochemical Medicine and Metabolic Biology*, 45, 6–15.

71. Ricciotti, E., and FitzGerald, G. A. (2011). Prostaglandins and inflammation. *Arteriosclerosis, Thrombosis, and Vascular Biology*, 31(5), 986–1000.

72. Rowley, D., Gutteridge, J.M., Blake, D., Farr, M.; Halliwell, B. (1984). Lipid peroxidation in rheumatoid arthritis: thiobarbituric acid-reactive material and catalytic iron salts in synovial fluid from rheumatoid patients. *Clinical Science*, 66, 691–695.

73. Rubin, K., Oldberg, A., Hook, M., Obrink, B. (1978). Adhesion of rat hepatocytes to collagen. *Experimental Cell Research*, 117, 165–177.

74. Sanmugapriya, E., Venkataraman, S. (2006) Studies on hepatoprotective and antioxidant actions of Strychnos potatorum Linn. seeds on CCl4-induced acute hepatic injury in experimental rats. *Journal of Ethnopharmacology*, 105(1–2), 154–160.

75. Saqib, A., & Karigar, C. (2008). *Cyclooxygenase isoforms in health and disease. The Internet Journal of Pharmacology,* 7 (1).

76. Shimizu, T., Kondo, K., Hayaishi, O. (1981). Role of prostaglandin endoperoxidases in the serum thiobarbituric acid reaction. *Archives of Biochemistry and Biophysics*, 206, 271–276.

77. Shouda, T., Yoshida, T., Hanada, T., Wakioka, T., Oishi, M., Miyoshi, K., Komiya, S., Kosai, K., Hanakawa, Y., Hashimoto, K., Nagata, K., & Yoshimura, A. (2001). Induction of the cytokine signal regulator SOCS3/CIS3 as a therapeutic strategy for treating inflammatory arthritis. *The Journal of Clinical Investigation*, 108(12), 1781–1788.

78. Somasundaran, S., Sadique, J., Subramoniam, A. (1983) Influence of extra-intestinal inflammation on the in vitro absorption of 14C-glucose and the effects of anti-inflammatory drugs in the jejunum of rats. *Clinical and Experimental Pharmacology and Physiology*, 10(2), 147–152.

79. Song, H. P., Li, X., Yu, R., Zeng, G., Yuan, Z. Y., Wang, W., Huang, H. Y., & Cai, X. (2015). Phenotypic characterization of type II collagen-induced arthritis in Wistar rats. *Experimental and Therapeutic Medicine*, 10(4), 1483–1488.

80. Song, Y.S., Park, E.H., Hur, G.M., Ryu, Y.S., Kim, Y.M., Jin, C. (2002). Ethanol extract of propolis inhibits nitric oxide synthase gene expression and enzyme activity. *Journal of Ethnopharmacology*, 80(2–3):155–161.

81. Sreekutty, M. S., & Mini, S. (2016). Ensete superbum ameliorates renal dysfunction in experimental diabetes mellitus. *Iranian Journal of Basic Medical Sciences*, 19(1), 111–118.

82. Srivastava, S., Singh, P., Jha, K. K., Mishra, G., Srivastava, S., & Khosa, R. L. (2012). Evaluation of anti-arthritic potential of the methanolic extract of the aerial parts of Costus speciosus. *Journal of Ayurveda and Integrative Medicine*, 3(4), 204–208.

83. Steel RGD, Torrie JH and Dickey DA. Principles and Procedures of Statistics: A Biometrical Approach, 3rd Edition. McGraw-Hill: New York 1997.

84. Thyagarajan, S. P., Jayaram, S., Gopalakrishnan, V., Hari, R., Jeyakumar, P., & Sripathi, M. S. (2002). Herbal medicines for liver diseases in India. *Journal of Gastroenterology and Hepatology*, 17 Suppl 3, S370–S376.

85. 85 Usha, S.S., Vilasrao, J.K., Rumi, G. (2008). Hepatoprotective Activity of Livobond A Polyherbal Formulation against CCl₄ Induced Hepatotoxicity in Rats. *International Journal of Pharmacology,* 4: 472–476.

86. Venkatesh, B. K.C., and Krishnakumari, S. (2006). Cardiospermum halicacabum suppresses the production of TNF-alpha and nitric oxide by human peripheral blood mononuclear cells. *African Journal of Biomedical Research,* 9, 95–99.

87. Vikrant, A., Vivek, K., Ranjeet, K. (2011). A review on plants having anti-arthritic potential. *International Journal of Pharmaceutical Sciences Review and Research*, 7(2), 133–136.

88. Viji, V., Luxumy, S., Helen, A. (2011) Betulinic acid inhibits endotoxin stimulated phosphorylation cascade and proinflammatory prostaglandin E2 production in human peripheral blood mononuclear cells. *British Journal of Pharmacology*, 162(6), 1291–1303.

89. Wang, X., He, X., Zhang, C.F., Guo, C.R., Wang, C.Z., Yuan, C.S. (2017). Anti-arthritic effect of berberine on adjuvant-induced rheumatoid arthritis in rats. *Biomed Pharmacotherapy*, 89:887–893. Weissmann, G. (1966). Lysosomes and joint disease. *Arthritis and Rheumatism*, 9, 834.

90. Weissman, G. (1967). Role of lysosomes in inflammation and diseases. *Annual Review of Medicine,* 18, 97–112.

91. Winder, C.V., Lembke, L.A., Stephens, MD. (2005). Comparative bioassay of drugs in adjuvant induced arthritis in rats: flufenamic acid, mefenamic acid and phenylbutazone. *Arthritis & Rheumatism*, 12(5), 472–482.

92. Wooley, P.H., Luthra, H.S., Stuart, J.M., David, C.S. (1981). Type II collagen-induced arthritis in mice. I. Major histocompatibility complex (I region) linkage and antibody correlates. *Journal of Experimental Medicine*, 154, 688–700.

93. Xia, J., Wang, H., Zhang, Q., & Han, Z. (2018). Modulation of P2X purinoceptor 3 (P2X3) in pentylenetetrazole-induced kindling epilepsy in rats. *Medical Science Monitor* 24, 6165–6177.

94. Xu, Q., Zhou, Y., Zhang, R., Sun, Z., & Cheng, L. F. (2017). Antiarthritic activity of Qi-Wu rheumatism granule (a Chinese herbal compound) on complete Freund's adjuvant-induced arthritis in rats. *Evidence-based Complementary and Alternative Medicine: eCAM, 2017*, 1960517.

95. Yimam, M., Lee, Y. C., Moore, B., Jiao, P., Hong, M., Nam, J. B., Kim, M. R., Kim, T. W., Kim, H. J., Hyun, E. J., Chu, M., Brownell, L., & Jia, Q. (2016). UP1304, a botanical composition containing two standardized extracts of Curcuma longa and Morus alba, mitigates pain and inflammation in adjuvant-induced arthritic rats. *Pharmacognosy Research*, 8(2), 112–117.

96. Zarghi, A., & Arfaei, S. (2011). Selective COX-2 Inhibitors: A Review of Their Structure-Activity Relationships. *Iranian Journal of Pharmaceutical Research,* 10(4), 655–683.

97. Kiritikar, K.R., Basu, B.D. (2005). *Indian Medicinal Plants. International Book Distributors*: Dehra Dun, India.

CHAPTER 9

Epigenetic Changes Caused by Contaminants Present in Groundwater and Their Reversal Using Natural Compounds

RUNJHUN MATHUR[1], SHEO PRASAD SHUKLA[2], GAURAV SAINI[3], and ABHIMANYU KUMAR JHA[4,*]

¹A. P. J. Abdul Kalam Technical University, Lucknow, Uttar Pradesh, India

²Rajkiya Engineering College, Banda, Uttar Pradesh, India

³Department of Civil Engineering, Sharda University, Greater Noida, Uttar Pradesh, India

⁴Professor and Head in Department of Biotechnology, School of Engineering and Technology, Sharda University, Greater Noida, Uttar Pradesh, India

*Corresponding author. E-mail: abhimanyu2006@gmail.com

ABSTRACT

Cancer is known to be a multistep process that involves different stages such as initiation, promotion, progression, and metastasis. Chemical carcinogens including arsenic, chromium, lead, mercury, chloroform, polycyclic aromatic hydrocarbon, and trihalomethanes elements can change any of these processes to induce their carcinogenic effects. The molecular cause of cancer is deregulation of cell cycle, cell death, and DNA repair pathways. One of the possible mechanisms for the deregulation of these pathways by various contaminants could be promoter hypermethylation, which is a covalent modification in which DNA is methylated by DNA methyltransferases at the 5-position (C5) of the cytosine ring resulting in the formation of 5-methylcytosine. Epigenetics is the study of heritable changes in gene expression that occur without causing

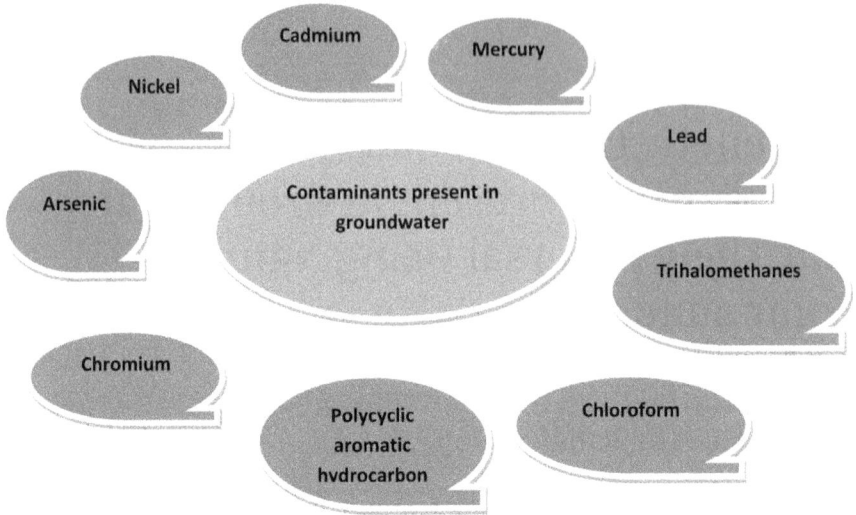

FIGURE 9.1 Inorganic and organic contaminants present in groundwater.

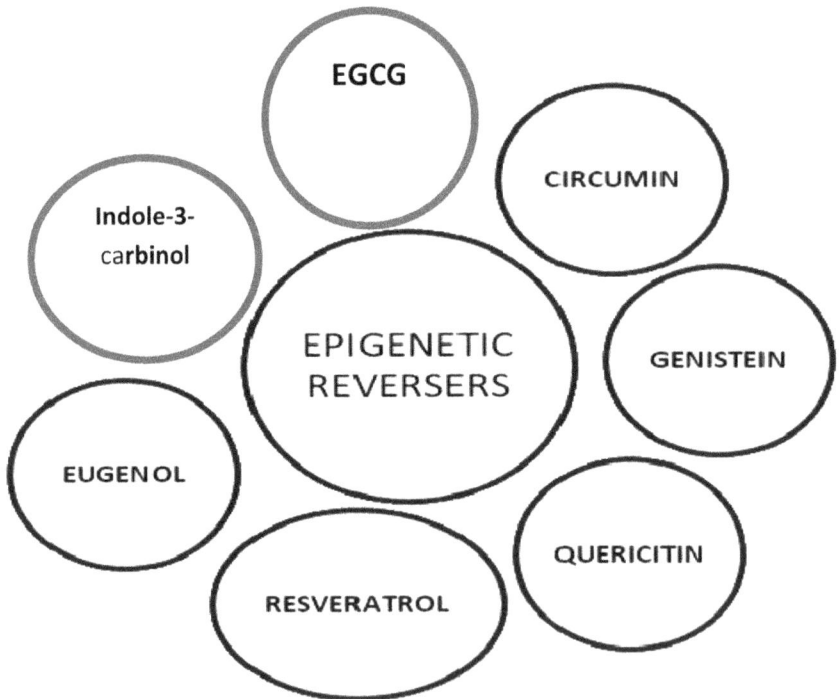

FIGURE 9.2 Reversal of epigenetics through natural compounds.

any change in DNA sequence. Epidemiological studies show that exposure to these contaminants leads to gene-specific DNA hypermethylation in some genes such as p53, DAPK, there may be a possible correlation between the presence of groundwater contaminants and promoter hypermethylation promoting increased incidence of cancer cases. Many anticancer drugs are derived from natural compounds and there have been reports of natural compounds modulating epigenetic activity for different types of cancers. These include curcumin, resveratrol, etc. Accumulating evidence clearly shows toxic metal exposure, which leads to alteration and induction of epigenetic marks in epidemiological and experimental studies. Since promoter hypermethylation is reversible, this will also provide very important therapeutic target in case there emerges a positive correlation between contaminants, promoter hypermethylation, and cancer.

9.1 INTRODUCTION

Gorakhpur, Uttar Pradesh is receiving nearly 80% of India's rural drinking water from underground sources. According to a 2012 study, arsenic contamination has been widely reported in Uttar Pradesh, Haryana, Punjab, etc. In the lower Ganga plain of West Bengal, Bangladesh, and the Terai region of Nepal, groundwater arsenic contamination has also been reported. Various activities such as soldering, mining, emissions from vehicles, processes involved in metal treatment, burning of coal, combustion of petroleum, plastics, textile manufacturing, pulp and paper manufacturing, and leakage of industrial wastes lead to the soil contamination, which, in turn, contaminate the groundwater. Increased concentration of arsenic leads to numerous kinds of hematological changes, that is, anemia, eosinophilia, hearing loss. Fluoride, arsenic, and iron are known to have caused encephalitis, jaundice, and typhoid, mostly among the poor who live in dismal sanitation conditions.

Most of the water contamination is triggered by anthropogenic factors such as industrial effluents leaching into the ground. According to previous reports, after the setup of an industrial area, the quality of groundwater has been deteriorating. Groundwater pollution is tough but once polluted, it can be extremely difficult to get rid of. There may be the presence of possible carcinogens such as arsenic, chromium, lead, mercury, nickel, chloroform, polyaromatic hydrocarbon, and trihalomethanes in the industrial wastes that might be leading to different types of cancer namely stomach, liver, skin, blood, and gut-related cancer in this area. The prolonged unchecked industrialization and urbanization has polluted the two major water bodies such as the Hindon and Yamuna rivers that flow through the crowded floodplains in

Uttar Pradesh. In Yamuna Floodplain Project, it was studied that millions of tones of sewage from Delhi and Ghaziabad cause the contamination in these two primary water bodies.

Population explosion leads to the overexploitation of groundwater resources that have made the problem more tedious.

9.2   POLLUTANTS AND THEIR CARCINOGENICITY

Elevated levels of heavy metals in water and sediments in river Ganges downstream have been reported [8]. Arsenic is not contained so much in the earth's crust, but greatly concentrated in some ores such as pyrite, hydrous Fe oxides, and sulfur compounds [4]. It is known that As would be easily solubilized in water from these minerals depending on pH, redox conditions, and temperature [4]. Nickson et al. [7] suggested that As may be released from As-rich Fe oxyhydroxides into groundwater under reductive conditions in alluvial sediments in Bangladesh and West Bengal. Increased usage of groundwater for drinking in these areas has caused serious health problems [6, 7] because inorganic As is carcinogenic and causes skin and various internal cancers (IARC, 1980; [5]). Arsenic distribution is also affected by anthropogenic activities such as mining and smelting operations, coal-fired combustion, and use of agricultural herbicides, pesticides, and medicinal and cosmetic products [17]. But, the major source of arsenic, in general, is chemical weathering of rocks [16]. A recent survey from rural Gangetic basin, North India, cluster analysis revealed a positive correlation of nickel, cadmium, and chromium in water with high prevalence of gallbladder diseases in adjacent villages in Vaishali district, Bihar [9]. Cr^{6+} was detected in about one-third of 7000 drinking water sources surveyed by the state of California. Cr^{6+} contamination of groundwater can be due to natural conditions or to discharges from industrial activity such as chromium ore processing, metal plating, and use of Cr^{6+} as an anticorrosion agent in cooling water [12, 13]. A study published in 1987 found elevated mortality rates for total cancer, stomach cancer, and lung cancer in communities with Cr^{6+} contaminated water in Liaoning Province, China [15]. Chronic ingestion of As-contaminated drinking water produces lesions to the skin, skin cancer, and various other types of cancer (lung, kidney, liver, and bladder). Because inorganic As has a half-life in the body for few days (it has been reported that 45%–85% of arsenic ingested in the human body are excreted in urine within 1–3 days), its presence in the urine has been used as biomarker of recent exposure (Crecelius, 1977; Hwang et al., 1997; Calderon et al., 1999; Karagas et al., 2001;). The heavy metals such as Cd, Ni, Pb, and U are known to have a number of negative impacts on human health such as DNA damage, cancer, and damage of the central nervous system. Lead is a "possible human carcinogen" because of inconclusive evidence of human and sufficient evidence of animal carcinogenicity [19]. Nickel is a "probable human carcinogen" (International Committee on Nickel Carcinogenesis in Man). Lead is a contaminant in food and water. Total diet studies in industrial countries indicate a daily intake of lead of the order of 200–300 µg. Intake from drinking water provides about 20 µg and inhalation of city air about another 20 µg/day. The unregulated discharge of industrial wastes is also seen to pose significant risks to the food system [21]. Not all villages have abandoned agricultural practices, but the scarcity of freshwater has led many farmers toward the irrigation of food crops such as cereals and vegetables with wastewater that can contain industrial pollutants. The main contaminants identified within the effluents of these industries include high levels of organic pollutants as well as high concentrations of heavy metals. Human risk was assessed in people exposed to trace metals using exposure risk assessment model indicated arsenic was the most important pollutant causing noncarcinogenic and carcinogenic concerns, particularly for sensitive children. As, Sb, and Se were the largest contributors to chronic risk, while Ni, Al, Fe, and Ba were the least contributors in both the dry and rainy seasons. The levels of these contaminants in the river and groundwater are consistently above permissible limits and as a result, the water is considered unfit for recreational activity and the sustenance of aquatic organisms. High values of heavy metals are frequently documented in the periurban and can be extremely toxic to aquatic organisms as well as to humans, where long-term ingestion of water polluted with heavy metals can be devastating leading to the development of a number of cancers, neurological disorders, and even death. In Arthala colony, lead has been found in the groundwater in concentrations more than three times the permissible limits of the WHO [23].

Synthetic chemicals disperse into lakes and streams from atmospheric fallout, for example, natural seepage problems of oil and polycyclic aromatic hydrocarbons (PAHs) into the continental shelf and beaches pose a health problem. Wilson et al. [18] and his coworkers estimate the release of carcinogenic PAH into the marine environment to occur at the rate of 0.2×10^6 to 6×10^6 metric tons per year. Trihalomethanes (THMs) are widely found at concentrations ranging from less than one part to several hundred parts per billion, usually at much higher levels than other halogenated hydrocarbon contaminants [1]. Disinfection by chlorination has been used in most large US cities with surface water supplies since the early 20th century [2]. Formation and escalation of levels of the suspected carcinogen, chloroform, from a few micrograms per liter concentration in raw water to several 100 µg/L in drinking water, an enhancement attributed to the effect of chlorination on humic acids. The geographical correlation studies appeared to show a stronger association than chloroform with certain cancer mortality rates, especially bladder cancer. The brominated alkanes have not been extensively bioassayed in experimental animals for carcinogenic activity [38].

Dichlorodiphenyltrichloroethane (DDT) was the first synthetic insecticide used in our country [26]. In India, 234 pesticides are registered for use at present. Long persistence of some agrochemicals in the environment sets in a series of undesirable effects through contamination of food and water. In India, DDT and benzene hexachloride (BHC) were the two major chemicals used in agriculture and public health programs. Our biggest concern is that these molecules are stable in the environment. It is suspected that most of our water bodies and soils are contaminated with these chemicals or with their degradation products. Residues of organochlorine pesticides (OCPs), namely isomers of hexachlorocyclohexane (HCH) and endosulfan and DDT and its metabolites, aldrin, dieldrin, were analyzed in water of river Yamuna along its 346 km stretch passing through Haryana–Delhi–Haryana and the canals originating from it. β-HCH, p,p'-DDT, p,p'-dichlorodiphenyldichloroethylene (DDE), and p,p'-DDD had maximum traceability in test samples (95–100%) followed by γ-HCH, α-HCH, and o,p'-DDD (60–84%) and o,p'-DDT, δ-HCH, and o,p'-DDE (7%–30%) while aldrin, dieldrin, and α and β endosulfan remained below detection limits (BDL). The concentration of ΣHCH and ΣDDT (i.e., their mean values) at different sites of the river ranged between 12.76 and 593.49 ng/L (with a mean of 310.25 ng/L) and 66.17 and 722.94 ng/L (with a mean of 387.9 ng/L), respectively. In canals, the values were found between 12.38 and 571.98 ng/L and 109.12–1572.22 ng/L for ΣHCH and ΣDDT, respectively [44]. Mahantesh and Singh [34] in their findings on groundwater quality assessment in the village of Lutfullapur Nawada, Loni, district Ghaziabad, India resulted that levels of electrical conductivity, alkalinity, chloride, calcium, sodium, potassium, and iron exceeding their permissible limits. The pesticide residue was major cause of these abnormalities in groundwater quality. Chaudhary et al. [35] assessed ground drinking water in some parts of Meerut district, Uttar Pradesh, India. The study reveals that some groundwater samples had marginally high concentration of sodium, calcium, and potassium. N-nitroso compounds are well-recognized carcinogens in animals and are considered potentially carcinogenic in humans [32, 33, 36].

9.3 EXPOSURE TO POTENTIAL CARCINOGENS AND HUMAN HEALTH

Exposure to pesticides and heavy metals both occupationally and environmentally causes a range of human health problems. It has been observed that the pesticide exposure is increasingly linked to immunosuppression, hormone disruption, diminished intelligence, reproductive abnormalities, and cancer. There are now some evidences available that some of these chemicals has adverse effect on environment, do pose a potential risk to humans, other life forms [28–30]. In today's scenario, no one in this world is completely protected against exposure to heavy metals and pesticides and has potentially deleterious effects on their health, though much of this is confined to the people of developing countries and by high-risk group of peoples in each country (for more details refer Table 9.1). It is estimated that nearly 10,000 deaths occur annually due to use of chemical pesticide worldwide with about three-fourths of these occurring in developing countries [27].

When any contaminated water is compared to drinking water guidelines established by the WHO, China, and the USEPA, much greater attention should be paid to Al, As, Cd, Pb, Sb, and Se (Refer to Table 9.2) and these chemicals are above the critical values in the different sampling time.

Nowadays, drinking water pollution is an important issue in cities across the world as contamination of drinking water is hazardous to human's health. In cities of China, drinking water is mainly supplied by tap water treatment plants (TWTPs). Besides, purified water, mineral water, as well as drinking water from street water fountain (collectively referred to as "other drinking waters" herein) are also consumed as drinking water by indigenes. Unfortunately, the inorganic and organic contaminants were not completely removed by the technological process that is employed during water purification in TWTPs. For example, the presence of heavy metals and organic compounds has been observed previously in tap water samples [39].

Ensuring safe drinking water availability for the public is a major livelihood issue and should be given all the attention it deserves. Despite the sudden increase in the case of cancer that has been reported in these villages, no study till date has been done to find the responsible contaminant, its source, and the remedy for this situation. Exposure to these contaminants in one way or another can cause epigenetic changes and since these changes are potentially reversible, anticancerous drugs that are derived from

TABLE 9.1 Documented Research on Contamination by Various Organic and Inorganic Compounds and Analyzing their Effects on Human Beings

Issues	References
Contamination by arsenic and other trace elements in tube-well water and its risk assessment to humans has been reported	Agusa et al. [3]
The relation between the bladder cancer and levels of arsenic was established	Bates et al. [10]
Chronic arsenic poisoning in Mexico has been reported	Cebrian [11]
Cancer mortality in a Chinese population exposed to hexavalent chromium in drinking water has been reported	Beaumont et al. [14]
Environmental risk assessment of arsenic and fluoride in the Chaco Province, Argentina was studied	
Exposure to inorganic arsenic in drinking water and total urinary arsenic concentration in a Chilean population were reported	Caceres et al. (2004)
A proposed mechanism of action by means of which the exposures related to environment may cause such epigenetic changes was proved in case of some metals	Hou et al. (2012)
Role of cobalt, iron, lead, manganese, mercury, platinum, selenium, and titanium in carcinogenesis was reported	Kazantzis [40]
Epigenetic alterations induced by genotoxic occupational and environmental human chemical carcinogen were investigated	
Epigenetic changes induced by nanomaterials and possible impact on health were investigated	Smolkova et al. [41]
Risk assessment and seasonal variations of dissolved trace elements and heavy metals in the Upper Han River, China	Li et al. [39]
Health risk assessment of polycyclic aromatic hydrocarbons was confirmed	Kumar et al. [42]
In-vitro profiling of epigenetic modifications underlying heavy metal toxicity of tungsten-alloy and its components was proved	Verma et al. [43]
The impact of PAH on biological health parameters of soils of an Indian refinery and adjoining agricultural area was investigated	
Blood levels of polycyclic aromatic hydrocarbons in children of Lucknow, India were investigated	
Study on water quality assessment of river Hindon at Ghaziabad, India: impact of industrial and urban wastewater environmental monitoring and assessment was done	Sharma et al. [39]
Water quality index of surface water quality in an industrial area in Kanpur City was measured	Shukla et al. [31]
Promoter hypermethylation of *p73* and *p53* genes in cervical cancer patients among north Indian population was investigated	Jha et al. [37]

natural compounds provide us the opportunities for primary prevention of environmentally-induced disease or by oligonucleotide therapies targeting microRNA regulatory circuitries. Since epigenetic modifications were induced by multiple environmental exposures, epigenetic biomarkers may provide better readouts of one's past exposome to predict future disease risk and devise effective counter measures.

TABLE 9.2   Abbreviations/Symbols

Sr. No.	Name of Elements	Symbol
1	Arsenic	As
2	Lead	Pb
3	Chromium	Cr
4	Nickel	Ni
5	Mercury	Hg
6	Cadmium	Cd
7	Polycyclic aromatic hydrocarbons	PAHs
8	Trihalomethanes	THMs
9	Indole-3-carbinol	I3C
10	Dichlorodiphenyltrichloroethane	DDT
11	Hexachlorocyclohexane	HCH
12	Dichlorodiphenyldichloroethane	DDD
13	Organochlorine pesticides	OCPs
14	Benzene hexachloride	BHC
15	Dichlorodiphenyldichloroethylene	DDE
16	Electrical conductivity	EC
17	Below detection limit	BDL
18	Principal component analysis	PCA

9.4   REVERSAL OF PROMOTER HYPERMETHYLATION USING NATURAL COMPOUNDS

Cancer is caused by genetic as well as epigenetic changes. Genetic changes such as mutation cannot be reversed, but epigenetic changes can be reversed. Epigenetic changes include promoter hypermethylation of tumor suppressor genes, which lead to inactivation of these genes. These changes have been shown to be reversed after using natural compounds. Some of the compounds are:

Epigallocatechin-3-gallate (EGCG): EGCG is the major active components of green tea. Recently, its intake has increased suddenly due to its potential anticarcinogenic property. It has good source of antioxidants, which can reduce the risk of various types of cancer such as prostate cancer, colorectal cancer, and breast cancer. Partial reversal of hypermethylation has been shown in *RECK* gene in oral cancer cells [45].

Eugenol: Clove is excellent source of eugenol. It has the capacity to prevent the cancer. It has phenolic structure and antioxidant properties that play an important role against cancer. It has already been proved that eugenol exhibits the toxicity against HeLa cell lines.

Curcumin: It is the phenolic component of *Curcuma longa* traditionally known as turmeric. It shows its anticancerous activities by apoptosis/cell cycle regulation and is considered as good epigenetic modulator [46]. Change in methylation status of colorectal cell lines HCT116 and HT29 has been observed while treating the cell with curcumin [47].

Genistein: It is found abundantly in soya beans. It shows its anticancerous properties through cell signaling, cell cycle regulation, and angiogenesis. Genistein can act directly or through steroid-dependent process and, thus, acts as a potent modulator of epigenetic markers. Reversal of promoter hypermethylation through genistein is already been known in KYSE510 esophageal squamous carcinoma cells resulting in reversal of promoter hypermethylation of *p16*, *RARβ2*, and *MGMT* genes [48].

Resveratrol: It is mainly present in grapes. Resveratrol causes programmed cell death in HL60 cells and T47D breast cancer cells through cell signaling pathway [49]. It is also found in red berries, peanuts, and possesses antioxidant activities against cancer [50]. It can also protect the cancer by modifying mRNA.

Quercetin: It is natural antioxidant found mainly in onions, citrus foods, parsley, red wine, etc. Mitogenic signaling, cell cycle regulation, and apoptosis are the main pathways to show its anticancerous activities. In human leukemia, it induces histone hyperacetylation [51]. It is known to have proapoptotic and antiproliferative activity in HeLa cell lines [52].

Indole-3-carbinol: It is found in cruciferous vegetables such as broccoli, cabbage, cauliflower, and radish. Indole-3-carbinol has been reported to induce programmed cell death in several neoplastic cell lines by nuclear receptor-mediated signaling [53].

9.5 FUTURE ASPECTS

On the basis of previous work, it may be suggested that the water from contaminated sites should not be used for drinking without treatment and Government may provide drinking water alternatives to these areas. Previous studies concluded that various anthropogenic factors such as urbanization, industrialization, agricultural practices, and constructional activities are responsible for deterioration of water quality, but the degree to which these factors are responsible is still unclear. Thus, it is necessary to decrease this uncertainty by extracting latent pollution sources. The information extracted facilitates water quality managers to prioritize and take coherent decisions for implementation of the best action plan for water.

Study needs to be carried out which clearly indicate the efficacy of multivariate techniques to assess the surface water quality and facilitate decision-makers to determine priorities for any pollution management program. Moreover, principal parameters responsible for significant variations identified by the principal component analysis, a statistical tool that can further be used to incorporate into the water quality index calculation which would give a more precise picture of water quality at the monitoring stations.

DNA methylation as a therapeutic target—inactivation of tumor suppressor genes by genetic and epigenetic mechanisms are, in many ways, functionally equivalent in tumorigenesis; there are some fundamental differences that may be potentially significant for anticancer therapy. First of all, while genetic hits confer a fixed, irreversible state of gene inactivation, epigenetic events do not interfere with the information content of the affected genes and are potentially reversible. The suppressing activity of epigenetic defects may be alleviated at two different levels: by inhibition of DNA methylation and inhibition of histone deacetylation. Potent inhibitors of DNA methylation or histone deacetylase are available that can modulate gene transcription in vitro and in vivo at nontoxic concentrations. A very potent specific inhibitor of DNA methylation, 5-aza-2'-deoxycytidine, has been widely used as a demethylating agent in vitro and is used clinically in the treatment of acute leukemias and myelodysplasia. Likewise, cell culture experiments have shown that histone deacetylase inhibitors (e.g., trichostatin A) can reactivate a range of epigenetically silenced genes and several of these agents are now in clinical trial.

KEYWORDS

- cancer
- carcinogens
- THM
- PAH
- epigenetics
- hypermethylation

REFERENCES

1. Symons, J. M. (1975). National organics reconnaissance survey. In: Preliminary assessment of suspected carcinogens in drinking water (pp. 12–100).
2. Wolman, A. and Enslow, L. H. (1919). Chlorine absorption and the chlorination of water. *J Ind Eng Chem.* 11: 209–213.
3. Agusa, T., Kunito, T., Fujihara, J., Kubota, R., Minh, T. B., Trang, P. T. M., Subramanian, H. I. A., Viet, P. H. and Tanabe, S. (2006). *Environ Pollut.* 139: 95–106.
4. Smedley, P. L. and Kinniburgh, D. G. (2002). A review of the source, behavior, and distribution of arsenic in natural waters. *Appl Geochem.* 17: 517–568.
5. WHO. (2001). Environmental health criteria 224: Arsenic and arsenic compounds, 2nd edition. World Health Organization, Geneva.
6. Bagla, P. and Kaiser, J. (1996). India's spreading health crisis draws global arsenic experts. *Science.* 274: 174–175.
7. Nickson, R., McArthur, J., Burgess, W., Ahmed, K. M., Ravenscroft, P. and Rahman, M. (1998). Arsenic poisoning of Bangladesh groundwater. *Nature.* 395: 338–345.
8. Singh, V. K., Singh, K. P. and Mohan, D. (2005). Status of heavy metals in water and bed sediments of river Gomti—a tributary of the Ganga River, India. *Environ Monit Assess.* 105: 43–67.
9. Unisa, S., Jagannath, P., Dhir, V., Khandelwal, C., Sarangi, L. and Roy T. K. (2011). Population-based study to estimate prevalence and determine risk factors of gallbladder diseases in the rural Gangetic basin of North India. *HPB (Oxford).* 13: 117–125.
10. Bates, M. N., Smith, A. H. and Hopenhayn, R. C. (1992). Arsenic ingestion and internal cancers: a review. *Am J Epidemiol.* 135: 462–476.
11. Cebrián, M. E., Albores, A., Aguilar, M. and Blakely E. (1983). Chronic arsenic poisoning in the north of Mexico. *Hum Toxicol.* 2: 121–133.
12. Ball, J. W. and Izbicki, J. A. (2004). Occurrence of hexavalent chromium in groundwater in the western Mojave Desert, California. *Appl Geochem.* 19: 1123–1135.
13. Fryzek, J. P., Mumma, M. T., McLaughlin, J. K., Henderson, B. E. and Blot, W. J. (2001). Cancer mortality in relation to environmental chromium exposure. *J Occup Environ Med.* 43: 635–640.

14. Beaumont, J. J., Sedman, R. M., Reynolds, S. D., Sherman, C. D., Li, L. H., Howd, R. A., Sandy, M. S., Zeise, L. and Alexeeff, G. V. (2008). Cancer mortality in a Chinese population exposed to hexavalent chromium in drinking water. *Epidemiology.* 19: 12–23.

15. Zhang, J. D. and Li, X. L. (1987). Chromium pollution of soil and water in Jinzhou. *Zhonghua Yu Fang Yi Xue Za Zhi.* 21: 262–264.

16. Bhattacharya, P., Welch, A. H., Stollenwerk, K. G., McLaughlin, M. J., Bundschuh, J. and Panaullah, G. (2007). Arsenic in the environment: biology and chemistry. *Sci Total Environ.* 379: 109–120.

17. Orloff, K., Mistry, K. and Metcalf, S. (2009). Biomonitoring for environmental exposures to arsenic. *J Toxicol Environ Health B.* 12: 509–524.

18. Wilson, R. D., Monoghan, P. H., Osanik, A., Price, L. C. and Rogers, M. A. (1974). Natural marine oil seepage. *Science.* 184: 857–865.

19. WHO. (1996). Guidelines for drinking-water quality, Vol 2: Health criteria and other supporting information, 2nd edition. WHO, Geneva.

20. Report of the International Committee on nickel carcinogenesis in man. (1990). *Scand J Work Environ Health.* 16(1): 9–74.

21. Marshall, F. M., Holden, J., Ghose, C., Chisala, B., Kapungwe, E., Volk, J., Agrawal, M. and Agarwal, R. (2007). Contaminated irrigation water and food safety for the urban and peri-urban poor: appropriate measures for monitoring and control from field research in India and Zambia. *Research.* 5: 18–20.

22. Waldman, L., Bisht, R., Saharia, R., Kapoor, A., Rizvi, B., Hamid, Y., Arora, M., Chopra, I., Sawansi, K. T., Priya, R. and Marshall, F. (2017). Peri-Urbanism in globalizing India: a study of pollution, health and community awareness. *Int J Environ Res Public Health.* 14(9): 980–997.

23. Lewis, H. (2007). Hindon river: gasping for breath. Janhit Foundation, Meerut, Uttar Pradesh.

24. Suthar, S., Sharma, J., Chabukdhara, M. and Nema, A. K. (2010). Water quality assessment of river Hindon at Ghaziabad, India: impact of industrial and urban wastewater. *Environ Monit Assess.* 165(1–4): 103–112.

25. Singh, S. and Kumar, M. (2006). Heavy metal load of soil, water and vegetables in periurban Delhi. *Environ Monit Assess.* 3: 79–91.

26. Joshi, M. (2005). Perils of pesticides. Centre for Environmental Education, Ahmedabad, ISBN: 81-7596-263-1.

27. Horrigan, L., Lawrence, R. S. and Walker, P. (2002). How sustainable agriculture can address the environmental and human heath harms of industrial agriculture. *Environ Health Perspect.* 110(5): 445–456.

28. Forget, G. (1993). Balancing the need for pesticides with the risk to human health. In: Impact of pesticide use on health in developing countries. IDRC, Ottawa, p. 2.

29. Igbedioh, S. O. (1991). Effects of agricultural pesticides on humans, animals, and higher plants in developing countries. *Arch Environ Health.* 46: 218–225.

30. Jeyaratnam, J. (1985). Health problems of pesticide usage in the third world. *BMJ.* 42: 505–525.

31. Shukla, S. P., Agrawal, V., Singh, N. B., Shukla, R., Bhargava, D. S. and Behera, S. N. (2011). Water quality index of surface water quality in an industrial area in Kanpur City. *J Environ Eng.* 19: 18–22.

32. Bartsch, H., Ohshima, H., Pignatelli, B. and Camels, S. (1989). Human exposure to endogenous nitroso compounds: quantitative estimate in subjects at high risk for cancer of the oral cavity, esophagus, stomach, and urinary bladder. *Cancer Surv*. 8: 335–362.

33. Mirvish, S. S. (1995). Role of N-nitroso compounds (NOC) and N-nitrosation in etiology of gastric, esophageal, nasopharyngeal, and bladder cancer and contribution to cancer of known exposures to NOC. *Cancer Lett*. 93: 17–48.

34. Mahantesh, N. and Singh, A. (2012). A study on farmers' knowledge, perception and intensity of pesticide use in vegetable cultivation in Western Uttar Pradesh. *Pusa Agri Sci*. 32: 63–69.

35. Chaudhary, R., Chaudhary, V., Mancini, F., Van Bruggen, A. H. and Jiggins, J. (2012). Assessment of cationic composition in ground drinking water in some parts of Meerut district, Uttar Pradesh, India. *Progress Agricul*. 3: 376–380.

36. Walker, R. (1990). Nitrates, nitrites and N-nitroso compounds: a review of the occurrence in food and diet and the toxicological implications. *Food Addit Contam*. 7: 717–718.

37. Jha A. K., Nikbakht, M., Jain, V., Sehgal, A., Capalash, N. and Kaur, J. (2012). Promoter hypermethylation of *p73* and *p53* genes in cervical cancer patients among north Indian population. *Mol Biol*. 39: 9145–9157.

38. Cantor, K. (1976). Aquatic pollutants and biological effects with emphasis on neoplasia. *Ann N Y Acad Sci*. 298: 27–29.

39. Li, S. and Zhang, Q. (2010). Risk assessment and seasonal variations of dissolved trace elements and heavy metals in the Upper Han river, China. *J Hazard Mater*. 181: 1051–1058.

40. Kazantzis, G. (1981). Role of cobalt, iron, lead, manganese, mercury, platinum, selenium, and titanium in carcinogenesis. *Environ Health Perspect*. 3: 143–161.

41. Smolkova, B., Yamani, N. E., Collins, A. R., Gutleb, A. C. and Dusinska, M. (2015). Nanoparticles in food: epigenetic changes induced by nanomaterials and possible impact on health. *Food Chem Toxicol*. 77: 64–73.

42. Kumar, S. N., Verma, P., Bastia, B. and Jain, A. K. (2014). Health risk assessment of polycyclic aromatic hydrocarbons. *J Pathol Toxicol*. 1: 16–30.

43. Verma, R., Xu, X., Jaiswal, M. K., Olsen, C., Mears, D., Caretti, G. and Galdzicki, Z. (2011). *In vitro* profiling of epigenetic modifications underlying heavy metal toxicity of tungsten-alloy and its components. *Toxicol Appl Pharmacol*. 253: 178–187.

44. Kaushik, C. P., Sharma, H. R., Jain, S., Dawra, J. and Kaushik, A. (2008). Pesticide residues in river Yamuna and its canals in Haryana and Delhi, India. *Environ Monit Assess*. 144: 329–340.

45. Baatout, S., Jacquet, P., Derradji, H., Ooms, D., Michaux, A. and Mergeay, M. (2004). Study of the combined effect of X-irradiation and epigallocatechin-gallate (a tea component) on the growth inhibition and induction of apoptosis in human cancer cell lines. *Oncol Rep*. 12(1): 159–167.

46. Dicato, M. and Diederich, M. (2013). Curcumin as a regulator of epigenetic events. *Mol Nutr Food Res*. 57: 1619–1629.

47. Link, A., Balaguer, F., Shen, Y., Lozano, J. J., Leung, H. C., Boland, C. R. and Goel, A. (2013). Curcumin modulates DNA methylation in colorectal cancer cells. *PLoS One*. 8: e57709.

48. Fang, M., Chen, D. and Yang, C. S. (2007). Dietary polyphenols may affect DNA methylation. *J Nutr*. 137(Suppl 1): 223S–228S.

49. Wheat, J. and Currie, G. (2008). Herbal medicine for cancer patients: an evidence-based review. *Int J Altern Med.* 5(2): 18–20.
50. Savouret, J. F. and Quesne, M. (2002). Resveratrol and cancer: a review. *Biomed Pharmacother.* 56: 84–87.
51. Lee, W. J., Chen, Y. R. and Tseng, T. H. (2011). Quercetin induces FasL-related apoptosis, in part, through promotion of histone H3 acetylation in human leukemia HL-60 cells. *Oncol Rep.* 25: 583–591.
52. Xiang, T., Fang, Y. and Wang, S. X. (2014). Quercetin suppresses HeLa cells by blocking PI3K/Akt pathway. *J Huazhong Univ Sci Technolog Med Sci.* 34: 740–744.
53. Banerjee, S., Kong, D., Wang, Z., Bao, B., Hillman, G. G. and Sarkar, F. H. (2011). Attenuation of multi-targeted proliferation-linked signaling by 3,30-diindolylmethane (DIM): from bench to clinic. *Mutat Res.* 728: 47–66.

CHAPTER 10

Medicinal Mushrooms in Supportive Cancer Therapy: A Review

C. R. MEERA

Department of Microbiology, St Mary's College, Thrissur, Kerala, India; E-mail: meera_mahes@yahoo.com.

ABSTRACT

Cancer is the second largest cause of death throughout the world. Conventional therapies of cancer include surgery, r\s, particularly greatest on hematopoietic tissue. Injury to hematopoietic tissue causes severe immunosuppression which negatively affects therapy by making the host more prone to different opportunistic and pathogenic microbial infections. Nowadays much more concern is also given to the patient's quality of life (QOL) rather than the treatment. Mushrooms are natural resources of least toxic bioactive components with immunopotentiating and anticancer properties. Many potential compounds have been isolated from mushrooms which include polysaccharides (PLs), polysaccharopeptides (PSP), polysccharide proteins, and proteins. Mushrooms also contain other pharmacologically active compounds like triterpenes, lipids, and phenols. Consumption of mushrooms or their bioactive components can improve the host immune system, renovate homeostasis, and increase resistance to diseases. Hence they can improve the QOL and survival of the host. Mushroom-derived compounds are now extensively used in cancer adjuvant therapy in countries like Japan, Korea, and China. Lentinan, Schizophyllan, PSK (Krestin), and PSP (Ppolysaccharide peptide) are the most widely used mushroom derived drugs with significant inhibitory action on human cancers and are considered as biological response modifiers. The most encouraging observation is that these drugs can considerably reduce the side effects of conventional therapies if administered prior to or during treatment. Also the toxicity studies of mushroom components showed no evidence of toxicity.

Thus, mushrooms can be promising candidates in adjuvant immunotherapy and for safe and effective drug development in cancer.

10.1 INTRODUCTION

Cancer is the second largest cause of death around the world which affects people irrespective of their age group and racial background. This awareness has led to a hike in anticancer studies and is now a hot spot of research [28]. Common methods of cancer treatment include surgery, radiation, and chemotherapy. However, cancer treatment by conventional therapies is known to have adverse side effects. The adverse effects are greatest on hematopoietic tissue, gastrointestinal mucosa, gonads, and skin. Damage to the hematopoietic tissue of the host considerably weakens the immune system and adversely affects therapy by leaving the host susceptible to infections by opportunistic and pathogenic microorganisms. Hence, nowadays much importance is also given to the quality of life of the patients which is being considerably affected by the classical treatment methods. Recent investigations have been focused on immunotherapy as well as on agents which can act like immunomodulators or biological response modifiers (BRMs) and by thus preventing and curing various forms of cancer [174, 175]. These agents could be also beneficial in adjunct cancer therapy if they do not hinder the efficacy of conventional cancer treatment methods. Macrofungi are considered as an excellent natural repertoire for immunopotentiating and antineoplastic agents. Applying such immunomodulatory agents of natural origin is vital as the increase in diseases like cancer, immune dysfunction, and autoimmune conditions are alarming in recent years.

Mushrooms are major group of macrofungi with profound nutritional and medicinal properties. Medicinal mushrooms can be edible or nonedible. The majority of medicinal mushrooms come from edible species. Edible mushrooms are widely consumed all over the world owing to their attractive taste, aroma, and nutritional values. The culinary and commercial value of edible mushrooms are mainly due to their organoleptic properties such as their texture, flavor, and also because of their characteristic odor or aroma. Mushrooms are rich in essential nutrients like proteins, carbohydrates, vitamins, especially vitamins B1 and B2, vitamin D, A, C, E, H, K, and PP (Pantothenic acid). The vitamin content of mushrooms is found to be much higher than in most of vegetables. Also, mushrooms have a very low-fat content ranging between 5% and 8%, and in most species less than 1%, except few species which contains up to 15%. Mushroom fruiting bodies are rich in a variety of biologically active compounds and the medicinal use of mushroom PLs has a very long tradition. Other widely studied groups of compounds found in mushrooms are phenolic compounds, terpenoids, indole compounds, and bioelements (e.g., selenium). Mushrooms contain biologically and therapeutically active primary and secondary metabolites that are used to treat serious ailments such as cardiovascular diseases, diabetes, atherosclerosis, and cancer [7, 137]. The host immune mechanisms are improved by the intake of mushroom compounds which restore homeostasis and enhance resistance to disease. Several major substances with immunomodulatory and/or antitumor activity have been isolated from mushrooms. Five BRMs isolated from mushrooms have been widely used against human cancers in different parts of the world. These include lentinan, D-fraction, schizophyllan, PSK (Krestin), and PSP (PL peptide). The first three compounds are derived from *L. edodes*, *G. frondose,* and *S. commune,* respectively. Both PSK and PSP are derived from *T. versicolor.* All these anticancer agents are mainly β-D-glucans or protein-bound β-D-glucans. Thus mushroom PLs are of great hope for patients having carcinomas and other devastating diseases [20].

10.2 ETIOLOGY OF CANCER

Cancer is a disease that develop through multiple stages and is caused by multiple agents. The exact etiology of this disease is still partially known. Many factors, including exposure to viruses, xenobiotic (foreign) chemicals, and radiation contribute to cancer development [187].

10.2.1 CHEMICAL CARCINOGENESIS

Chemical carcinogenesis is usually induced by a chemical carcinogen. A chemical carcinogen is any chemical agent, process, or habit which in humans or animals promotes the chance of cancer development in a particular age group. Cancer development is the unique and extreme response of tissues to chemical toxins [139]. Clinical observations in humans themselves were the first evidence of chemical carcinogenesis. In 1775, Percival Pott, an eminent English physician, and surgeon observed that the occurrence of cancer of the scrotum was linked to soot exposure in English chimney sweeps. In 1918, Yamagiwa and Ichikawa produced tumors by the repeated painting of coal tar on the skin of rabbits. This breakthrough provided the foundation for the isolation, identification, synthesis, and biological testing of chemical carcinogens [127].

Most chemicals that were identified as carcinogens in early research are by-products of industrial processes. Combustion of petroleum or tobacco release chemical carcinogens like Benzo [a] pyrene (BP) and related polycyclic aromatic hydrocarbons. Benzidine and other aromatic amines were also present in the workplace, as was vinyl chloride. Food products and the environment are also other sources of chemical carcinogens. Examples include aflatoxin B1, a potent liver carcinogen formed by molds that contaminate improperly stored grains, and 2-amino-3-methylimidazo [4, 5-f] quinoline (IQ), a heterocyclic amine derived from amino acids during high-temperature cooking [1]. In addition to organic compounds, inorganic compounds are found to be carcinogenic in both animals and humans [107]. At least 10 elements or their compounds, including beryllium, iron, cobalt, zinc, lead, and platinum, have been shown to be carcinogenic in experimental animals. However, it has been estimated that chemical pollution causes only less than 1% of cancers in man. Some important chemical carcinogens associated with the workplace, lifestyle, and medical therapy are given in Tables 10.1–10.3.

Chemical carcinogenesis is a cumulative process. During cancer development, chemical carcinogens interfere with different stages and modify processes at the cellular and molecular levels.

Some chemical carcinogens are genotoxic agents that directly damage DNA and cause mutation in affected cells. Another group of chemical carcinogens are nongenotoxic in action and act through non-DNA/indirect-DNA reaction mechanisms. However, their exact mode of action is not known, yet it is assumed that these compounds modulate cell growth and cell death [169].

10.2.1.1   THE MULTISTEP PROCESS OF CHEMICAL CARCINOGENESIS

Clinical studies and in vivo experiments have proved that chemical carcinogenesis is a multistage mechanism including initiation, promotion, and progression, and each stage is characterized by different underlying mechanisms [79, 166]. Initiation of carcinogenesis usually occurs through a nonlethal mutation in DNA followed by at least one round of synthesis process of DNA which would fix the error generated by mutation. Initiation is an irreversible change, however, all initiated cells do not develop to tumor as many will undergo apoptosis eventually.

TABLE 10.1 Exposures to Chemicals in the Workplace

Agent	Industries and Trades with Proved Excess Cancers and Exposure	Primary Affected Site
p-Aminodiphenyl	Chemical manufacturing	Urinary bladder
Asbestos	Construction, asbestos mining, and milling, production of friction products and cement	Pleura, peritoneum, bronchus
Arsenic	Copper mining and smelting	Skin, bronchus, liver
Alkylating agents (mechloroethamine hydrochloride and bis[chloromethyl]ether)	Chemical manufacturing	Bronchus
Benzene	Chemical and rubber manufacturing, petroleum refining	Bone marrow
Benzidine, b-naphthylamine, and derived dyes	Dye and textile production	Urinary bladder
Chromium and chromates	Tanning, pigment making	Nasal sinus, bronchus
Isopropyl alcohol manufacture	Chemical manufacturing	Cancer of paranasal sinuses
Nickel	Nickel refining	Nasal sinus, bronchus
Polynuclear aromatic hydrocarbons from coke, coal tar, shale, mineral oils, and creosote	Steel making, roofing, chimney cleaning	Skin, scrotum, bronchus
Vinyl chloride monomer	Chemical manufacturing	Liver
Wood dust	Cabinetmaking, carpentry	Nasal sinus

Modified from Cullen et al. [27].

TABLE 10.2   Carcinogenic Factors Associated with Lifestyle

Chemical, Physiological Condition, or Natural Process	Associated Neoplasm
Alcoholic beverages	Esophagus, liver, oropharynx, larynx
Aflatoxins	Liver
Betel chewing	Mouth
Dietary intake (fat, protein, calories)	Breast, colon, endometrium, gallbladder
Reproductive history	Breast
Late age at first pregnancy	Ovary
Zeo or low parity	
Tobacco smoking	Mouth, pharynx, laryns, lung, esophagus, bladder

Modified from Pitot (1986).[134].

TABLE 10.3   Carcinogenic Risks of Chemical Agents Associated with Medical Therapy and Diagnosis

Chemical or Drug	Associated Neoplasms
Alkylating agents (cyclophosphamide, melphalan)	Bladder, leukemia
Inorganic arsenicals	Skin, liver
Azathioprine (an immunosuppressive drug)	Lymphoma, reticulum cell sarcoma, skin, Karposi's sarcoma
Chlornaphazine	Bladder
Chloramphenicol	Leukemia
Diethylstibesterol	Vagina (clear cell carcinoma)
Estrogens	Liver cell adenoma
Premenopausal	Endometrium
Postmenopausal	
Methoxypsoralen with ultaviolet light	Skin
Oxymetholone	Liver
Phenacetin	Renal pelvis (carcinoma)
Phenytoin (diphenyhydantoin)	Lymphoma, neuroblastoma
Thorotrast	Liver (angiosarcoma)

On the other hand, tumor promotion may be modulated by various environmental factors, including diet, age, hormonal balance, and sex. At the stage of tumor promotion constant presence of tumor promotion stimuli is necessary and hence it is considered as a reversible phenomenon [100]. Promotion is that stage in the neoplastic development that is characterized by the reversible expansion and alternation of initiated cells and genetic expression. The third and final stage of carcinogenesis is called progression [79]. The stage of progression is characterized by changes at the cellular and molecular levels leading to neoplasia from the preneoplastic stage. Irreversible benign and malignant neoplasms are characteristic of this stage of neoplastic development. Progression has been defined as that stage of carcinogenesis exhibiting measurable morphological karyotypic changes in the structure of the cell genome [134]. However, it is clear that this entire process does not always compartmentalize neatly into these three classic stages and multiple sequential mutations are required in order to convert a typical cell into a cancerous one [10, 80].

10.2.1.2 TARGETS OF CHEMICAL CARCINOGENS

Proto-oncogenes and tumor suppressor genes are the usual targets for mutagenesis by carcinogens. Mutation in proto-oncogenes activates them and the cell growth signals are elevated whereas, in tumor suppressor genes, mutation leads to loss of their function [127].

10.2.1.2.1 Oncogenes

Commonly found mutations in chemically induced tumors in rodents are those which activate the *ras* family of oncogenes. For example, rat mammary tumors induced by *N*-methyl-*N*-nitrosourea (MNU) contain H-*ras* genes that have been activated by a single point mutation (G-to-A transition) at codon 12 of the gene [190]. In mouse skin papillomas and carcinomas produced by 7,12-dimethylbenz[*a*]anthracene, mutation occurred in codon 61 by A-to-T transversion of the H-*ras* gene [135]. Genomic analysis of cells derived from neuroblastoma has revealed frequent amplification of the c-myc family member, N-myc. Similar analysis of small cell lung carcinoma showed amplification of all three transforming members of the *myc* gene family, C-myc, N-myc, and L-myc [130]. Examples of amplification of other oncogenes include the epidermal growth factor receptor in glioblastomas, Her-2/ NEU, and Cyclin D1 found in carcinoma of breast and C-abl in Chronic Myeloid Leukemia. Bcl-2 oncogene translocation was identified in human follicular lymphomas that juxtaposed the Bcl-2 gene to the immunoglobulin heavy chain gene leading to over expression of Bcl-2. Over expression of Bcl-2 protein has also been observed in other leukemias, such as B-cell chronic lymphocytic leukemia, acute myeloid leukemia, multiple myeloma, and solid tumors of the breast, lungs, skin, and intestine [129].

10.2.1.2.2   *Antioncogenes (Tumor Suppressor Genes)*

The first identified human tumor suppressor gene was retinoblastoma (Rb) gene which on mutation causes familial Rb, a rare form of pediatric eye tumor. In addition to Rb, mutations of Rb can be found in other human malignancies, including osteosarcoma, small cell lung carcinoma, prostate, and breast cancer [144, 176]. More than 50% of human tumors are found to be associated with mutations in p53 tumor suppressor gene. The evidence linking particular chemical exposures to cancer has been greatly strengthened by the observation that chemicals leave molecular signatures in the form of characteristic patterns of mutation in p53 and other genes. For example, tumorous as well as normal tissues of lungs from smokers identified with lung cancer are found to have a high mutational rate at codons 157, 248, and 249 in the *p53* gene [62]. Most p53 mutations in lung cancer are G-to-T transversions, a type of mutation also observed in hepatocellular carcinoma, but rare in other tumors. In Africa and China, more than 50% of the aflatoxin-exposed hepatocellular carcinomas have a G-to-T transversion of the p53 gene at codon 249 [143, 150]. Phosphatase and Tensin Homolog Deleted on Chromosome 10 (PTEN) was discovered as a candidate tumor suppressor gene deleted at human chromosome 10q23 in a number of advanced tumors [95]. Mutations of BRCA1, located on human chromosome 17q21, and BRCA-2, located on 13q12–13, account for a majority of familial breast cancer cases. Besides breast cancers, mutations of BRCA1 have been found in familial ovarian cancer and prostate cancer, whereas BRCA2 mutations can be found in ovarian, prostate, pancreatic, gall bladder, bile duct, and stomach cancer [178].

10.3   RADIATION AND CANCER

Cancer induction may arise from exposure to sufficient doses of ionizing radiation and tissue susceptibility to radiation differs considerably. However, all tissues appear to be at risk [8]. The first observed cancer was skin cancer and radiation-induced leukemia was suspected only some years later. The information about radiation-induced leukemogenesis in humans and animals is now extensive, partly because the latent period for leukemia is shorter than that for solid cancers [164, 167]. Sunlight is a major etiologic factor and exposure to greater intensities of sunlight leads to skin cancer. In 1928, ultraviolet radiation (UVR) induced skin cancer in experimental animals was demonstrated; later, the carcinogenic effect was found to be restricted to wavelengths shorter than 320 nm. Recognition of the role of UVR in the induction of this disease and the degradation of the ozone layer, which absorbs UV in sunlight, has led to the promotion of reduced levels of sun exposure and more extensive use of sun screen preparations [127].

10.4   VIRUSES AND CANCER

Viruses are found to be involved in around 15% of all cancers. Oncogenes and tumor suppressor genes were initially discovered through the studies on these viruses. Tumor suppressor genes like p53 and Rb were identified through studies with simian virus 40 [138]. Cervical cancer, the third most common cancer in women, is associated with human papilloma viruses (HPV) types including HPV16, 18, 31, 33, and 45, and are found in about 90% of all cervical cancers [192]. Epstein–Barr virus (EBV) infection is associated with three lymphoproliferative diseases of B-cell origin including infectious mononucleosis, Burkitt's lymphoma, and lymphoma of the immunocompromised host. Undifferentiated nasopharyngeal carcinoma and Hodgkin's disease are also found to be associated with EBV infection [177]. EBV may also be associated with some gastric carcinomas [159]. Chronic infection with Hepatitis B virus (HBV) is found in above 80% of patients with liver cancer. Only two viral genes, HBx and M (perS2/S) are usually retained intact after viral DNA integration which stimulate gene transcription for growth and survival [32, 56]. HBx is reported to sequester the tumor suppressor, p53, within the cytoplasm, which again has a supportive role in oncogenesis [165, 171].

Only retroviruses that are known to cause human cancers are HTLV-1 and HTLV-2 (Human T-Cell Leukemia Viruses). HTLV-1 by itself can cause adult T-cell leukemia, a rare but virulent cancer [185]. Hairy cell leukemia is caused by HTLV-2 which is less common than HTLV-1. The related Human Immunodeficiency Viruses (HIV) are associated with tumorigenesis through immune suppression and subsequent reactivation of many of the DNA-containing viruses. Immunodebiliating nature of HIV can cause different types of cancers during the late stages of infection, even though they do not cause any malignancy directly [140].

10.5 ROLE OF FREE RADICALS IN CANCER

Reactive oxygen species (ROS) and reactive nitrogen species (RNS) are a constant source of attack for our genetic material. In all aerobic organisms, ROS is generated continuously which is either enhanced or partly reduced by hormonal, nutritional, and environmental factors. Sometimes overproduction of ROS and RNS occurs through endogenous and exogenous insults which is harmful to living cells and is termed as oxidative and nitrosative stress [169].

10.5.1 SOURCES AND REACTIONS OF ROS AND RNS

Generation of ROS and RNS takes place in the environment through irradiation of UV light, gamma rays, and X-rays, through metal-catalyzed reactions, and also from pollutants present in the atmosphere. In a living system, they are generated by neutrophils and macrophages during inflammation, through mitochondrial electron transport chain, and by other reactions [16]. Both exogenous and endogenous free radicals are deleterious to living organisms. Nonenzymatic and enzymatic antioxidant agents can diminish the adverse effects caused by ROS [49]. Irrespective of the presence of antioxidant enzymes in the cells, accumulation of free radicals occurs which leads to damaging effects on the important biomolecules like DNA, proteins, and lipids. Damage to these biomolecules plays a crucial part in the development of diseases like cancer, neurodegenerative diseases, arthritis, arteriosclerosis, and other age-related conditions.

Primary ROS are usually the superoxide anion ($O_2^{\cdot-}$) which is generated through metabolic activities or through the activation of oxygen by physical irradiation. They further interact with other molecules in the living system and generate secondary ROS [38]. The direct action of superoxide radical ions on biomolecules is not evident and also its effect on lipids is controversial.

Redox-active metals are closely associated with the production of different free radicals in the living system [168]. In vivo studies show that under stress conditions if superoxide ions are present in excess amount, they could release "free iron" from iron-containing molecules. The released Fe(II) will participate in the Fenton reaction and thus highly reactive hydroxyl radical is generated. $O_2^{\cdot-}$ is also known to facilitate hydroxyl radical ($\cdot$OH) generation from H_2O_2 under stressed conditions by making Fe (II) available for the Fenton reaction [92, 157]. $\cdot$OH is highly reactive with a half-life of less than 1ns in an aqueous solution [133]. Thus when hydroxyl radicals are produced with in the system, they react with the biomolecules that are close to their site of formation. DNA strand breaks are produced if ·OH free radicals are generated in their vicinity as the ·OH free radicals attack the bases and deoxyribosyl backbone of DNA.

Peroxyl radicals (ROO·) are the characteristic additional radicals formed from oxygen in living systems. They are high energy free radical species. The most important property of peroxyl radicals is their ability to participate in diverse biological reactions. Peroxyl radicals are found to attack lipid molecules leading to lipid peroxidation which is frequently associated with the pathophysiology of human diseases [17, 47]. Peroxyl radicals can also cause harm to DNA, protein molecules and are also implicated in the enhancement of DNA damage by superoxide.

Nitric oxide (NO·) is a small molecule containing an unpaired electron in its orbital and is also an abundant reactive species that act as an oxidative biological signaling molecule in different physiological processes like neurotransmission, immune defense mechanisms, regulation of blood pressure, and relaxation of smooth muscles [2, 37]. When the generation of RNS in living cells exceeds the neutralizing ability of the system, nitrosative stress may occur leading to harmful effects.

10.5.2 OXIDATIVE DAMAGE TO BIOMOLECULES

ROS can cause considerable damage to DNA. It can produce modifications in purine, pyramidine, or deoxyribose, cause strand breaks and cross-links in DNA. These assaults may lead to inhibition or induction of transcription, induction of signal transduction, replication errors, and thus genomic instability, all of which contribute to carcinogenesis [24, 105]. DNA damage can be induced not only by ROS but also by RNS [15]. Peroxynitrites react with guanine to form 8-nitroguanine and because of its structure, it can induce G: C to T: A transversions. ROS are also known to attack other biomolecules like proteins and lipids. 8-OH-G lesions are the extensively studied DNA lesion produced by ROS. These easily formed lesions are highly mutagenic and hence considered as the important biomarker of carcinogenesis [169].

Lipid peroxidation is a process that includes steps like initiation, propagation, and termination. Endoperoxides are the precursors of malondialdehyde (MDA) and are formed through the cyclisation reaction of Peroxyl radicals (ROO·). MDA is the end product of peroxidation and is carcinogenic to human beings. MDA can react with DNA bases guanine (G), adenine (A), and cytosine (C) to form adducts M_1G, M_1A, and M_1C, respectively [106].

Amino acid side chain residues of all proteins are highly susceptible to the action of ROS and RNS [155]. The polypeptide backbone of protein is transformed into carbon-centered radical by the action of hydroxyl free radicals. Under aerobic conditions, peroxyl radicals are formed by the reaction of carbon-centered radical with dioxygen [156]. The peroxyl radicals are then converted to alkyl peroxides by protonated superoxide (HO_2). Cysteine and methionine residues are found to be highly sensitive to ROS oxidation [93]. Oxidation of protein by free radicals has the close association with the process of aging and also with the development of age-related diseases [154].

10.5.3   *ANTIOXIDANT DEFENSE MECHANISMS IN CARCINOGENESIS*

Maintenance of a particular electron concentration in different cellular constituents is a characteristic property of each cell. The fluctuation of this redox state of a cell determines cellular differentiation [33, 119]. Usually this redox balance is impaired in cancer cells due to oncogenic stimulation. The damaging effects of ROS and RNS are usually nullified by the activity of nonenzymatic and enzymatic antioxidants. They are involved in the direct removal of pro-oxidants from biological systems and thus are extremely important in protection against free radical-generated damages in cells and tissues. Superoxide dismutase, catalase, and glutathione peroxidase are the most important enzymatic antioxidants [109]. Other compounds like Vitamin C, Vitamin E, carotenoids, thiol antioxidants (glutathione, thioredoxin, and lipoic acid), natural flavonoids, and melatonin are examples of nonenzymatic antioxidants [111]. Altered levels of enzymatic and nonenzymatic antioxidants and the resulting changes in the related pathways are evident in various human malignancies [112].

10.6   ASSOCIATION BETWEEN INFLAMMATION AND NEOPLASIA

The process of inflammation can be acute or chronic. Acute inflammation lasts only for few days and is considered to be a natural defense mechanism, beneficial to the host. Acute inflammation usually clears the pathogenic agents through activation of the humoral and cell-mediated immune system. On clearance of pathogenic stimulation, the immune cells return to their inert state. In contrast, chronic inflammation lasts for a long time, extending to weeks, months, or even indefinite with persisting inflammatory stimulus. The prolonged inflammation as an attempt to heal and repair the tissue damage produced, inevitably causes harm to host tissue. The magnitude of the struggle between the causative agent and innate and adaptive immune mechanisms of the host determines the nature and duration of chronic inflammation [6].

The inter-relationship between the inflammatory process and cancer is multifaceted. It is dependent on various factors including type and site of origin of the tumor and other components in the microenvironment of the tumor. In many cancers, an intimate association of inflammation with initiation and progression of tumors is found. However, it is advocated that inflammatory responses at tumor sites are actually the earlier attempts of the host to suppress the arising tumor. The failure in defense mechanisms of host gradually leads to uncontrolled chronic inflammatory responses in which the inflammatory mediators turn into the "enemies within" [9].

Chronic inflammation related to malignancy may be the result of normal protective mechanisms against pathogens. It may also be induced by conditions such as exposure to agents like asbestos fibers or due to consumption of alcohol and also may result directly from infection of the host cells [25, 141, 163]. The microenvironment of tumor usually consists of resident tissue cells, such as fibroblasts, endothelial cells, and also the host leukocytes that have infiltrated the tumor. The host leukocytes mainly consist of the macrophages that are ample in many tumors, as well as other cells like neutrophils, lymphocytes, dendritic cells, natural killer (NK) cells, and eosinophils [131, 170]. As the inflammatory process progresses, there will be a considerable rise in the amount of released proinflammatory mediators of different types, including cytokines, chemokines, prostaglandins, and reactive oxygen/nitrogen species. These events are supposed to be self-limiting, however, at times the control over inflammatory process is lost which will eventually lead to neoplasia [9]. Acceleration of neoplastic process by chronic inflammation was clearly observed in many malignant diseases. Inflammation due to *Helicobacter pylori* infection is closely associated with gastrointestinal carcinoma, Schistosomiasis with bladder carcinoma, HBV with hepatocellular carcinoma, alcohol abuse with pancreatic cancer, asbestos, smoking, and silica with lung carcinoma [88, 102, 126].

Many of the mediators, which are released in deregulated chronic inflammation, have been found to promote cell growth, invasion, mutagenesis, and angiogenesis which in turn supported the initiation and transformation of cancer. In addition, many of the factors released by inflammatory cells that are excessively present at the inflammatory milieu induce direct as well as indirect suppression of immune responses that would have effectively eliminated the evolving tumor [5, 14, 91, 186]. As such, chronic inflammation increases the risk of cancer in inflamed tissues and has a significant association with cancer development.

10.7   APOPTOSIS AND CANCER

Regulation of cell number plays a crucial role in the development and structural integrity maintenance of organs as well as in sustaining homeostasis. The fundamental feature of this regulation is maintaining a balance between proliferation and death of cells. Programmed cell death which is also known as apoptosis is a phenomenon of loss of cells that is dependent on protein synthesis both pre-existing and de novo [161, 180]. Apoptosis has a key role in development, metamorphosis, and also in disease development [64]. In mammalian cells apoptosis can be triggered in response to endogenous stimuli (such as growth factor deprivation) as well as to exogenous stimuli such as UV and γ-irradiation or other DNA damaging agents (chemotherapeutic drugs). Apoptosis can also be induced in response to inadequate cell-matrix interactions and is called *anoikis* [39].

The tumor suppressor genes like p53, PTEN, and oncogenes like AKT, Bcl-2 have direct involvement in the mechanism of apoptosis which is a clear indication for the requirement of tight regulation of this cellular process. Apoptosis regulation occurring in mammalian cells is considered to be complex and involves a variety of molecules including both antiapoptotic proteins such as Bcl-2 and Bcl-X_L and proapoptotic proteins such as Apaf-1 and caspases [46, 55]. In the early stages of apoptosis, mitochondria are known to possess significant role by liberating factors such as cytochrome *c* and apoptosis inducing factors which trigger apoptotic pathways [48].

Diseases like cancer, neurodegenerative, and autoimmune diseases usually arise from deregulation of cellular pathways which results in either weakening or boosting of apoptosis [65]. In the multistep tumorigenesis, acquired mutations result in deregulation of fundamental cellular pathways including cell cycle, apoptosis, and repair of DNA damage [51]. Loss of expression of the proapoptotic genes *caspase-8* or *Apaf-1* and over expression of the antiapoptotic *Bcl-2* gene are among the defects of apoptosis associated with human cancers. The loss of caspase-8 expression has been found frequently in neuroblastomas and is associated with amplification of the oncogene N-myc [160]. In human melanomas, Apaf-1 expression is normally silenced [152]. In contrast, Bcl-2 is overexpressed in various types of tumors including human follicular B-cell lymphomas [120].

Research focused on apoptosis is gaining much importance nowadays as it plays a very important role in the clinical management of human cancers. Selective triggering of apoptosis in cancerous cells could be an excellent way of disease control. Apoptosis in cancer cells is triggered through induction of proapoptotic molecules, activation of antiapoptotic proteins, or restoration of function of tumor suppressor genes. Death receptors on the malignant cells have been considered as probable targets for cancer therapy [36]. Also, activation of mitochondria plays a vital role in apoptosis [162], so manipulation of mitochondria activation to proapoptotic initiation is a possible therapeutic strategy.

10.8 THE PHARMACOLOGICAL POTENTIAL OF MUSHROOMS

Mushrooms are considered as the major source of novel pharmacological agents but yet mostly unexplored resource [172]. According to Chang and Miles, mushrooms are macrofungus with a unique fruiting body that can grow either above the soil (hypogeous) or below the soil (epigeous). The fruiting bodies are large enough, easily visible to the naked eyes, and can be picked by hands [18]. Mushrooms mainly belong to the taxonomic groups including basidiomycetes and ascomycetes. In latin, mushrooms are known as "Macromycetes" which means fungi that are visible with the naked eye [118]. It is estimated that there are around 140,000 mushroom species on earth and only 10% are known yet. It is assumed that 5% of useful mushrooms are still among the undiscovered and unexamined mushrooms, which implies that around 7000 yet undiscovered species are likely to benefit to mankind [53].

Fungi have been used in medicine since 3000 BC and after the discovery of Penicillin in 1929, they were recognized as a rich source of bioactive and antibiotic compounds of natural origin. The use of fungal metabolites to cure human ailments was widely established thereafter, especially in traditional oriental therapies. In China, Japan, Korea, and Slav regions, mushrooms like *Ganoderma lucidum, L. edodes, Fomes fomentarius, Fomitopsis officinalis*, and many others have been used for several years to treat various illnesses [172]. Several bioactive primary and secondary metabolites with therapeutic properties have been separated from macrofungi which include PLs, proteoglycans, glycoproteins, proteins, fatty acids, terpenoids, lectins, etc (Table 10.4). The major immunomodulating and antitumor effects have been associated with PLs, glycopeptide/protein complexes, proteoglycans, proteins, and triterpenoids [118].

TABLE 10.4 The Different Groups of Bioactive Compounds Isolated from Mushrooms

Main Compound Group	Example	Medical Potentiality
Polysaccharides	Grifolan, Lentinan, Schizophyllan	Immunomodulator, antitumor, antiviral, antimicrobial
Polysaccharide-peptide	PSP, PSK	Antitumor, antiviral, antimicrobial, cytotoxic
Proteins	Fips, Ganoderic acids, Ganoderiol, Ganoderenic acids, Lucidenic acids	Immunomodulator, Anti-HIV activity, antitumor, cytotoxic
Terpenoids	Ganolucidic acids, Lucidumols, Ganoderols, Applanoxidic acids	Histamine release inhibition, antihypertension, anti-inflammatory
Steroids	Polyoxygenated derivatives of ergosterol	Cytotoxic, antitumor, antibacterial
Fatty acids	Linoleic acid, palmitic acid, 11-Octadecanoic acid	Antimutagenic, antibacterial
Organic germanium	Bis-β-carboxyethyl germanium sesquioxide	Antitumor, immunomodulating
Nucleotides	Adenosine	Platelet aggregate inhibition
Polyacetylenic compounds	Biformyne, Agrocybin, Nemotinic acid, Marasmin, Quadrifidins	As antibiotic

Many traditionally used mushrooms are reported to have promising pharmacological effects [128] which include the species like *Auricularia, Flammulina, Ganoderma, Grifola, Lentinus, Pleurotus, Trametes, Schizophyllum, Tremella* [172], and *Phellinus* [23, 71]. Metabolites derived from mushrooms need not have to go through phases I, II, and III clinical trials like other conventional medicines as they are safe in short- and long-term use with no adverse effects. Mushroom parts like fruiting bodies, mycelia, and also mycelial culture broth can be used for the isolation of active principles [26]. Around 651 species of basidiomycete mushrooms contain antitumor or immunomodulating metabolites [172]. A lot of scientific investigations have been performed to discover possible functional properties of mushroom metabolites and found to be useful in the treatment of diseases like allergic asthma [96, 97, 99], food allergy [60], atopic dermatitis [87], inflammation [67, 72, 77], rheumatoid arthritis [73], atherosclerosis [11, 181], thrombosis [184], hyperglycemia [44], HIV infection [123, 124], listeriosis [84], tuberculosis [104], septic shock [74], and cancer [35, 43, 52, 57, 70, 89, 103, 121, 146]. Various *Phellinus* mushrooms like *P. igniarius, P. hartigii, P. gilvus, P. pini,* etc., have shown medicinal properties such as anticancer and immuno-stimulating activities [3, 68, 75, 136, 145, 149]. *Phellinus baummi* extracts are reported to possess high antioxidant and free radical scavenging activity [148]. PLs isolated from *Phellinus gilvus* significantly inhibited benzo(a) pyrene-induced forestomach carcinogenesis in mice by down-regulating mutant p53 expression [4]. *P. linteus* is a well-known species for its potent antitumor effect and other medicinal values. A novel protein bound PL from *Phellinus rimosus* (Berk) Pilat exhibited significant antioxidant, anti-inflammatory, and antiarthritic activity in in vitro and animal systems [15, 16]. Prominent antioxidant and antitumor activities are found to be possessed by aqueous extracts of mushrooms like *Lentinula edodes* and *Pleurotus sajor-caju* [34].

10.9 MUSHROOM DERIVED PLS IN CANCER TREATMENT

Biologic response modifiers (BRM) are the compounds that can interact with the immune system and promote the humoral and cell-mediated immune response of the host. They are also known as immunomodulators or immunopotentiators. Ability of different compounds to enhance or suppress immune responses can be influenced by various factors including the dose of drug, route of administration as well as the timing of administration. The type of activity can also depend on their mechanism of action or the site of activity [172]. These compounds influence different cells of hematopoietic system and thus enhance innate and adaptive immune systems, cytokine networks, and signaling pathways. Many immunomodulators have been isolated from mushrooms and the most potent ones are PLs and protein-bound PLs. These immunomodulators are also effective as anti-infective and antitumor agents [118].

Immunomodulatory PLs are widespread among higher basidiomycetes with unique structures in each species. Moreover, PLs with different properties are produced by different strains of the same Basidiomycetes species [172]. Mushroom PLs have been reported to be efficient in eliminating esophageal, stomach, prostrate, and lung carcinomas. Antitumor effect of higher basidiomycete like *Boletus edulis* was demonstrated by Lucas et al. [101]. Isolated compounds from the mushroom *Lampteromyces japonicus* (kowamura) Sing were found to be effective against Ehrlich carcinoma of the mouse [182]. More than 7000 cultures of higher basidiomycetes have been experimented on for antitumor activity against rodent tumor systems and promising results were obtained against sarcoma 180, mammary adenocarcinoma 755, and leukemia L-1210 [45]. Remarkable antitumor activity against induced cancers in animals such as sarcoma 180 by essence obtained from the fruiting body of edible mushrooms was reported by Ikekawa et al. [63]. The edible mushroom *Pleurotus Ostreatus,* cultivated on date waste also possessed potent antitumor activity against Ehrlich ascites carcinoma (EAC) [29, 30]. Further research carried out by the authors was on the biochemical analysis of essence isolated from the mushrooms which produced significant growth inhibition on the tumors transplanted in mice. The antitumor essence was later identified to be a type of β-D-glucan, which is a PL yielding D-glucose only by acid hydrolysis [117]. Chen et al. [19] reported the growth inhibitory effect of *Pleurotus citrinopileatus* against U937 leukemia cells. The active principle involved in the process was found to be a glycoprotein. Most of the mushroom PLs are glucans, linked by β-(1–3), (1–6) glycosidic bonds, and α-(1–3) glycosidic bonds but many are true heteroglycans. Above 50 mushroom species have been investigated for potential immunoceuticals and found to have anticancer activity in in vitro and in vivo models. Six of these PLs that have shown efficacy against human malignancies are Lentinan, Schizophyllan, Active hexose correlated compounds, Maitake D-fraction, PL-K (PSK), and PL-P (PSP) (Table 10.5) [28, 122].

TABLE 10.5 Some Antitumor Polysaccharides Isolated from Macrofungi

Compound	Origin	Molecular Structure
Lentinan	*Lentinus edodes*	1,6-Monoglucosylbranched 1,3-β-D-glucan
Schizophyllan	*Schizophyllum commune*	1,6-Monoglucosylbranched 1,3-β-D-glucan
AHCC	A proprietary extract from several species of basidiomycete mushrooms, including *Lentinus edodes*	1,3-α-D-glucan
Maitake D-fraction	*Grifola frondosa*	1,6-Monoglucosylbranched 1,3-β-D-glucan
PSK	*Coriolus versicolor*	1,3 and 1,6-monoglucosylbranched 1,4-β-D-glucan with binding to aspartic, glutamic and other acidic amino acids
PSP	*Coriolus versicolor*	Resemble to PSK structure but is riched in glutamic and aspartic acids

10.9.1 LENTINAN FROM L. EDODES

Lentinan is an antitumor PL isolated from the fruiting bodies of *L. edodes*, commonly known as the Shiitake mushroom. This mushroom is widely consumed as a nutritional health food throughout the world, particularly in Asia, and is known to have very strong host-mediated anticancer activity via activation of the human immune system [191]. Lentinan is a β- (1→3)-D-glucan having two β-(1→6)-D-glucopyranoside branches for every five β-(1→3)-D-glucopyranoside linear linkages, with a moderate molecular weight of $5–15×10^5$ Da [188, 189]. The molecular weight and a triple-helical conformation play key role in the immune-stimulating activity of lentinan [12]. The anticancer activity of lentinan was decreased considerably when confirmation of the molecule changed from triple-helical structure to a single-flexible chain, indicating strong correlation between the biological properties with structure and molecular weight of lentinan [158]. The first anticancer study of lentinan was against Sarcoma 180 cell line as reported by Chihara et al. [21, 22]. Lentinan has been reported to produce stimulatory effect on cell-mediated immunity and thus inhibited cancer cell development [58, 174]. The immunomodulatory effects of lentinan have been associated with activation of numerous immune cells and elevation of the release of cytokines and messengers, such as NO, and thus promoting the scavenging ability of immune cells [59]. Lentinan-induced cytokine production in immune cells was found to be dose-dependent and could inhibit the expression of caspase-3 in mice with liver cancer which resulted in reduced tumor growth [40]. Clinical studies have confirmed the anticancer effect of lentinan against gastric, ovarian, or colorectal carcinoma and also have shown to prolong the life span of cancer patients [13, 41].

10.9.2 SCHIZOPHYLLAN FROM S. COMMUNE

Schizophyllan (Sizofiran or SPG) produced by the mushroom *S. commune* is another extensively studied mushroom-derived PL with immunomodulatory activity. This compound is widely used in the management of cancer in several Asian countries [42, 172]. The molecular weight of Schizophyllan is ~450,000 Da and by structure it is β-(1→3)-D-glucan with β-(1→6)-D-glucopyranoside side branches at every three repeating units [183]. Composition and antitumor activity of schizophyllan is similar to lentinan [66]. Schizophyllan has shown promising antitumor activity against several carcinomas and sarcoma cell lines [172] and has been used for anticancer immunotherapy of stage II/III cervical cancers in combination with radiotherapy [42, 147]. Also, clinical evaluation of schizophyllan as an immunosupportive agent has shown increased recovery rate in patients with head and neck cancers [78].

10.9.3 MAITAKE D-FRACTION FROM G. FRONDOSA

G. frondosa (Maitake) is a mushroom widely consumed as food in Japan for many years and well-known for its medicinal properties [117]. Maitake D-fraction is a mixed β-D-glucan fraction prepared from *G. frondosa* fruiting bodies and contains mainly β-D-glucan with β-(1→6) main chains and β-(1→4) branches and the more common β- (1→3) main chains and β-(1→6) branches [110]. Maitake- D-Fraction was also found to enhance immune system and induce apoptosis in cancer cells [82, 83, 85, 108]. Maitake D-fraction has been shown to induce programmed cell death or apoptosis in breast cancer cell lines by upregulation of BAK-1 gene activation and with the involvement of cytochrome C [151]. Phase II clinical trials of Maitake D fraction on patients with advanced stage of breast and prostate carcinomas were done in 1998 with the permission of Food and Drug Administration [85]. Maitake fraction is shown to improve the efficacy of chemotherapy by reducing the immunosuppressive effect of chemotherapeutic drugs and thus reduce possible side effects of conventional cancer treatment [83].

10.9.4   KRESTIN FROM T. VERSICOLOR

Krestin produced by the mushroom *T. versicolor* is a polysaccharopeptide (PSP) with D-glucose as the major monosaccharide and α-(1→4) and β- (1→3) glucosidic linkages. Krestin prevents multistep progression of tumor metastasis by inhibiting adhesion and invasion through suppression of cell matrix-degrading enzyme production by malignant cells as evidenced by animal model systems [81]. PSP krestin has been reported as a promising BRM for clinical use of cancer patients in Japan [70], which remarkably prolonged the survival rate and reduced the recurrence of tumors. Randomized trials with krestin as adjuvant immune-chemotherapy in patients with gastric cancer improved the survival of patients [125]. Also, adjuvant treatment with krestin on nonsmall cell lung cancer patients after radical radiotherapy revealed satisfactory tumor shrinkage as compared to the control group [54].

10.9.5   PLS FROM GANODERMA

Genus *Ganoderma* is one of the ancient medicines and particularly the species *G. lucidum* (Reishi or Ling-Zhi) has been a part of traditional medicine in China as a tonic for good health, eternal youth, strength, and longevity. Intensive research has been carried out on this particular mushroom species in recent years because of its powerful antitumor and immune-stimulating properties [98, 142]. The PLs isolated from its fruiting bodies contain (1→3)/β- (1→6)-D-glucans [61]. *Ganoderma* PLs are found to enhance the cytotoxic activity of NK cells, also increased the tumor necrosis factor-α (TNF-α) and interferon-γ release from macrophages and lymphocytes, respectively [86]. PLs from *G. lucidum* have also shown to prevent cancer invasion and metastasis through the modulation of kinase signaling and subsequent activator protein-1 and NF-κB supression [179].

10.9.6   PLS FROM PHELLINUS

Ikekawa et al. [63] first reported the antitumor activity of the PLs isolated from *Phellinus linteus* mushroom fruiting body. Many research studies on the pharmacological property of this particular mushroom PL have been documented thereafter by several researchers [23, 69, 90]. *P. linteus* PL produced significant hypoglycemic effect in streptozotocin-induced diabetic rats. It could also decrease total cholesterol and triacylglycerol levels and aspartate aminotransferase activity [71]. Extract of *P. linteus* activated catalase activity by regulating its expression at the translational/transcriptional level [132]. PL produced an inhibition of 96.7% in Sarcoma 180 transplanted immuno competent ICR mice and found to be the most potent antitumor agent among all other PLs isolated from Basidiomycetes [153]. The PL isolated from the mycelial culture of *P. linteus* stimulated both humoral and cell-mediated immunity. Compared to all other PLs isolated from Basidiomycetes, PL was found to have a wider range of immunopotentiation and antitumor activity [76]. PL is also suggested as a suitable agent for immunochemotherapy of cancer because of its ability to prevent tumor growth and metastasis through immunostimulation without inducing any toxic effect on the host system [50]. A novel PL-protein complex (PPC-*Pr*) isolated from the wood-rotting mushroom *P. rimosus* inhibited growth of Dalton's lymphoma ascites and EAC murine cancer cell lines in vivo [113]. PPC-*Pr* was able to significantly inhibit the growth of HCT116 colon cancer cell line in a time and concentration-dependent manner [114].

10.10 MODE OF ACTION OF Β-GLUCANS OF MUSHROOMS

The mode of action of β-D-glucans is different from conventional chemotherapeutic agents. They prevent tumor growth via activation of host immune system. Lentinan, a pure β-D-glucan could affect and stimulate the key immune mechanisms of the host to mediate the destruction of tumor cells. Such immunomodulating mechanisms are also shown by protein linked of β-D-glucans. There are also other pathways and mechanisms through which mushrooms prevent tumor cell growth. It has been proved that different components of mushrooms have different modes of action. The assumed mechanisms of action include detoxification of carcinogens, enhancement of Phase II enzymes, inhibition of organ exposure to carcinogens, reduced activity of Phase I enzymes, prevention of toxic metabolite, and adduct formation with macromolecules. Free radical scavenging and antioxidant activities, anti-inflammation, induction of differentiation, direct cytotoxicity, induction of cell cycle arrest, antiproliferation and modulation of signaling transduction molecules, antiprogression, and tumor growth inhibition, anti-metastasis and antiangiogenesis, are also other modes of action [173].

According to literature, the mechanism behind antitumor action of *Phellinus* mushroom can be different. PL from *P. linteus* is found to stimulate the production of costimulatory molecules in B cells by regulating protein tyrosine kinase and protein kinase C signaling pathways [74]. Another study says that the tumoricidal activity of peritoneal macrophages (PM) cultured with PL was enhanced against B16 melanoma cells. This study concluded that PL act as an effective immunomodulator and enhances the antitumoal activity of PM through the up-regulation of NO and TNF-α [77]. Extract of *P. linteus* is reported to prevent cancer by inducing NAD (P)H: quinine oxidoreductase and glutathione S-transferase activities and can also prevent mutation [149]. Direct cytotoxicity against cancer cells was also exhibited by PL [94]. A study says that PL inhibited cellular proliferation of SW480 human colon cancer cells by induction of apoptosis and G_2/M phase arrest. The inhibition of HCT116 cell line proliferation by the protein-PL complex of *P. rimosus* was the result of apoptosis induction, as evidenced by the cell morphological analyses of HCT 116 cells by DAPI and AO/EB staining methods. The typical DNA fragmentation in the PPC-*Pr* treated cells was obtained in comet assay which further confirmed the apoptotic activity of PPC-*Pr* on HCT116 cells [114].

10.11 CONCLUSIONS

Mushrooms are rich in useful bioactive components and can be used as a resource for the least toxic natural drugs. Mushrooms are repertoire of biological compounds with a wide spectrum of pharmacological activities. Isolation and evaluation of pharmacologically active components from medicinal mushrooms as natural safe drugs for cancer treatment has become a hotspot of research.

In traditional oriental therapies, medicinal mushrooms have been used since ancient history. The knowledge of pharmacological use of mushrooms primarily originated from Far East where decoctions and essences from medicinal mushrooms were used as medicine [58, 172]. Medicinal mushrooms have been used to fight cancer in Korea, China, Japan, Russia, the USA, and Canada for a very long time. According to an old Japanese legend, wild monkeys very rarely experience cancer, high blood pressure, and diabetes. The legend says that these monkeys had the habit of consuming wild mushrooms in abundance. Mushrooms can be considered as immunoceutical agents by their mode of action. Nowadays, there is a considerable increase in diseases involving immune function debilitation, autoimmune diseases, and life-threatening conditions like cancer. Mushrooms are a natural resource of immunopotentiating and anticancer agents. In this scenario, it is vital and desirable to develop natural immunomodulatory and anticancer agents from medicinal mushrooms.

Mushrooms are rich in essential nutrients like proteins, carbohydrates, vitamins and have least fat content. They are cholesterol-free. They have been highly valued as a natural source of bioactive principles and their consumption have potential effect on promotion of human health [31]. Consumption of edible mushrooms or bioactive components of medicinal mushrooms can improve the host immune system, renovate homeostasis and thus increase resistance to diseases. The basic idea in oriental medicine is to rejuvenate the whole body homeostasis of diseased person to bring him back to normal and healthy state.

Several anticancer and immunomodulatory agents have been isolated from mushrooms. PLs, mainly β-D-glucans, PSP, PL–protein complexes, and proteins are the main active principles isolated from mushrooms. Other bioactive components derived from mushrooms like triterpenes, lipids, and phenols are also found to possess significant medicinal properties. Among all these components of mushrooms, PLs are the most powerful and best-known anticancer and immunostimulatory agents. Many of the isolated and purified mushroom PLs are already in a clinical trial in countries like China, Japan, and the USA for several years with no report of any adverse effects [20]. It has been proven that these compounds can be consumed for long periods as part of treatment as they cause no harm effects in the host. More than that mushroom PLs can considerably reduce the side effects of radiotherapy and chemotherapy. Thus medicinal mushrooms can be suitable candidates for safe drug development in cancer.

KEYWORDS

- **mushrooms**
- **polysaccharides**
- **anticancer activity**
- **carcinogens**
- **immunomodulators**

REFERENCES

1. Ames, B.N.; Profet, M.; Gold, L. Dietary pesticides (99.9% all natural). *Proc. Natl. Acad. Sci. USA.* 1990, 87, 7777–7781.
2. Archer, S. Measurement of nitric-oxide in biological models. *FASEB J.* 1993, 7, 349–360.
3. Ayer, W.A.; Muir, D.J.; Chakravarty, P. Phenolic and other metabolites of *Phellinus pini*, a fungus pathogenic to pine. *Phytochemistry.* 1996, 42, 1321–1324.
4. Bae, J.S.; Jang, K.H.; Park, S.C.; Jin, H.K. Inhibitory effects of polysaccharides isolated from *Phellinus gilvus* on benzo(a)pyrene-induced forestomach carcinogenesis in mice. *World J. Gastroenterol.* 2005, 11(4), 577–579.
5. Balkwill, F.; Mantovani, A. Inflammation and cancer: back to Virchow? *Lancet.* 2001, 357, 539.
6. Baniyash, M. Chronic inflammation, immunosuppression and cancer: new insights and outlook. *Sem. Cancer Biol.* 2006, 16, 80–88.
7. Barros, L.; Cruz, T.; Baptista, P.; Estevinho, L.M.; Ferreira, I.C.F.R. Wild and commercial mushrooms as source of nutrients and nutraceuticals. *Food Chem. Toxicol.* 2008, 46, 2742–2747.
8. Beebe, G.W. 1982. Assessment of health risks from exposure to ionizing radiation. In: *Evironmental Epidemiology: Risk Assessment*; Prentice, R.L.; Whittemore, A.S. Eds; Philadelphia, PA: SIAM, 1982; pp. 3–21.
9. Ben-Baruch, A. Inflammation-associated immune suppression in cancer: the roles played by cytokines, chemokines and additional mediators. *Sem. Cancer Biol.* 2006, 16, 38–52.
10. Bertram, J.S. The molecular biology of cancer. *Mol. Aspects Med.* 2001, 21, 167–223.
11. Bobek, P.; Galbavy, S. Hypocholesterolemic and antiatherogenic effect of oyster mushroom (*Pleurotus ostreatus*) in rabbits. *Nahrung.* 1999, 43(5), 339–342.
12. Bohn, J.A.; BeMiller, J.N. β-(1→3)-D-glucan as biological response modifiers: a review of structure–functional activity relationships. *Carbohyd. Polym.* 1995, 28, 3–14.
13. Borchers, A.T.; Stern, J.S.; Hackman, R.M.; Keen, C.L.; Gershwin, M.E. Mushrooms, tumors, and immunity. *Proc. Soc. Exp. Biol. Med.* 1999, 221, 281–293.
14. Brigati, C.; Noonan, D.M.; Albini, A.; Benelli, R. Tumors and inflammatory infiltrates: friends or foes? *Clin. Exp. Metastasis.* 2002, 19, 247.
15. Brown, G.C.; Borutaite, V. Nitric oxide, mitochondria and cell death. *IUBMB Life.* 2001, 52, 189–195.
16. Cadenas, E. Biochemistry of oxygen toxicity. *Ann. Rev. Biochem.* 1989, 58, 79–110.
17. Cadenas, E.; Sies. H. The lag phase. *Free Rad. Res.* 1998, 28, 601–609.
18. Chang, S.T.; Miles, P.G. Mushrooms biology— a new discipline. *Mycologist.* 1992, 6, 64–65.
19. Chen, J.N.; Wang, Y.T.; Wu, J.S.B. A glycoprotein extracted from golden oyster mushroom *Pleurotus citrinopileatus* exhibiting growth inhibitory effect against U937 leukemia cells. *J. Agric. Food Chem.* 2009, 57, 6706–6711.
20. Chihara, G. 1992. Immunopharmacology of Lentinan, a polysaccharide isolated from *Lentinus edodes*: its application as a host defence potentiator. *Int. J. Orient. Med.* 1992, 17, 57–77.
21. Chihara, G.; Hamuro, J.; Maeda, Y.; Arai, Y.; Fukuoka, F. Fractionation and purification of the polysaccharides with marked antitumour activity, especially lentinan, from *Lentinus edodes* (Berk.) Sing, an edible mushroom. *Cancer Res.* 1970, 30, 2776–2781.

22. Chihara, G.; Maeda, Y.; Hamuro, J.; Sasaki, T.; Fukuoka, F. Inhibition of mouse sarcoma 180 by polysaccharides from *Lentinus edodes* (Berk.) Sing. *Nature*. 1969, 222, 687–688.

23. Chung, K.S.; Kim, S.S.; Kim, H.S.; Kim, K.Y.; Han, M.W.; Kim, K.H. Effect of Kp, an anti-tumor protein polysaccharide from mycellial culture of *Phellinus linetus* on the humoral immune response of tumor bearing ICR mice to sheep red blood cells. *Arch. Pharmacol. Res*. 1993, 16, 336–338.

24. Cooke, M.S.; Evans, M.D.; Dizdaroglu, M.; Lunec, J. Oxidative DNA damage: mechanisms, mutation and disease. *FASEB J*. 2003, 17, 1195–1214.

25. Coussens, L.M.; Werb, Z. Inflammation and cancer. *Nature*. 2002, 420, 860.

26. Cristina, L; Harry, J.W.; Huub, F.J.; Savelkoul. Antiinflammatory and immunomodulating properties of fungal metabolites. *Mediat. Inflamm.,* 2005, 2, 63–80.

27. Cullen, M.R.; Cherniack, M.G.; Rosenstock, L. Medical progress: occupational medicine. *New Engl. J. Med.,* 1990, 322, 594–601.

28. Daba, A.S.; Ezeronye, O.U. Anti-cancer effect of polysaccharides isolated from higher basidiomycetes mushrooms. *Afr. J. Biotechnol*. 2003, 2(12), 672–678.

29. Daba, A.S. Biochemical studies of effect of mushrooms and isolated polysaccharides on tumors transplanted in mice. *2nd International Conference of the Federation of African Society of Biochemists and Molecular Biologists August 1998,* Potshfostroom. 1998.

30. Daba, A.S.; Wissa, J.E.; Esmat, A.Y.; Rashad, M.; Fattah, A. Antitumor activity of polysaccharides from *Pleurotus ostreatus* fruiting bodies and mycelia cultivated on date waste media. *Egypt. J. Biochem. Mol. Biol*. 2002, 20(2), 23–40.

31. Dilani, D.De.S.; Sylvie R.; Françoise, F.; Ali, B.; Kevin, D.H. Medicinal mushrooms in supportive cancer therapies: an approach to anti-cancer effects and putative mechanisms of action. *Fungal Divers*. 2012, 55, 1–35

32. Feitelson, M.A. Hepatitis B virus in hepatocarcinogenesis. *J. Cell Physiol*. 1999, 181, 188–202.

33. Filomeni, G.; Rotilio, G.; Ciriolo, M.R. Cell signaling and the glutathione redox system. *Biochem. Pharmacol*. 2002, 64, 1057–1064.

34. Finimundy, T.C.; Gambato, G.; Fontana, R.; Camassola, M.; Salvador, M.; Moura, S.; et al. Aqueous extracts of *Lentinula edodes* and *Pleurotus sajor-caju* exhibit high antioxidant capability and promising *in vitro* antitumor activity. *Nutr. Res*. 2013, 33, 76–84.

35. Fisher, M., Yang, L.X. Anticancer effects and mechanisms of polysaccharide-K (PSK): implications of cancer immunotherapy. *Anticancer Res*. 2002, 22(3), 1737-1754.

36. Fleischer, A.; Ghadiri, A.; Dessauge, F.; Duhamel, M.; Rebollo, M.P.; Alvarez-Franco, F.; Rebollo, A. Modulating apoptosis as a target for effective therapy. *Mol. Immunol*. 2006, 43, 1065–1079.

37. Forstermann, U.; Boissel, J.P.; Kleinert, H. Expressional control of the 'constitutive' isoforms of nitric oxide synthase (NOS I and NOS III). *FASEB J*. 1998, 12, 773–790.

38. Fridovich, I. Biological effects of the superoxide radical. *Arch. Biochem. Biophys*. 1986, 247, 1–11.

39. Frisch, S.M.; Screaton, R.A. Anoikis mechanisms. *Curr. Opin. Cell Biol*. 2001, 13, 555–562.

40. Fu, H.; Guo, W.Y.; Yin, H.; Wang, Z.X.; Li, R.D. Inhibition of *Lentinus edodes* polysaccharides against liver tumour growth. *Int. J. Phys. Sci*. 2011, 6, 116–120.

41. Fujimoto, K.; Tomonaga, M.; Goto, S. A case of recurrent ovarian cancer successfully treated with adoptive immunotherapy and lentinan. *Anticancer Res*. 2006, 26, 4015–4018.

42. Furue, H. Biological characteristics and clinical effect of sizolilan (SPG). *Med. Actual.* 1987, 23, 335–346.

43. Gao, Y.H.; Zhou, S.F. Cancer prevention and treatment by *Ganoderma*, a mushroom with medicinal properties. *Food Rev. Int.* 2003, 19, 275–325.
44. Gray, A.M.; Flatt, P.R.; Insulin-releasing and insulin like activity of *Agaricus campestris* (mushroom). *J. Endocrinol.* 1988, 157(2), 259–266.
45. Gregory, F.J. Studies on antitumor substances produced by Basidomycetes. *Mycologia.* 1966, 58, 80–90.
46. Gross, A.; McDonnell, J.M.; Korsmeyer, S.J. BCL-2 family members and the mitochondria in apoptosis. *Genes Dev.* 1999, 13, 1899–1911.
47. Gutteridge, J.M.C. Lipid-peroxidation and antioxidants as biomarkers of tissue-damage. *Clin. Chem.* 1995, 41, 1819–1828.
48. Hakem, R.; Harrington, L. Cell Death. In: *The Basic Science of Oncology*; 4th ed. Tannock, I.F.; Hill, R.P.; Bristow, R.G.; Harrington, L., Eds; Singapore: McGraw-Hill, 2005, 194–204.
49. Halliwell, B. Antioxidants in human health and disease. *Ann. Rev. Nutr.* 1996, 16, 33–50.
50. Han, S.B.; Lee, C.W.; Jeon, Y.J.; Hong, N.D.; Yoo, I.D.; Yang, K.H., Kim, H.M. The inhibitory effect of polysaccharides isolated from *Phellinus linteus* on tumor growth and metastasis. *Immunopharmacology.* 1999, 41, 157–164.
51. Hanahan, D.; Weinberg, R.A. The hallmarks of cancer. *Cell.* 2000, 100, 57–70.
52. Hattori, T.S.; Komatsu, N.; Shichijo, S.; Itoh, K. Protein-bound polysaccharide K induced apoptosis of the human Burkitt lymphoma cell line, Namalwa. *Biomed. Pharmacother.* 2004, 58(4), 226–230.
53. Hawksworth, D.L. Mushrooms: the extent of the unexplored potential. *Int. J. Med. Mushrooms.* 2001, 3, 333–337.
54. Hayakawa, K.; Mitsuhashi, N.; Saito, Y.; Takahashi, M.; Katano, S.; Shiojima, K.; Furuta, M.; Nibe, H. Effect of Krestin (PSK) as adjuvant treatment on the prognosis after radical radiotherapy in patients with non small cell lung cancer. *Anticancer Res.* 1993, 13, 1815-1820.
55. Hengartner, M.O. The biochemistry of apoptosis. *Nature.* 2000, 407, 770–776.
56. Hildt, E.; Saher, G.; Bruss, V.; et al. The hepatitis B virus large surface protein (LHBs) is a transcriptional activator. *Virology.* 1996, 225, 235–239.
57. Ho, J.C.; Konerding, M.A.; Gaumann, A.; Groth, M.; Liu, W.K. Fungal polysaccharopeptide inhibits tumor angiogenesis and tumor growth in mice. *Life Sci.* 2004, 75(11), 1343–1356.
58. Hobbs, C.; Medicinal value of *Lentinus edodes* (Berk) Sing (Agaricomycetideae). *Int. J. Med. Mush.* 2000, 2(4), 287–302.
59. Hou, X.J.; Chen, W. Optimization of extraction process of crude polysaccharides from wild edible BaChu mushroom by response surface methodology. *Carbohyd. Polym.* 2008, 72, 67-74.
60. Hsieh, K.Y.; Hsu, C.I., Lin, J.Y.; Tsai, C.C., Lin, R.H. Oral administration of an edible-mushroom-derived protein inhibits the development of food-allergic reactions in mice. *Clin. Exp. Allergy.* 2003, 33(11), 1595-1602.
61. Hung, W.T.; Wang, S.H.; Chen, C.H.; Yang, W.B. Structure determination of β-Glucans from *Ganoderma lucidum* with matrixassisted laser desorption/ionization (MALDI) Mass Spectrometry. *Molecules.* 2008, 13, 1538–1550.
62. Hussain, S.P.; Amstad, P.; Raja, K.; et al. Mutability of p53 hotspot codons to benzo[a] pyrene diol epoxide (BPDE) and the frequency of p53 mutations in nontumorous human lung. *Cancer Res.* 2001, 61, 6350–6355.

63. Ikekawa, T.; Nakanishi, M.; Uehara, N.; Chihara, G.; Fukuoka, F. Antitumor action of some Basidiomycetes, especially *Phellinus lintens*. *Gann.* 1968, 59, 155–157.

64. Jacobson, M.D.; Weil, M.; Raff, M.C. Programmed cell death in animal development. *Cell.* 1997, 88, 347–354.

65. Johnstone, R.W.; Ruefli, A.A.; Lowe, S.W. Apoptosis: a link between cancer genetics and chemotherapy. *Cell.* 2002, 108, 153–164.

66. Jong, S.C.; Birmingham, J.M.; Pai, S.H. Immunomodulatory substances of fungal origin. *J. Immun. Immunopharmacol.* 1991, 11, 115–122.

67. Jose, N.; Ajith, T.A.; Janardhanan, K.K. Methanol extractof the oyster mushroom, *Pleurotus florida*, inhibits inflammation and platelet aggregation. *Phytother. Res.* 2004, 18(1), 43–46.

68. Jung, I.C.; Kim, S.H.; Kwon, Y.I.; Kim, S.Y.; Lee, J.S.; Park, S. Cultural condition for the mycelial growth of *Phellinus igniarius* on chemically defined medium and grains. *Korean J. Mycol.* 1997, 25, 133–42.

69. Kang, T.S.; Lee, D.G.; Lee, S.Y. Isolation and mycelial submerged cultivation of *Phellinus* sp. *Korean J. Mycol.* 1997, 25, 257–67.

70. Kidd, P.M. The use of mushroom glucans and proteoglycans in cancer treatment. *Altern. Med. Rev.* 2000, 5(1), 4–27.

71. Kim, D.H.; Yang, B.K.; Jeong, S.C.; Park, J.B.; Cho, S.P.; Das, S. Production of a hypoglycemic, extracellular polysaccharide from the submerged culture of mushroom. *Phellinus linetus. Biotechnol. Lett.* 2001, 23, 513–517.

72. Kim, G.Y.; Choi, G.S.; Lee, S.H.; Park, Y.M. Acidic polysaccharide isolated from *Phellinus linteus* enhances through the up-regulation of nitric oxide and tumor necrosis factor- α from peritoneal macrophages. *J. Ethnopharmacol.* 2004a, 95, 69–76.

73. Kim, G.Y.; Kim, S.H.; Hwang, S.Y. et al. Oral administration of proteoglycan isolated from *Phellinus linteus* in the prevention and treatment of collagen-induced arthritis in mice. *Biol. Pharm. Bull.* 2003a, 26(6), 823–831.

74. Kim, G.Y.; Roh, S.I.; Park, S.K. et al. Alleviation of experimental septic shock in mice by acidic polysaccharide isolated from the medicinal mushroom *Phellinus linteus. Biol. Pharm. Bull.* 2003b, 26(10), 1418–1423.

75. Kim, G.Y.; Park, S.K.; Lee, M.K.; Lee, S.H.; Oh, Y.H.; Kwak, J.Y.; Yoon, S.; Lee, J.D.; Park, Y.M. Proteoglycan isolated from *Phellinus linteus* activated murine B lymphocytes via protein kinase C and protein tyrosine kinase. *Int. Immunopharmacol.* 2003c, 3, 1281–1292.

76. Kim, H.M.; Han, S.B.; Oh, G.T.; Kim, Y.H.; Hong, D.H.; Hong, N.D.; Yoo, I.D. Stimulation of humoral and cell mediated immunity by polysaccharide from mushroom *Phellinus linteus. Int. J. Immunopharmacol.* 1996, 18, 295-303.

77. Kim, S.H.; Song, Y.S.; Kim, S.K.; Kim, B.C.; Lim, C.J.; Park, E.H. Anti-inflammatory and related pharmacological activities of the n-BuOH subfraction of mushroom *Phellinus linteus. J. Ethnopharmacol.* 2004a, 93(1), 141–146.

78. Kimura, Y.; Tojima, H.; Fukase, S. Clinical evaluation of sizofilan as assistant immunotherapy in treatment of head and neck cancer. *Acta Otolaryngol.* 1994, 511, 192–195.

79. Klaunig, J.E.; Kamendulis, L.M. The role of oxidative stress in carcinogenesis. *Ann. Rev. Pharmacol. Toxicol.* 2004, 44, 239–267.

80. Knudson, A.G. Two genetic hits (more or less) to cancer. *Nat. Rev. Cancer.* 2001, 1, 157–162.

81. Kobayashi, H.; Matsunaga, K.; Oguchi, Y. Antimetastatic effects of PSK (Krestin), a protein-bound polysaccharide obtained from basidiomycetes: an overview. *Cancer Epidemiol. Biomarkers Prev.* 1995, 4, 275–281.

82. Kodama, N.; Harada, N.; Nanba, H. A polysaccharide, extract from *Grifola frondosa*, induces Th-1 dominant responses in carcinoma-bearing BALB/c mice. *Jpn. J. Pharmacol.* 2002a, 90, 357-360.

83. Kodama, N.; Komuta, K.; Nanba, H. Can Maitake MD-fraction aid cancer patients? *Altern. Med. Rev.* 2002b, 7, 236-239.

84. Kodama, N.; Yamada, M.; Nanba, H. Addition of maitake D-fraction reduces the effective dosage of vancomycin for the treatment of *Listeria*-infected mice. *Jpn. J. Pharmacol.* 2001, 87(4), 327–332.

85. Konno, S. Maitake D-fraction: apoptosis inducer and immune enhancer. *Altern. Complementary Ther.* 2001, 17, 102-107.

86. Kuo, M.C.; Weng, C.Y.; Ha, C.L.; Wu, M.J. *Ganoderma lucidum* mycelia enhance innate immunity by activating NF-κB. *J. Ethnopharmacol.* 2006, 103, 217-222.

87. Kuo, Y.C.; Huang, Y.L.; Chen, C.C.; Lin, Y.S.; Chuang, K.A.; Tsai, W.J. Cell cycle progression and cytokine gene expression of human peripheral blood mononuclear cells modulated by *Agaricus blazei. J. Lab. Clin. Med.* 2002, 140, 176-187.

88. Kuper, H.; Adami, H.O.; Trichopoulos, D. Infections as a major preventable cause of human cancer. *J. Intern. Med.* 2000, 248, 171.

89. Lee, I.S.; Nishikawa, A. *Polyozellus multiplex*, a Korean wild mushroom, as a potent chemopreventive agent against stomach cancer. *Life Sci.* 2003, 73, 3225-3234.

90. Lee, J.H.; Cho, S.M.; Kim, H.M.; Hong, N.D.; Yoo, I.D. Immunostimulating activity of polysaccharides from mycelia of *Phellinus linteus* grown under different culture conditions. *J. Microbiol. Biotechnol.* 1996, 6, 52-55.

91. Leek, R.D.; Harris, A.L. Tumor associated macrophages in breast cancer. *J. Mammary Gland Biol. Neoplasia.* 2002, 7, 177.

92. Leonard, S.S.; Harris, G.K.; Shi, X.L. Metal-induced oxidative stress and signal transduction. *Free Rad. Biol. Med.* 2004, 37, 1921–1942.

93. Levine, R.L.; Mosoni, L.; Berlett, B.S.; Stadtman, E.R. Methionine residues as endogenous antioxidants in proteins. *Proc. Natl. Acad. Sci. USA.* 1996, 93, 15036–15040.

94. Li, G.; Kim, D.H.; Kim, T.D.; Park, B.J.; Park, H.D.; Park, J.T. Protein bound polysaccharide from *Phellinus linteus* induces G2/M phase arrest and apoptosis in SW480 human colon cancer cells. *Cancer Lett.* 2004, 216, 175–181.

95. Li, J.; Yen, C.; Liaw, D. et al. PTEN, a putative protein tyrosine phosphatase gene mutated in human brain, breast and prostate cancer. *Science,* 1997, 275, 1943–1947.

96. Li, X.M.; Huang, C.K.; Zhang, T.F.; et al. The Chinese herbal medicine formula MSSM-002 suppresses allergic airway hyperreactivity and modulates TH1/TH2 responses in a murine model of allergic asthma. *J. Allergy Clin. Immunol.* 2000, 106(4), 660–668.

97. Liu, Y.H.; Kao, M.C.; Lai, Y.L.; Tsai, J.J. Efficacy of local nasal immunotherapy or Dp2-induced airway inflammation in mice: using Dp2 peptide and fungal immunomodulatory peptide. *J. Allergy Clin. Immunol.* 2003a, 112(2), 301–310.

98. Liu, Y.W.; Gao, J.L.; Guan, J.; Qian, Z.M.; Feng, K.; Li, S.P. Evaluation of antiproliferative activities and action mechanisms of extracts from two species of Ganoderma on tumor cell lines. *J. Agric. Food Chem.* 2009, 57, 3087-3093.

99. Liu, Y.H.; Tsai, C.F.; Kao, M.C.; Lai, Y.L.; Tsai, J.J. Effectiveness of Dp2 nasal therapy for Dp2-induced airway inflammation in mice: using oral *Ganoderma lucidum* as an immunomodulator. *J. Microbiol. Immunol. Infect.* 2003b, 36(4), 236–242.

100. Loft, S.; Poulsen, H.E. Cancer risk and oxidative DNA damage in man. *J. Mol. Med.* 1996, 74, 297–312.

101. Lucas, E.H.; Montesano, R.; Pepper, M.S.; Hafner, M.; Sablon, E. Tumor inhibitors in *Boletus edulis* and other holobasidiomycetes. *Antibiot. Chemother.* 1957, 7, 1–4.

102. Lucia, M.S.; Torkko, K.C. Inflammation as a target for prostate cancer chemoprevention: pathological and laboratory rationale. *J. Urol.* 2004, 171, S30–S35.

103. Mahajan, R.G.; Patil, S.I.; Mohan, D.R.; Shastry, P. *Pleurotus eous* mushroom lectin (PEL) with mixed carbohydrate inhibition and antiproliferative activity on tumor cell lines. *J. Biochem. Mol. Biol. Biophys.* 2002, 6(5), 341–345.

104. Markova, N.; Kussovski, V.; Drandarska, I.; Nikolaeva, S.; Georgieva, N.; Radoucheva T. Protective activity of lentinan in experimental tuberculosis. *Int. Immunopharmacol.* 2003, 3(10–11), 1557–1562.

105. Marnett, L.J. Oxyradicals and DNA damage. *Carcinogenesis.* 2000, 21, 361–370.

106. Marnett, L.J. Lipid peroxidation–DNA damage by malondialdehyde. *Mut. Res.-Fund. Mol. Mech. Mutagen.* 1999, 424, 83–95.

107. Martell, A.E. Chemistry of carcinogenic metals. *Environ. Health Prospect.* 1981, 40, 207.

108. Masuda, Y.; Ito, K.; Konishi, M.; Nanba, H. A polysaccharide extracted from *Grifola frondosa* enhances the anti-tumor activity of bone marrow-derived dendritic cell-based immunotherapy against murine colon cancer. *Cancer Immunol. Immun.* 2010, 59, 1531–1541.

109. Mates, J.M.; Perez-Gomez, C.; De Castro, I.N. Antioxidant enzymes and human diseases. *Clin. Biochem.* 1999, 32, 595–603.

110. Matsui, K.; Kodama, N.; Nanba, H. Effects of maitake (*Grifola frondosa*) D-fraction on the carcinoma angiogenesis. *Cancer Lett.* 2001, 172, 193–198.

111. McCall, M.R.; Frei, B. Can antioxidant vitamins materially reduce oxidative damage in human? *Free Rad. Biol. Med.* 1999, 26, 1034–1053.

112. McEligot, A.J.; Yang, S.; Meyskens, F.L. Redox regulation by intrinsic species and extrinsic nutrients in normal and cancer cells. *Ann. Rev. Nutr.* 2005, 25, 261–295.

113. Meera, C.R.; Janardhanan, K.K. Antitumor activity of a polysaccharide-protein complex isolated from a wood-rotting polypore macrofungus *Phellinus rimosus* (Berk) Pilat. *J. Environ. Pathol. Toxicol. Oncol.* 2012, 31(3), 223–232.

114. Meera, C.R.; Janardhanan, K.K.; Karunagaran, D. Anti-proliferative and apoptotic activities of the medicinal mushroom *Phellinus rimosus* (Berk) Pilat on HCT 116 human colon cancer cells. *Int. J. Med. Mushrooms.* 2018, 20(10), 935–945.

115. Meera, C.R.; Janardhanan, K.K.; Nitha, B.; Viswakarma, R.A. Anti-inflammatory and free radical scavenging activities of polysaccharide-protein complex isolated from *Phellinusrimosus* (Berk) Pilat. *Int. J. Med. Mushrooms.* 2009a, 11, 365–373.

116. Meera, C.R.; Smina, T.P.; Nitha, B.; Mathew J.; Janardhanan, K.K.; Anti-arthritic activity of a polysaccharide-protein complex isolated from *Phellinusrimosus* (Berk) Pilat (Aphyllophoromycetideae), in Freund's complete adjuvant induced arthritic rats. *Int. J. Med. Mushrooms.* 2009b, 11, 21–28.

117. Mizuno, T. The extraction and development of antitumor active polysaccharides from medicinal mushrooms in Japan (Review). *Int. J. Med. Mushrooms.* 1999, 1, 9–29.

118. Moradali, M.F.; Mostafavi, H.; Ghods, S.; Hedjaroude, G.A. Immunomodulating and anti-cancer agents in the realm of macromycetes fungi (macrofungi). *Int. Immunopharmacol.* 2007, 7, 701–724.

119. Moran, L.K.; Guteridge, J.M.C.; Quinlan, G.J. Thiols in cellular redox signaling and control. *Curr. Med. Chem.* 2001, 8, 763–772.

120. Mullauer, L.; Gruber, P.; Sebinger, D. Mutations in apoptosis genes: a pathogenetic factor for human disease. *Mutat. Res.* 2001, 488, 211–231.

121. Nakamura, T.; Matsugo, S.; Uzuka, Y.; Matsuo, S.; Kawagishi, H. Fractionation and anti-tumor activity of the mycelia of liquid-cultured *Phellinus linteus. Biosci. Biotechnol. Biochem.* 2004, 68(4), 868–872.

122. Nanba, H. Results of non-controlled clinical study for various cancer patients using Maitake D-fraction. *Explore.* 1995, 6, 19–21.

123. Nanba, H.; Kodama, N.; Schar, D.; Turner, D. Effects of Maitake (*Grifola frondosa*) glucan in HIV-infected patients. *Mycoscience.* 2000, 41, 293–295.

124. Ngai, P.H.; Ng, T.B. Lentin, a novel and potent antifungal protein from Shiitake mushroom with inhibitory effects on activity of human immunodeficiency virus-1 reverse transcriptase and proliferation of leukemia cells. *Life Sci.* 2003, 73(26), 3363–3374.

125. Oba, K.; Teramukai, S.; Kobayashi, M.; Matsui, T.; Kodera, Y.; Sakamoto, J. Efficacy of adjuvant immunochemotherapy with polysaccharide K for patients with curative resections of gastric cancer. *Cancer Immunol. Immunother.* 2007, 56, 905–911.

126. Ohshima, H.; Tatemichi, M.; Sawa, T. Chemical basis of inflammation induced carcinogenesis. *Arch. Biochem. Biophys.* 2003, 417, 3.

127. Okey, A.B.; Harper, P.A.; Grant, D.M.; Hill R.P. Chemical and radiation carcinogenesis. In *The Basic Science of Oncology*; 4th ed. Tannock, I.F.; Hill, R.P.; Bristow, R.G.; Harrington, L.; Eds; Singapore: McGraw-Hill, 2005; pp. 25–48.

128. Ooi, V.E.C.; Liu, F. Immunomodulation and anti-cancer activity of polysaccharide-protein complexes. *Curr. Med. Chem..* 2000, 7, 715–729.

129. Oster, S.; Penn, L.; Stambolic, V. 2005. Oncogenes and tumor suppressor genes. In: *The Basic Science of Oncology*; 4th ed. Tannock, I.F.; Hill, R.P.; Bristow R.G.; Harrington L.; Eds; Singapore: McGraw-Hill, 2005; pp. 123–141.

130. Oster, S.K.; Ho, C.S.; Soucie, E.L.; Penn, L.Z. The myco oncogene; Marvelous IY Complex. *Adv. Cancer Res.* 2002, 84, 81–154.

131. Park, C.C.; Bissell, M.J.; Barcellos-Hoff, M.H. The influence of the microenvironment on the malignant phenotype. *Mol. Med. Today.* 2000, 6, 324.

132. Park, J.; Lee, B.R.; Jin, L.H.; Kim, C.K.; Choi, K.S.; Bahn, J.H.; Lee, K.S.; Kwon, H.Y.; Chang, H.W.; Baek, N.I.; Lee, E.H.; Kang, J.H.; Cho, S.W.; Choi, S.Y. The stimulatory effect of *Ganoderma lucidum* and *Phellinus linteus* on the antioxidant enzyme catalase. *J. Biochem. Molecul. Biol.* 2001, 34, 144–149.

133. Pastor, N.; Weinstein, H.; Jamison, E.; Brenowitz, M. A detailed interpretation of OH radical footprints in a TBP-DNA complex reveals the role of dynamics in the mechanism of sequence-specific binding. *J. Mol. Biol.* 2000, 304, 55–68.

134. Pitot, H.C. *Fundamentals of Oncology*, 3rd ed. New York, NY: Marcel Dekker, 1986.

135. Quintanilla, M.; Brown, K.; Ramsden, M.; Balmain, A. Carcinogen specific mutation and amplification of Ha-ras during mouse skin carcinogenesis. *Nature.* 1986, 322, 78–80.

136. Rew, Y.H.; Jo, W.S.; Jeong, K.C.; Yoon, J.T.; Choi, B.S. Cultural characteristics and fruit body formation of *Phellinus gilvus. Korean J. Mycol.* 2000, 28, 6–10.

137. Ribeiro, B.; Guedes de Pinho, P.; Andrade, P.B.; Baptista, P.; Valentão, P. Fatty acid composition of wild edible mushrooms species: a comparative study. *Microchem. J.* 2009, 93, 29–35.

138. Richardson, C.D. Viruses and cancer. In: *The Basic Science of Oncology*; 4th ed. Tannock, I.F.; Hill, R.P.; Bristow, R.G.; Harrington, L.; Eds; Singapore: McGraw-Hill, 2005; pp. 100–122.

139. Saffiotti, U. Identifying and defining chemical carcinogens. In: *Origins of Human Cancer;* Hiatt, H.H.; Watson, J.D.; Winsten, J.A. Eds; New York, NY: Cold Spring Harbor, 1977; Books A-C; pp. 1311–1326.

140. Scadden, D.T.; AIDS-related malignancies. *Annu. Rev. Med.* 2003, 54, 285–303.

141. Schwartsburd, P.M. Chronic inflammation as inductor of pro-cancer microenvironment: pathogenesis of dysregulated feedback control. *Cancer Metastasis Rev.* 2003, 22, 95.

142. Shang, D.; Li, Y.; Wang, C. A novel polysaccharide from Se-enriched *Ganoderma lucidum* induces apoptosis of human breast cancer cells. *Oncol Rep.* 2011, 25, 267–272.

143. Shen, H-M.; Ong, C-N. Mutations of the p53 tumor suppressor gene and ras oncogenes in aflatoxin hapatocarcinogenesis. *Mut. Res.* 1996, 366, 23–44.

144. Sherr, C.J. Cancer cell cycles. *Science,* 1996, 274, 1672–1677.

145. Shibata, S.; Nishikawa, Y.; Mei, C.F.; Fukoka, F.; Nakanishi, F. Anti-tumor studies on some extracts of Basidiomycetes. *Gann.* 1968, 59, 159–161.

146. Shibata, Y.; Kurita, S.; Okugi, H.; Yamanaka, H. Dramatic remission of hormone refractory prostate cancer achieved with extract of the mushroom, *Phellinus linteus.* *Urol. Int.* 2004, 73(2), 188–190.

147. Shimizu, Y.; Chen, J.T.; Hirai, Y.; Nakayama, K.; Hamada, T.; Fujimoto, I.; Hasumi, K. Augmentation of immune responses of pelvic lymph node lymphocytes in cervical cancer patients by sizofiran. *Nihon Sanka Fujinka Gakkai Zasshi.* 1989, 41, 2013-2014.

148. Shon, M.Y.; Kin, T.H.; Sung, N.J. Antioxidants and free radical scavenging activity of *Phellinus baummi (Phellinus of Hymenochaetaceae)* extracts. *Food Chem.* 2003, 82, 593–597.

149. Shon, Y.H.; Nam, K.S. Antimutagenicity and induction of anticarcinogenic phase II enzymes by basidiomycetes. *J. Ethnopharmacol.* 2001, 77, 103–109.

150. Smela, M.E.; Currier, S.S.; Bailey, E.A.; Essigmann, J.M. The chemistry and biology of aflatoxin B1: from mutational spectrometry to carcinogenesis. *Carcinogenesis.* 2001, 22, 535–545.

151. Soares, R.; Meireles, M.; Rocha, A.; Pirraco, A.; Obiol, D.; Alonso, E.; Joos, G.; Balogh, G. Maitake (D Fraction) mushroom extract induces apoptosis in breast cancer cells by BAK-1 gene activation source. *J. Med. Food.* 2011, 14, 563-572.

152. Soengas, M.S.; Capodieci, P.; Polsky, D. Inactivation of the apoptosis effector Apaf-1 in malignant melanoma. *Nature.* 2001, 409, 207–211.

153. Song, K.S.; Cho, S.M.; Lee, J.H.; Kim, H.M.; Han, S.B.; Ko, K.S.; et al. B-lymphocyte-stimulating polysaccharide from mushroom *Phellinus linteus*. *Chem. Pharm. Bull.* 1995, 43, 2105–2108.

154. Stadtman, E.R. Protein oxidation in aging and age-related diseases. *Ann. New York Acad. Sci.* 2001, 928, 22–38.

155. Stadtman, E.R. Role of oxidant species in aging. *Curr. Med. Chem.* 2004, 11, 1105–1112.

156. Stadtman, E.R. Protein oxidation and aging. *Science.* 1992, 257, 1220–1224.

157. Stohs, S.J.; Bagchi, D. Oxidative mechanisms in the toxicity of metal-ions. *Free Rad. Biol. Med.* 1995, 18, 321–336.

158. Surenjav, U.; Zhang, L.; Xu, X.; Zhang, X.; Zeng, F. Effects of molecular structure on antitumor activities of β-(1→3)-D-glucans from different *Lentinus edodes*. *Carbohyd. Polym.* 2006, 63, 97–104.

159. Takada, K. Epstein-Barr virus and gastric carcinoma. *Mol. Pathol.* 2000, 53, 255–261.

160. Teitz, T.; Wei, T.; Valentine, M.B. Caspase 8 is deleted or silenced preferentially in childhood neuroblastomas with amplification of MYCN. *Nat. Med.* 2000, 6, 529–535.

161. Thompson, C.B. Apoptosis in the pathogenesis and treatment of disease. *Science.* 1995, 267, 1456.

162. Thornberry, N.A.; Lazebnik, Y. Caspases: enemies within. *Science.* 1998, 281, 1312–1316.

163. Thun, M.J.; Henley, S.J.; Gansler, T. Inflammation and cancer: an epidemiological perspective. *Novartis Found Symp.* 2004, 256, 6.

164. Tolle, D.V.; Fritz, T.E.; Seed, T.M.; et al. Leukemia induction in beagles exposed continuously to ^{60}Co gamma irradiation: Hematology. In: *Experimental Hematology Today*; Baum, S.J.; Ledney, G.D.; Theirfedler, S.; Eds, Basel: S Karger, 1982; pp. 241–249.

165. Truant, R.; Antunovic, J.; Greenblatt, J.; et al. Direct interaction of the hepatitis B virus HBx protein with p53 leads to inhibition by HBx of p53 response element-directed transactivation. *J. Virol.* 1995, 69, 1851–1859.

166. Trueba, G.P.; Sanchez, G.M.; Guilani, A. Oxygen free radical and antioxidant defense mechanism in cancer. *Front. Biosci.* 2004, 9, 2029–2044.

167. Upton, A.C.; Randolph, M.L.; Conklin, J.W. Late effects of fast neutrons and gamma rays in mice as influenced by the dose rate of irradiation: Induction of neoplasia. *Radiat. Res.* 1970, 41, 467–491.

168. Valko, M.; Morris, H.; Cronin, M.T.D. Metals, toxicity and oxidative stress. *Curr. Med. Chem.* 2005, 12, 1161–1208.

169. Valko, M.; Rhodes, C.J.; Moncol, J.; Izakovic, M.; Mazur, M. Free radicals, metals and antioxidants in oxidative stress-induced cancer. *Chemico-Biol. Interact.* 2006, 160, 1–40.

170. Vicari, A.P.; Treilleux, I.; Lebecque, S. Regulation of the trafficking of tumor-infiltrating dentritic cells by chemokines. *Semin. Cancer Biol.* 2004, 14, 161.

171. Wang, X.W.; Forrester, K.; Yeh, H.; et al. Hepatitis B virus X protein inhibits p53 sequence-specific DNA binding, transcriptional activity and association with transcription factor ERCC3. *Proc. Natl. Acad. Sci. USA.* 1994, 91, 2230–2234.

172. Wasser, S.P. Medicinal mushrooms as a source of antitumour and immunomodulating polysaccharides. *Appl. Microbiol. Biotechnol.* 2002, 60, 258–274.

173. Wasser, S.P. Reishi or Ling Zhi (Ganoderma lucidum). *Encyclop. Diet. Suppl.* 2005, 1, 603–622.

174. Wasser, S.P.; Weis A. Medicinal properties of substances occurring in higher basidiomycetes mushrooms: current perspective (review). *Int. J. Med. Mush.* 1999a, 1, 31–62.

175. Wasser, S.P.; Weis, A. Therapeutic effects of substances occurring in higher basidiomycetes mushrooms, a modern perspective (review). *Crit. Rev. Immunol.* 1999b, 19, 65–96.

176. Weinberg, R.A. The retinoblastoma protein and cell cycle control. *Cell.* 1995, 81, 323–330.

177. Weinreb, M.; Day, P.J.; Niggli, F.; et al. The consistent association between Epstein-Barr virus and Hodgkin's disease in children in Kenya. *Blood.* 1996, 87, 3828–3836.

178. Welsch, P.L.; King, M.C. BRCA1 and BRCA2 and the genetics of breast and ovarian cancer. *Hum. Mol. Genet.* 2001, 10, 705–713.

179. Weng, C.J.; Yen, G.C. The in vitro and in vivo experimental evidences disclose the chemopreventive effects of Ganoderma lucidum on cancer invasion and metastasis. *Clin Exp Metastasis.* 2010, 27, 361–369.

180. Williams, G.T.; Smith, C.A. Molecular regulation of apoptosis: genetic controls on cell death. *Cell.* 1993, 74, 777–779.

181. Yamada, T.; Oinuma, T.; Niihashi, M. et al. Effects of *Lentinus edodes* mycelia on dietary-induced atherosclerotic involvement in rabbit aorta. *J. Atheroscler. Thromb.* 2002, 9(3), 149–156.

182. Yohida, T.O. A tumor inhibitor in *Lampteromyces japonica. P.S.E.B.M.* 1962, 3, 676–679.

183. Yoneda, K.; Ueta, E.; Yamamoto, T.; Osaki, T. Immunoregulatory effects of Sizofiran (SPG) on lymphocytes and polymorphonuclear leukocytes. *Clin. Exp. Immunol.* 1991, 86, 229–235.

184. Yoon, S.J.; Yu, M.A.; Pyun, Y.R. et al. The nontoxic mushroom *Auricularia auricula* contains a polysaccharide with anticoagulant activity mediated by antithrombin. *Thromb. Res.* 2003, 112(3), 151–158.

185. Yoshida, M. Expression of the HTLV-1 genome and its association with a unique T-cell malignancy. *Biochem. Biophys. Acta.* 1987, 907, 145–161.

186. Yu, J.L.; Rak, J.W. Host microenvironment in breast cancer development: inflammatory and immune cells in tumor angiogenesis and arteriogenesis. *Breast Cancer Res.* 2003, 5, 83.

187. Yuspa, S.H; Overview of carcinogenesis: past, present and future. *Carcinogenesis.* 2000, 21, 341–344.

188. Zhang, L.; Zhang, X.; Zhou, Q.; Zhang, P.; Zhang, M.; Li, X. Triple helix of β-glucan from *Lentinus edodes* in 0.5 M NaCl aqueous solution characterized by light scattering. *Polym. J.* 2001, 33, 317–321.

189. Zhang, P.; Zhang, L.; Cheng, S. Chemical structure and molecular weight of $(1\rightarrow3)$-α-D-glucan from *Lentinus edodes. Biosci. Biotechnol. Biochem.* 1999, 63, 1197–1202.

190. Zhang, R.; Haag, J.D.; Gould, M.N. Quantitating the frequency of initiation and cH-ras mutation in *in situ* N-methyl-N-nitrosourea-exposed rat mammary gland. *Cell Growth Differ.* 1991, 2, 1–6.

191. Zhang, Y.; Li, S.; Wang, X.; Zhang, L.; Cheung, P.C.K. Advances in lentinan: isolation, structure, chain conformation and bioactivities. *Food Hydrocolloid.* 2011, 25, 196–206

192. zur Hausen, H. Papilloma viruses causing cancer: evasion from host-cell control in early events in carcinogenesis. *J. Natl. Cancer Inst.* 2000, 92, 690–698.

CHAPTER 11

Sthoulya: A Holistic Approach to Obesity Through Ayurveda

M. L. AADITHYA LAKSHMI

Government Ayurveda Medical College, Kottar, Nagercoil, Kanyakumari District, Tamil Nadu, India; E-mail: aaadithyalakshmi1@gmail.com

ABSTRACT

The preventive aspect of Ayurveda emphasizes on the fact that, becoming healthy and being thus is the best decision anyone can make. But in the process, one may slow down when incurred with hurdles in the form of communicable diseases as well as lifestyle diseases like obesity, type-2 diabetes, hypertension, cardiovascular ailments. While the former need social co-operation, the latter needs only self-awareness and adaptation of better lifestyle modifications. Obesity being one of the most commonly faced lifestyle disorder among the world population, is dealt in this chapter. Ayurvedic literature describes the same as "sthoulya" which has it's own set of causative factors, pathogenesis, symptoms, and treatment protocol. Each of these points has been comprehensively mentioned below aided with the citations from long established scriptures like Charaka Samhita, Susruta Samhita, and Ashtanga Hridayam. Obesity may have either primary or secondary origin nevertheless needs physical as well as mental therapy. The subsequently referred role of psyche, rejuvenation and daily routines are tectonic towards improving the quality of life. On the whole, this chapter gives a clearer picture of the ailment along with paving an insight to it's management.

11.1 INTRODUCTION

Ayurveda is known as the science of *Ayu,* that is, life. It depicts the *sama avastha* (balanced state) of three *saririka dosa (bio-humors-vata, pitta,* and *kapha),* the *manasika guna (satwa)* and *dosa (rajas and tamas),* all types of *agni,* seven *dhathus,* three *malas,* and the pleasant state of *atma* (soul), *indriya* (the sensory faculty), and *manas* (mind) as *swastha* (health) [1]. According to *Acharyas* of Ayurveda, health is the best source of virtue, wealth, gratification, and emancipation while diseases are the destroyers of this source, welfare, and life itself [2]. That is why this science has set an aim to provide measures to maintain the health of a healthy person along with bringing a sick one back to his physical and mental well-being. This enhances the holistic approach of this classical system of medicine toward assuring the four dimensions of the health-physical, mental, social, and spiritual well-being of a person.

In the present era, physical and mental lifestyle disorders are common. Lifestyle disorders are ailments primarily based on the day-to-day habits of people and can be considered as the outcome of unhealthy choices made by them. A person develops a lifestyle based on his physical and physiological capacity and shapes a unique behavior and habits, follow a dietary and living pattern based on his childhood, parental genes, friends, and the environment he is surrounded by. But factors like improper food habits, sedentary routine, emotional stress, irregular sleep pattern, addictions like smoking and alcohol, etc., may lead to the development of lifestyle disorders like obesity, depression, hypertension, atherosclerosis, cardiovascular disease, diabetes, chronic obstructive pulmonary disease, chronic liver disease, varicose veins, or different types of carcinoma. Basically, lifestyle disorders can be considered as the result of improper relation of a person with his environment.

Ayurveda suggests several principles and routines to be followed on a daily basis as well as seasonally. *Samhitas* enlist different types of *ahara dravya, dinacarya, rtucarya* to successfully lead a healthy life. Acharyas also emphasize *siddhanta* of *nidana parivarjana* [3].

11.2 LIFESTYLE DISORDERS IN AYURVEDA

Classically, Ayurveda describes three major causes of illness being *kala parinama, pragyaparadha,* and *asatmendriyartha samyoga.* Kala parinama signifies the impact of change of seasons like increasing industrialization and pollution which ultimately lead to the changes in the normal pattern of seasons. Pragyaparadha is entirely responsible for the production of lifestyle disorders. It is defined as the *vibhramsh* (destruction) of *dhi* (intellect), *dhriti* (patience), and *smriti* (memory) [4]. It is the improper actions of body, mind, and speech by which a person does things which he should not do.

The third one is the overuse, less use, or misuse of sense organs that lead to many ailments like mental disorders. The *asamyak yoga* (improper use) of *rasanendriya* (gustatory sense organ) leads to lifestyle disorders which includes nonjudicious use of *shadrasas* (the six tastes—*madhura* (sweet), *amla* (sour), *lavana* (salt), *katu* (pungent), *tikta* (bitter), *kashaya* (astringent)) and following the wrong diet.

Obesity which is one of the leading lifestyle disorders currently can also be considered as the stepping stone to another set of dreadful disorders hidden in a body system. Many chronic noncommunicable diseases like diabetes mellitus, hypertension, varicose veins, and cardiovascular disorders are increasing among the world population for which obesity is traced to be a major risk factor. Obesity is the condition of abnormal and excessive fat accumulation in adipose tissue that leads to an increase in the body mass index. It is correlated with *sthoulya* in Ayurveda. *Sthoulya* is prevalent worldwide in all age groups, especially in urban communities. This is a complex or multifactorial disease as it triggers the above-mentioned diseases along with endocrine abnormalities, obstetric complications, trauma to weight-bearing joints, weakens the immunological resistance to diseases along with posing a mental pressure on the affected person who values the cosmetic physical appearance. Morbidity and mortality rates are higher among obese/*sthoola* people than lean people. As WHO has found obesity as a global epidemic of recent times, it has coined the term "globesity" to highlight the issue.

11.3 OBESITY IN AYURVEDA—STHOULYA

A person in whom the excessive and abnormal increase of *medo dhathu* and *mamsa dhathu* is found resulting in bulkiness and heaviness of the body is called *sthoola*. *Sthoulya* is referred to as "*sthulasya bhava*" being bulky. It has been mentioned under *ashtanindita purusha* (the eight undesirable physical appearances), *kapha pradhanaja vyadhi* (predominantly caused due to vitiated *kapha dosa*), *medopradoshaja* (as *medas* is the mainly affected *dhathu*), *santarpanajanyavyadhi* (caused due to defective anabolism), and as a *bahudosavasta* (multifactorial condition) [5].

The need for proper diagnosis of disease before planning its management is emphasized as per Ayurveda which tells that *rogapareeksha* (observation and study of the disease and its factors) is the primary task of the physician after which he must prescribe the medicines [6]. The conclusive diagnosis and treatment in Ayurveda are possible only after understanding the etiology, prodromal symptoms, symptomatology, the relieving and aggravating factors, and the pathogenesis of disease [7].

11.3.1 NIDANA (ETIOLOGY)

The knowledge of the etiological factor allows the physician to choose the apt treatment protocol and also helps to provide the *pathyaapathya* (the suitable and unsuitable) in *sthoulya*. Generally, the factors may be *ahara-viharaja* (exogenous), *bijadosaja* (endogenous), miscellaneous, or *manasika* (psychogenic).

Exogenous: This includes the imbalance between diet and energy expenditure. The increased intake of *guru* (heavy), *madhura* (sweet), *amla* (sour), *slesmala* (which increase *kapha dosa*), and fatty foods, *adhyashana* (intake of a meal before the previous meal has been completely digested), *avyayama* (physical inactivity), *avyavaya* (sexual abstinence), and *divaswapna* (day-time sleep) [8]. Addictive habits like alcoholism and smoking are also contributive factor.

Endogenous: This involves *bijadosaja sthoulya* (hereditary predisposition) constituting the development of a stout but a weak body. Hormonal imbalance is manifested here which associates the individual to conditions like hypothyroidism, hypogonadism, hypopituitarism, or Cushing's syndrome according to modern science.

Miscellaneous: This includes sthoulya seen in women during postmenopausal age, sedentary occupation, and increased occurrence among higher income group due to increased satiety. It also highlights the effects of certain medications as the reason for *sthoola prakruthi.*

Psychogenic: Acharyas have mentioned *harshanithyatvad* (uninterrupted cheerfulness) and *achinthanat* (absence of mental stress) as one of the reasons causing obesity [9]. But this subsequently ends up in anxiety, depression, depletion of *dhathus* and sleeplessness.

11.3.2 SAMPRAPTI (PATHOGENESIS) [10]

Pathogenesis is the process by which a disease or disorder develops. It can include the causative factors which contribute to the onset of the disease or disorder and any other factor which leads to its progression and maintenance. Ayurveda describes the same as samprapti and the nidana, dosa, dusya, utbhava sthana (origin), etc., which ultimately lead to the diseases are called samprapti ghataka. Flowchart 11.3.2.1 shows the samprapti (pathogenesis) of sthoulya.

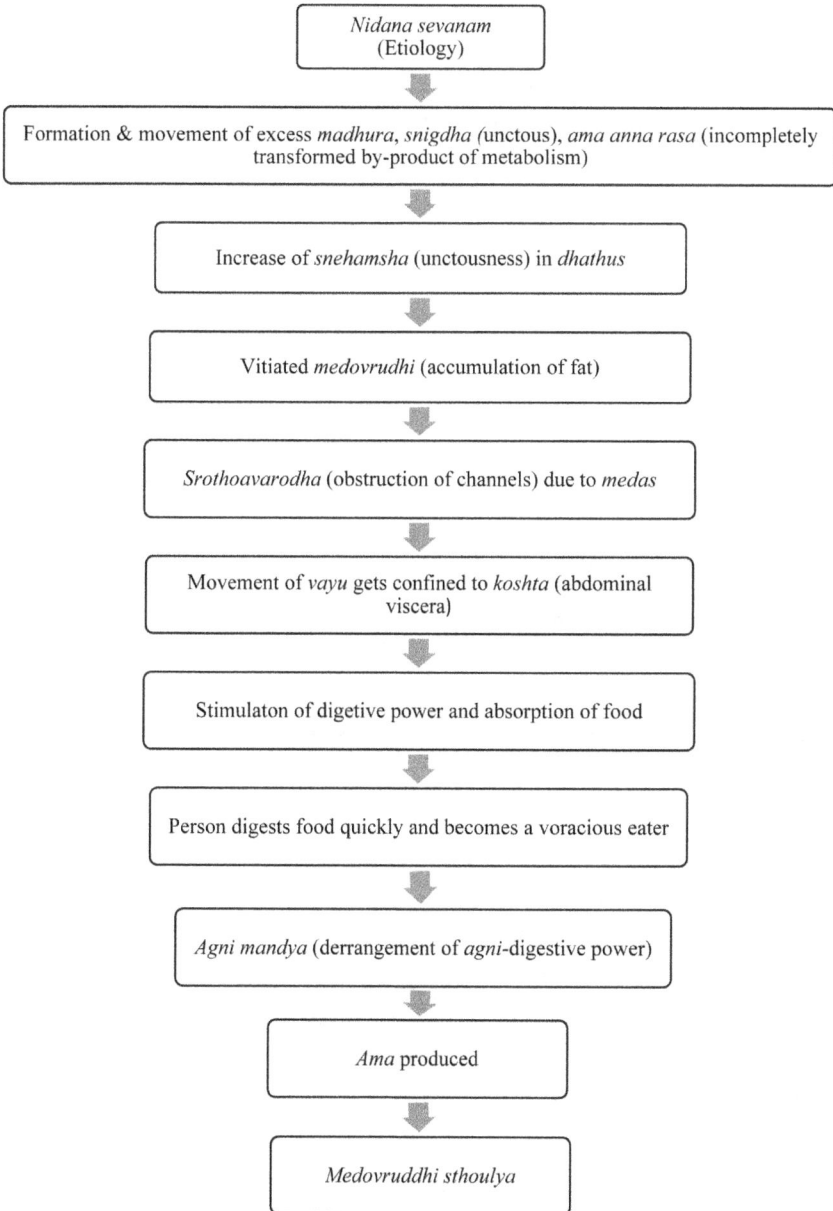

FIGURE 11.1 Samprapti (pathogenesis) of sthoulya.

By not following the rules of taking meals at specific times during the day, the *sthoola* person who has been transformed to a voracious eater gets afflicted by dreadful diseases. Agni (the component of *pitta dosa* responsible for digestion) and *vayu* are the two troublesome factors from the standpoint of obesity. These factors blight an obese person as a wildfire destroys a forest as per the *Acharyas*. Thus, *sthoulya* invites many complications resulting in rapid deterioration of life.

11.3.3   PURVARUPA (PRODROMAL SYMPTOMS)

These are the symptoms that appear before the complete manifestation of the disease. These include excessive sleep, drowsiness, laziness, and excessive body odor, heaviness of the body, and laxity of the body parts.

11.3.4   RUPA (SYMPTOMS)

The person is considered to be affected by *sthoulya roga* when

1. the excessive fat accumulation in the regions of buttocks, abdomen, and breasts make them pendulous, and
2. the person suffers from deficient metabolism and energy.

According to the classics, *atisthoola* person possess eight inherent defects in them:

1. reduced lifespan,
2. constricted or limited movement (hampered due to loose, tender, and heavy fat deposition),
3. reduced sexual activities or impotence (due to the small quantity of semen or obstruction of the channel of semen by *medas*),
4. debility (due to imbalance of *dhathus*),
5. profuse sweating (since *medas* and *kapha dosa* are vitiated),
6. emit bad body odor,
7. excessive hunger, and
8. excessive thirst.

The accumulation of fat leads to consequent tissue depletion [11].

11.3.5   UPADRAVA (COMPLICATIONS)

1. GIT.

2. *Atikshudha* (~excessive hunger), Polyphagia, *Atisara* (~diarrhoea), *Ajirna* (~indigestion), *Arsa* (~hemorrhoids), *Bhagandara* (~fistula), *Kamala* (~jaundice).
3. Respiratory system.
4. *Kasa* (~cough), *Swasa* (~dyspnoea).
5. Cardiovascular system.
6. *Kasa, Swasa, Sanyasa* (~coma), *Prana* and *Ojodushti.*
7. Neurological system.
8. Diseases due to *vata dosa* vitiation, *Urusthambha* (~stiffness of thighs).
9. Urinary system.
10. *Mutrakrucchra* (~disorders of urine), *Prameha* (~diabetes), *Pramehapidaka* (~diabetic carbuncle).
11. Integumentary system.
12. *Visarpa* (~cellulitis), *Jantuvaha* (~worm infestations), *Dourgandhya* (foul body odor).
13. Musculoskeletal system.
14. *Vata vyadhi* (disorders due to *vata*).

11.3.6 CHIKITSA (TREATMENT)

Chikitsa according to Ayurveda is not only prescribing medicines and removal of the etiological factors but also restoration of the equilibrium of *dosas* in the body. The therapeutics and lifestyle modifications are chosen based on the strength of the disease as well as the patient to undergo the treatment procedure.

11.4 GENERAL LINE OF TREATMENT

The general line of treatment is administration of *guru* (heavy) and *apatarpana* (nonsaturating) diet which possesses properties alleviating *vata dosa* and *kapha dosa*. It must also be chosen such that the diet does not increase medas further. This kind of heavy food satisfies the deranged *agni* by suppressing the excessive hunger of the patient. The nonsaturating diet leads to depletion of accumulated *medas* by preventing further nourishment. *Langhana* (measures of lightening) are advocated.

Kaphahara or *vatahara* (*kapha* or *vata* alleviating), *srotoshodhana* (to clear the blocked channels), *lekhana* (scraping) type of medicines, and measures are taken.

1. *Bahya chikitsa (external applications)*

- *Rukshana karma*

  It is the procedure of providing *rukshana* (dryness) to the body. It is attributed by many *oushadhas/aharas/viharas*.

- *Udwarttanam*

  It is the external application of medicated *curna* (powder) or pastes on the body with affordable pressure massage in retrograde direction (opposite to the direction of hair growth). This is more specific to *twak* and *medo dhatu*. This procedure cleanses the body, increases brightness, increases circulation, expansion, and dilatation of vessels. It relieves itching, imparts good complexion, enhances channel and circular even at the cellular level, and influences general metabolism, and has a stress-relieving property.

  Udwarttanam in combination with internal medication and *pancakarma* forms effective treatment for *sthoulya*.

2. *Abhyantara chikitsa (internal medications).*

Kashaya kalpana	*Guggulutiktaka ks, Rasonadi ks, Varanadi ks, Pancatiktaka ks, Asanadi gana ks, Varasanadi ks*
Arishta and *Asava kalpana*	*Guggulutiktarishta, Ayaskriti, Lodhrasava, Varanasavam, Nimbamrtasava*
Curna kalpana	*Pancakola curna, Shaddharana curna, Vyoshadi guggulu curna, Triphala curna, Vidangadi curna*
	For external use
	Kolakulathadi curna, Kottamchukadi curna
Guggulu kalpana	*Kancanara guggulu, Amrta guggulu, Triphala guggulu, Punarnava guggulu, Yogaraja guggulu*
Ghritha kalpana	*Guggulutiktaka ghritha, Pancatiktaka ghritha, Varanadi ghritha*
Lehya kalpana	*Dasamula haritaki, Gomutra haritaki*
Bhasma and *Kshara kalpana*	*Loha bhasma, Kalyanaka kshara*
Rasoushadhi	*Mahalakshmivilasa rasa, Rasa sindhura, Agnitundi vati*

11.5   AHARA (FOOD)

The three pillars needed to maintain a healthy life are considered as *ahara* (food), *nidra* (sleep), and *brahmacharya* (control of senses/celibacy) which constitute the *thrio-upasthambha* in Ayurveda. By the wisdom of well-regulated support of these three, one can own a properly grown body with strength, good complexion which will sustain till death provided, the person does not get involved in regimens that are detrimental to his health. This concept indicates the holistic approach of Ayurveda to deal with lifestyle disorders like *sthoulya*.

According to body constitutions and pathological conditions, *Acharyas* have mentioned specific food articles, drugs, and regimen which do not affect the body and mind adversely are brought under *Pathya* and in the same way, those which affect the body adversely are brought under *Apathya*. Table 11.1 shows the pathya ahara (therapeutic diet indicated in obesity) and apathya ahara (diet that is contraindicated in obesity).

11.6 IMPORTANCE OF NIDRA (SLEEP)

Sleep is the most under-rated pillar needed for a healthy state of both mind and body. It is necessary for maintaining synchronization of life. *Nidra* can be considered as a basic act provoked by *kapha dosa* in the body to maintain harmony with the other *vata* and *pitta dosas*. It is essential for biological drives like hunger and thirst. Many studies have shown that an adequate amount of good sleep at the proper time plays a role in maintaining the hormonal balance and blood sugar levels in the body.

In many cases, *sthoulya* has been viewed as an evident result of improper sleep patterns.

11.6.1 AYURVEDIC ASPECTS OF SLEEP

Physiologically, an individual falls asleep when his mind including the sensory and motor organs get exhausted and they dissociate themselves from their objects. According to Ayurveda, happiness and misery, nourishment and emaciation, strength and weakness, fertility and infertility, knowledge and ignorance, life and death depend upon proper and improper sleep [12].

Sleeping during daytime is contraindicated in seasons other than summer. People having excessive fat, those who are addictive to fatty substances, suffering from vitiated *kapha dosic* disorders must never sleep during the day-time [13]. Habit of staying up late at night causes roughness in the body and sleeping during the day causes unctuousness.

TABLE 11.1 Pathya Apathya Ahara for Sthoulya

Ahara varga	Pathya	Apathya
Shuka dhanya (cereal grains)	Purana shali (old rice-Oryza sativa), Yava (Hordeum vulgare), Laja (parched rice), Kodrava (Paspalum scrobiculatum), Navara rice	Godhuma (Triticum aestivum), Naveena shali (new rice)
Shami dhanya (pulses)	Mudga (Vigna radiata), Rajamasha (V.unguiculata), Kulattha (Dolichos biflorus), Chanaka (Cicer arietinum), Masur (Lens culinaris), Adhaki (Cajanus cajan), Makusthaka (V.aconitifolia)	Masha (V.mungo), Tila (Sesamum indicum)
Shaka varga (vegetables)	Patola (Trichosanthes dioica), shigru (Moringa oleifera), Vrunthaka (Solanum melongena), Ardraka (Zingiber officinale), Mulaka (Raphanus sativus), Surasa (Ocimum tenuiflorum)	Kanda shaka (root tubers), Madhura rasatmaka (of sweet taste)
Phala varga (fruits)	Kapitha (Feronia linonia), Jambu (Syzygium cumini), Amalaki (Emblica officinalis), Vibhithaki (Terminalia bellerica), Haritaki (T.chebula), Maricha (Piper nigrum), Pippali (Piper longum), Ela (Elettaria cardamomum), Eranda karkati (Carica papaya), Ankola (Alangium salvifolium), Narang (Citrus limetta), Bilvaphala (Aegle marmelos)	Madhura phala
Drava varga (liquids)	Madhu (honey), Takra (buttermilk), Ushnajala (~warm water), Tila and Sarshapa (Brassica compestris) taila (oil), Asava arishta, Sura, Jeerna madya	Milk preparations (Dugdha, Dhadhi, Sarpi), Ikshu (Saccharum officinarum) preparations
Mamsa varga (nonvegetarian)	Rohita matsya (Labeo rohita)	Anupa, Auduka, Gramya mamsa sevana

Along with a wholesome diet, sleep is also essential for happiness. Ayurvedic purificatory measures like *vamana* (emesis), *virecana* (purgation), and *nasya* helps in elimination of *dosas* and suppress *tamas* (*manasika dosa*). The emotions such as fear, anxiety, anger, habits, and activity such as medicated smoking, physical exercise, fasting, and environmental setting, such as uncomfortable bed help in overcoming excessive sleep/hypersomnolence [14]. Natural sleep at night is the best form of sleep that nurses all the living beings.

11.7 VYAYAMA (PHYSICAL EXERCISE)

Physical exercises or activities which produce exertion of the body are known as *vyayama* [15]. It is considered as an important component of *dinacarya*. Acharyas have advised that this is the best measure to reduce *sthoulya* and the persons who exercise daily are not afflicted by any diseases. Table 11.2 shows the pathya vihara (therapeutic physical activity regimen indicated in obesity) and apathya vihara (physical activity regimen that is contraindicated in obesity).

TABLE 11.2 *Pathya Apathya Vihara* for *sthoulya* (Physical Regimen)

Pathya	Apathya
Shrama (exhaustion)	Intake of cold water
Jagarana (staying awake at night)	*Diwaswapna* (Day-time sleep)
Vyayama (exercise)	Physical inactivity
Vyavaya (sexual intercourse)	Overeating/intake of a meal before the digestion of the previous meal
Nitya bhramana (regular brisk walking)	
Activities like horse riding	

11.7.1 SIGNS OF PROPER VYAYAMA [16]

1. Sweating.
2. Increased respiratory rate.
3. Increased heart rate (pulse rate).
4. Feeling of lightness in the body.
5. Dryness of mouth.
6. Exertion.

11.7.2　BENEFITS OF VYAYAMA [17]

1. Acts as an immune booster.
2. Produces well compact muscles.
3. Stimulates *agni*.
4. Increases tolerance to heat and cold.
5. Regulates dyslipidemia.
6. Aids as a treatment of *sthoulya*.
7. Delays ageing.
8. Provides mental stability and tolerance to various physical and psychological stresses.

The best time to follow *vyayama* is morning since the metabolism is at its peak.

Aerobic activities must be primly chosen since they help to expand more calories in a relatively short time. Exercise can be broken into smaller sections with duration of 10–20 min and practiced. A beginner must always be careful to start the routine slowly and increase the vigor and duration steadily and maintain it so as to avoid injury to tissues and excessive soreness and fatigue.

Moderately vigorous exercises like walking, brisk walking, treadmill, stair climbing, swimming, etc., with the duration of 30–60 min are adequate to maintain a healthy body and mind.

11.7.3　PRECAUTIONS NEEDED

The person who is aged 40 or above, those who experience pressure over the region of the chest along with pain and exertion, those who develop fatigue and shortness of breath easily, those who have developed the complications of sthoulya or have a history of cardiovascular or respiratory disorder, asthma, arthritis, osteoporosis, those who have a family history of cardiovascular problems, etc., must consult a physician before starting vyayama as a measure of precaution.

Adequate sleep and a balanced diet are quintessential to get the needed benefits of *vyayama*.

11.8　MANAS (PSYHE) IN STHOULYA

The *manas* (psyche), *atma* (soul), and *sharira* (body) are the tripods for existence of life. *Manas* has three tendencies called *satwa* (balance), rajas (arrogance), and *tamas* (indolence) like the *sharirika vata, pitta, and kapha dosas*. The relation between body and mind is compared to that of "a pot and an amount of ghee in it." Whenever the ghee is hot, it imparts its heat to the pot and in the same way, whenever the pot is heated in turns it melts the ghee in it. A change in any one of them affects the other in a similar manner. The psyche and the body are always interrelated. A vitiation of the body leading to metabolic disturbance ultimately culminates in a psychological disturbance and vice versa. This concept may have opened the *Sattvavajaya chikitsa* (psychotheraupeutic treatment) in Ayurveda.

Sthoulya patients usually find themselves filled with anxiety and many of them get worried about their cosmetic value in society ending up in depression and sleep disorders like insomnia. Table 11.3 shows the pathya vihara (therapeutic mental activities indicated in obesity) and apathya vihara (mental activities that are contraindicated in obesity) which are advised for the mental well-being and happiness.

TABLE 11.3 *Pathya Apathya Vihara* for Mental Health in *sthoulya*

Pathya*	Apathya
Chintha (here, it means thinking and practicing mental activities)	*Nitya harsha* (uninterrupted cheerfulness)
Shoka (worry)	*Achinthana* (being mentally inactive)
Krodha (anger)	*Manaso nivrutti* (absence of mind)

This pathya can be considered for those who have become sthoola due to overnourishment and lifestyle filled with comfort like higher economic class of the society.

11.8.1   COUNSELING

Sthoulya patients can be given encouragement and motivation to overcome their health problems and face their challenges with willpower. Social stigma about being obese and the chance of bullying and mental trauma must be dealt with in the best suitable manner.

Emotional support must be ensured and the patient must be educated about the possible health risks so as to make a decision to lose weight and regain his health.

11.8.2   SADVRITTA—RULES OF GOOD CONDUCT

The practices described for the promotion of mental health in Ayurveda include *sadvritta*. The *Acharyas* have described this schedule giving a comprehensive account of the mode of a healthy and happy life. A man is considered healthy only when he is in the state of biological balance and enjoys sensorial, mental, and spiritual well-being. Such a state of health can be achieved only by observing *sadvritta* that helps in the maintenance of positive health and control over sense organs [18].

11.8.3 YOGA AND PRANAYAMA [19]

Yoga means "joined together." It works on the body-mind complex. Millions practice *yoga* for its *asanas*, its physical exercises, which have been universally acclaimed by physicians.

It is different from exercise as it does not involve speedy movements, but instead very slow and steady movements. *Asana* is described as a posture that is stable and pleasant. It helps to achieve physical health, control over mind, and power of concentration. Some *yogasanas* for mitigating *sthoulya*:

1. Pawanamukthasana
2. Bhujangasana
3. *Ushtrasana*
4. *Paschimottasana*
5. *Veerabhadrasana*
6. *Naukasana*
7. *Shalabhasana*
8. *Gomukhasana*
9. *Suryanamaskara.*

Each *asana* has its own set of indications and contraindications. If *yoga* appeals to you, you will need to find a good teacher who can guide you properly.

Pranayama is "control of breath"; *Prana* means breath or bioenergy in the body and *ayama* means control. On subtle levels, *prana* represents the *pranic* energy responsible for life or life force. One can control the *pranic* energy with *pranayama* and achieve a healthy mind and body.

Proper care and guidance are necessary before practicing *pranayama* since it leads to unwanted health complications if practiced unscientifically.

11.9 PANCAKARMA (PURIFICATION THERAPY)

This is a set of five measures intended toward purification of the body. Ayurveda highlights this biocleansing regimen in its classics by naming them as *shodhana karma*. *Acharyas* have emphasized the importance and effect of *pancakarma* in the *rtucharya* (seasonal regimen) as well as therapeutics. The five measures are vamana (emesis), *virecana* (purgation), *vasti* (enema), *nasya* (instillation of medicine through nostrils) [20], and *rakthamokshana* (blood-letting).

11.9.1   BENEFITS OF PANCAKARMA

It covers a wide range of preventive and curative conditions. Pancakarma helps the body to prepare itself for better bioavailability of the pharmological therapies. It promotes the homeostasis of *dosas* through the elimination of accumulated *dosas* in the months of their vitiation as a preventive measure. The effects of the procedures may be generalized to be detoxifying, immune-modulating, and rejuvenating. It cleanses the macro- and microchannels in the body. It helps the early repair of tissues and improves nourishment by preventing early ageing.

The selection of *sodhana karma* is based on the disease characteristic and *dosa avastha* (state of *dosa*) and *sthana* (seat of *dosa*) in Ayurveda. The strength of the patient is also taken into account. The *sthoulya* patients with increased *dosa* and strength are subjected to *shodhana karma* [21].

11.9.2   PURVAKARMA (PREPARATORY PROCEDURES)

11.9.2.1   DIPANA-PACANA CHIKITSA

The first step of *shodhana* is the administration of on the patient. This improves the *agni* of the patient and reduces the consequences which may possibly arise due to *ama avastha* (due to improper metabolism).

11.9.2.2   SNEHANA

Snehana karma (intake of unctuous articles) is always restricted for patients of *sthoulya*. However, properties of *taila* (medicated oils) such as *lekhaniya* (scrapping) type, *medohara* (reducing *medas*) type, and those that tend to reduce accumulated fat can be used. [22]

11.9.2.3 SWEDANA

Swedana karma (induction of sweating) is indicated at a mild level. *Anagneya* (without fire) *sweda* like exercise, warm chamber, heavy clothing, application of poultice, induction of fear, anger hunger, excessive drinking, wrestling, exposure to sunrays, etc., can be used in the case *ofsthoulya*.

11.9.3 PRADHANA KARMA (THE MAIN PROCEDURES)

11.9.3.1 VAMANA

Vamana karma (emesis) is the expulsion of aggravated *dosas* through the upper route, that is, oral route following the administration of *vamanoushadhis* (medicines intended to induce emesis). It is contraindicated in *sthoulya* due to the inability to bear the potency of medicine and therapy. Therefore, it should be done according to the requirement and stage of the disease by taking sufficient precautions and care [23].

As an emergency treatment, it can be done by administering *snehana* on the first day, *kapha utkleshana ahara* (intake of food which increases *kapha dosa*) on the second day, and inducing *vamana* on the third day.

This procedure helps in the elimination of *kapha dosa*, helps to clear the blocked channels, and purifies the *dhathus* along with stimulating the *agni* [24].

11.9.3.2 VIRECHANA

Virechana karma (purgation) is the procedure in which the *dosas* are expelled through the lower route, that is, anal canal by the administration of medicines through oral route. It is also not recommended in *sthoulya* but the drugs with *medohara* property can be applied based on the strength of the patient and the stage of disease.

This procedure helps to eliminate accumulated *pitta dosa* and by-products of *kapha dosa*. It purifies the blood and enhances *agni* from the cellular level. It also helps in *vata anulomana* (movement of *vata dosa* in the proper direction, here it is downward) along with purification of blocked channels. [25].

11.9.3.3 *VASTI*

Vasti karma (enema) is the procedure in which the medicine is introduced through the anal canal, or urethra or vagina with the use of *vastiyantra* (instrument used for *vasti*). It is also called the *arddha chikitsa* as it is the most superior *karma* of Ayurveda. It has multidimensional action and is very much effective in lifestyle diseases, neuromuscular diseases, occupational stress, and related mental problems. *Vasti* with *ruksha* (dry), *ushna* (hot), and *tikshna* (sharp) are suggested for *sthoulya* treatment among which *lekhana vasti* and *kshara vasti* are found to be most effective [26].

Lekhana vasti contains:

1. *Triphala kwatha (Amalaki, Haritaki and Vibhitaki)*
2. *Gomutra (cow's urine)*
3. *Madhu (honey)*
4. *Yavakshara (carbonate of potash)*
5. *Shathapushpam (Anethum sowa)*
6. *Ushaka (Dorema ammoniacum)*
7. *Saindhava (Rock salt)*
8. *Shilajatu (Asphaltium punjabinum)*
9. *Kasisa (Ferrous sulfate)*
10. *Hingu (Ferula northax)*.
11. *Tuttha (Copper sulfate)*.

Kshara vasti contains:

1. *Saindhava*
2. *Guda (jaggery)*
3. *Chincha (Tamarindus indica)*
4. *Gomutra*
5. *Shathapushpam*

The *lekhana vasti* and *kshara vasti* are very effective in sthoulya treatment.

11.10 RASAYANA (REJUVENATION THERAPY)

One of the eight clinical specialties in Ayurveda is *rasayana* chikitsa. It includes administration of rejuvenating recipes, special diet regimen and health-promoting conducts for both body and mind. The good conducts are emphasized as a separate code of social behavior as per the classics. It includes worship of God (the supreme power), respecting the elders, and the able, holding on truth, nonviolence, avoiding anger, avoiding alcohol, unwanted sex and strain, maintenance of peace, speaking sweet words, practicing mantra, prayers, etc., being kind to the surrounding living beings, the practice of proper sleep schedule and diet, caring for the seasons, being humble, well-behaved and self-restrained, practicing meditation and religious literature, and respecting the followers of God.

11.10.1 BENEFITS OF RASAYANA

Rasayana chikitsa must be given to a person after he has been subjected to the most suitable *shodhana* therapy based on his strength, stage of disease, or the state of the three dosas in his body. By this *rasayana* treatment, one attains longevity, memory, intelligence, freedom from illness, youthfulness, excellence of luster, complexion and voice, optimum strength of physique and sense organs, perfection and deliberation, respectability, and brilliance. *Rasayana* is the means of attaining excellent qualities of all the seven *dhathus* starting from *rasa* [27].

11.11 LIFESTYLE IN AYURVEDA

Ayurveda has always been keen on the idea of maintenance of health and prevention of diseases through following proper diet and lifestyle rather than medicines and treatment. In order to achieve it, the science suggests a lifestyle based on a routine regimen called *swasthavritta* as a means to preserve and sustain a healthy state of body and mind. It can be described in terms of *dinacarya* [28], *ratricharya*, and *ritucharya* [29]. This proves the basic principle of Ayurveda which is to preserve the health of the healthy, rather than cure the diseases of the diseased [30].

11.11.1 DINACHARYA

This is the daily routine prescribed by the classics. It suggests that a healthy person must get up from bed at *brahma muhurta* (45 min before sunrise) to preserve his health in order to protect his life. Then, the individual should attend to his urges of eliminating urine and faeces. Then the benefits, procedure and the materials used, and the contraindications of *danta dhawana* (cleaning teeth) are elaborated. Next comes *anjana* (application of collyrium), which is followed by *navana* (nasal drops), *gandusha* (mouth gargles), *dhuma* (inhalation of smoke), and *tambula* (chewing betel leaves).

After the cleansing one must do *abhyanga* (oil massage) on his ears, head, and feet daily to improve his vision, nourishment of tissues, to get good sleep, improve skin tone, and delays ageing. The indications and contraindications must be carefully followed both in the case of *abhyanga* and the next routine which is *vyayama* (exercise). Next is *udwarttana* and *snana* (bathing). The importance of maintaining personal hygiene has been has been always specially mentioned.

11.11.2 RTUCHARYA

A person can lead a healthy and happy life full of strength and happiness only if he knows how to get accustomed to suitable changes in diet and behavior according to the seasons and can practice such habits accordingly. He must also make sure that his diet is flourished with all the *shadrasas*. Table 11.4 shows the relation between the six seasons according to Ayurveda and the subsequent variations in the dosic state of a healthy person.

Rtucharya describes the "dos and don'ts" (Regimen) during the six seasons. The seven days at the end of a season and at the commencement of the next is called the interseasonal period. During this time, the regimen should be discontinued gradually and that of the succeeding season should be gradually adopted. Sudden discontinuance or sudden adoption gives rise to diseases caused by *asatmya* (nonhabituation). Already known as the diabetes capital of the world, India is likely to get another title as the capital of lifestyle diseases as well. To prevent this and to safeguard our health and harmony, we must follow all the possible measures of preservation of mental, physical, and social health through Ayurveda. Table 11.5 shows the summary of dietary and physical activity regimen recommended according to seasons for maintaining a healthy body and mind.

11.12   CONCLUSIONS

The term lifestyle disorders themselves show the remedy to stay away from them, that is, people can overcome the disorders caused due to their improper lifestyle through maintenance of a systematic life filled with a healthy diet and an adequate amount of sleep. For a healthy life, people must balance a body with a happy mind because the mental entity is as equal as the external

A Holistic and Integrated Approach to Lifestyle Diseases

TABLE 11.4 Relation Between Seasons and State of a Healthy Person

Rtu (Seasons)	Months	Environmental Condition	Strength of a Healthy Person	Predominant *dosas* in the Body	Strength of agni of the Person
Shishira (winter)	Mid-January–Mid-March	Cold with cold wind	Less	Deposition of *kapha*	Remains high
Vasanta (spring)	Mid-March–Mid-May	Flowering, growth of new leaves	Medium	Vitiation of *kapha*	Less
Grishma (*summer*)	Mid-May–Mid-July	Intense heat, unhealthy wind, dried water bodies lifeless plants	Less	Pacification of previous state and deposition of *vata*	Less
Varsha (monsoon)	Mid-July–Mid-September	Rain clouds, rains with thunderstorm	Again less	Vitiation of *vata* and deposition of *pitta*	Vitiation of agni
Sharad (autumn)	Mid-September–Mid-November	Bright sun, clear sky with white clouds	Medium	*Vata* is pacified and *pitta* is vitiated	High
Hemanta (late autumn)	Mid-November–Mid-January	Cold wind starts and chillness is felt	Very high	*Pitta* is pacified	Very high

TABLE 11.5 Summary of Regimen of Diet and Physical Activity According to Seasons

Rtu (Seasons)	Diet		Physical Activity	
	Pathya	Apathya	Pathya	Apathya
Shishira (winter)	*Shali, Godhuma, Tila*, etc. Milk and milk products, *Ikshu* and its products, etc., fats, edible oils, flour products, green vegetables, *Sunti (Zingiber officinale), Lashuna Allium sativum), Haritaki, Pippali* etc.	Cold drinks, *Vata* aggravating foods like *Chanaka*, etc., too much of foods having *amla, tikta*, and *kashaya rasa*. Light foods like *Laja*	*Abhyanga*, Wearing warm cloths, *Snana* in hot water and Exposure to sunlight	Exposure to wind, Excessive walking, Staying awake at night
Vasanta (spring)	*Shali, Godhuma, Kulmasha (Zea mays), Yava, Mudga, Masur, Adhaki* etc. Honey, *Khadira (Acacia catechu), Musta (Cyprus rotandus), Sunti, Haridra (Curcuma longa), Tulsi*, etc.	Cold drinks, too much of foods having *madhura rasa* and *amla rasa*, fatty and oily foods, heavy foods like meats (in excess). New grains, *Masha*, etc	Use hot water for *snana* and drinking. *Udwarttanam* with *Chandana (Santalum album), Kesara (Crocus sativus), Agaru (Aquillaria agallocha), Kavala, Dhuma, Anjana, Vamana, Nasya*	Day-time sleep
Grishma (summer)	*Shali, Mudga*, etc., fruits such as *Amra (Mangifera indica), Watermelon (Citrulus vulgaris), fruit juices, Narikelambu* (coconut water), *Takra*, curd with pepper, etc.	Heavy and warm foods like new grains, *Masha, Sarshapa*, salt, chilli, etc.	Residing in cool places, application of paste of *Chandana*, Wearing garlands, white dresses. Day-time sleep is indicated only during this *rtu*	Exposure to moon rays and breeze, excessive exercise, physical work, sexual intercourse, and intake of alcohol
Varsha (monsoon)	Old *Yava*, old Rice, Old Wheat etc., meat soup, *Yasa* (porridge). *Pancakola-Pippali, Maricha, Sunti, Chavya (Piper chaba), Citraka (Plumbago zeylanica)*, etc.	Excessive liquid and wine, river water, churned and fermented preparations, etc. Heavy diet, excessive salts, etc.	*Snana* in hot water, application of oil on body after *snana, Vasti karma*	Exposure to the initial showers, Day-sleep, Excessive exercise, physical work and sexual intercourse

TABLE 11.5 *(Continued)*

Rtu (Seasons)	Diet		Physical Activity	
	Pathya	Apathya	Pathya	Apathya
Sharad (autumn)	Easily digestible cereals and pulses, *Sarkara* (sugar candy), *Jangala* mamsa, *Patola, Amalaki*, dates (*Phoenix sylvistris*), grapes (*Vitis vinifera*)	Amla rasa predominant and fermented foods such as curd, etc., fats and oils, meat of aquatic animals, etc.	Food must be taken only on feeling hungry. Application of *Chandana* on body, exposure to moon rays during first 3 h of appearance of moon. *Virecana, Raktamokshana*	Day-sleep. Excessive eating and exposure to sun
Hemanta (late autumn)	*Shali, Godhuma, Masha*, etc. Milk and milk products, *Ikshu* and its products, fats and oils, similar to that of *Shishira rtu*	Cold drinks, foods that aggravate vata such as *Chanaka* etc. light foods such as puffed rice, etc.	Exercise, *Abhyanga*, Hot water for *snana* and drinking, Sunbath, Use of *Agaru*, heavy clothing, Sexual intercourse, Residing in warm places.	Exposure to strong cold wind, Day-sleep

physical entity. Obesity in Ayurveda comes as *sthoulya* which tells that it is a result of improper diet, physical inactivity, and improper sleep, and possible emotional stress. Some procedures which come under *Sodhana* (purificatory) and *Samana* (palliative) modalities of Ayurveda can be effective against *sthoulya*. The importance of the dietary regimen and seasonal regimen is often neglected whereas the strict follow-up of these can bring a tremendous change in the world population. Lifestyle correction can hardly become late in anyone's health and nobody is too old to incorporate a healthy diet and exercise schedule into their daily life. With all these, one can enjoy mental stability, emotional balance, and necessary sleep which are often considered to be the most under-rated necessities of the growing urban lifestyle.

KEYWORDS

- **Ayurveda**
- **lifestyle disease**
- **obesity**
- **sthoulya**
- **Charaka Samhita**
- **Susruta Samhita**
- **Ashtanga Hridayam**
- **psyche**
- **rejuvenation**

REFERENCES

1. Trikamji, V. J. (2008). Charaka Samhita Sutra Sthana 2, Sloke no. 15. *Varanasi: Acharya Chaukhambha Surbharati Prakashana*.Agnivesha, Caraka Samhita, Sutrasthana 1/15 ed. Yadavji Trikamji Acharya Chowkambha Surbharathi Prakashan, Varanasi; 2008.
2. Shri Dalhana Acharya, Sushrutha Samhita, Uttarasthana 1/25 ed. Yadavji Trikamji Acharya Chowkambha Surbharathi Prakashan, Varanasi; 2008.
3. Agnivesha, Caraka Samhita, Sharirasthana 1/99 ed. Yadavji Trikamji Acharya Chowkambha Surbharathi Prakashan, Varanasi; 2008.
4. Agnivesha, Caraka Samhita, Sutrasthana 21/3 ed. Yadavji Trikamji Acharya Chowkambha Surbharathi Prakashan, Varanasi; 2008.
5. Agnivesha, Caraka Samhita, Sutrasthana 21/20 ed. Yadavji Trikamji Acharya Chowkambha Surbharathi Prakashan, Varanasi; 2008.

6. Sri Sudarshana Sastry, Madhavakara's Madhava Nidanam 1/4 with Madhukosha Commentery, Chowkambha Surbharathi Prakashan, Varanasi; 2008.
7. Agnivesha, Caraka Samhita, Sutrasthana 21/4 ed. Yadavji Trikamji Acharya Chowkambha Surbharathi Prakashan, Varanasi; 2008.
8. Agnivesha, Caraka Samhita, Sutrasthana 21/4 ed. Yadavji Trikamji Acharya Chowkambha Surbharathi Prakashan, Varanasi; 2008.
9. Agnivesha, Caraka Samhita, Sutrasthana 21/5 ed. Yadavji Trikamji Acharya Chowkambha Surbharathi Prakashan, Varanasi; 2008.
10. Agnivesha, Caraka Samhita, Sutrasthana 21/6 ed. Yadavji Trikamji Acharya Chowkambha Surbharathi Prakashan, Varanasi; 2008.
11. Agnivesha, Caraka Samhita, Sutrasthana 21/35 ed. Yadavji Trikamji Acharya Chowkambha Surbharathi Prakashan, Varanasi; 2008.
12. Agnivesha, Caraka Samhita, Sutrasthana 21/44 ed. Yadavji Trikamji Acharya Chowkambha Surbharathi Prakashan, Varanasi; 2008.
13. Agnivesha, Caraka Samhita, Sutrasthana 21/55 ed. Yadavji Trikamji Acharya Chowkambha Surbharathi Prakashan, Varanasi; 2008.
14. Shri Dalhana Acharya, Sushrutha Samhita, Chikitsasthana 24/38 ed. Yadavji Trikamji Acharya Chowkambha Surbharathi Prakashan, Varanasi; 2008.
15. Agnivesha, Caraka Samhita, Sutrasthana 7/33 ed. Yadavji Trikamji Acharya Chowkambha Surbharathi Prakashan, Varanasi; 2008.
16. Shri Dalhana Acharya, Sushrutha Samhita, Chikitsasthana 24/39 ed. Yadavji Trikamji Acharya Chowkambha Surbharathi Prakashan, Varanasi; 2008.
17. Agnivesha, Caraka Samhita, Sutrasthana 8/18 ed. Yadavji Trikamji Acharya Chowkambha Surbharathi Prakashan, Varanasi; 2008.
18. Rao Mangalagowri V. Textbook of Swasthavritta; Chaukambha Orientalia, Varanasi; 2007.
19. Agnivesha, Caraka Samhita, Sutrasthana 13/3 ed. Yadavji Trikamji Acharya Chowkambha Surbharathi Prakashan, Varanasi; 2008.
20. Vagbhata's Ashtanga Hridaya, Sutrasthana 14/12 ed. Acharya Hari Shastri Paradakara Vaidya; Chaukambha Orientalia, Varanasi; 2002.
21. Shri Dalhana Acharya, Sushrutha Samhita, Sutrasthana 45/112 ed. Yadavji Trikamji Acharya Chowkambha Surbharathi Prakashan, Varanasi; 2008.
22. Agnivesha, Caraka Samhita, Siddhisthana 2/8 ed. Yadavji Trikamji Acharya Chowkambha Surbharathi Prakashan, Varanasi; 2008.
23. Agnivesha, Caraka Samhita, Sutrasthana 16/10 ed. Yadavji Trikamji Acharya Chowkambha Surbharathi Prakashan, Varanasi; 2008.
24. Agnivesha, Caraka Samhita, Sutrasthana 16/15 ed. Yadavji Trikamji Acharya Chowkambha Surbharathi Prakashan, Varanasi; 2008.
25. Shri Dalhana Acharya, Sushrutha Samhita, Chikitsasthana 38/82 ed. Yadavji Trikamji Acharya Chowkambha Surbharathi Prakashan, Varanasi; 2008.
26. Agnivesha, Caraka Samhita, Chikitsasthana 1/6 ed. Yadavji Trikamji Acharya Chowkambha Surbharathi Prakashan, Varanasi; 2008.
27. Vagbhata's Ashtanga Hridaya, Sutrasthana 2/1 ed. Acharya Hari Shastri Paradakara Vaidya; Chaukambha Orientalia, Varanasi; 2002.
28. Vagbhata's Ashtanga Hridaya, Sutrasthana 3/3 ed. Acharya Hari Shastri Paradakara Vaidya; Chaukambha Orientalia, Varanasi; 2002.
29. Agnivesha, Caraka Samhita, Sutrasthana 30/26 ed. Yadavji Trikamji Acharya Chowkambha Surbharathi Prakashan, Varanasi; 2008.

CHAPTER 12

Marine Environment: A Reservoir of Natural Anticancer Drugs

ARUN M. SHANKREGOWDA[1*], and JESIYA SUSAN GEORGE[2]

[1]Faculty of Biosciences and Aquaculture, Nord University, Bodø, Norway

[2]School of Chemical Sciences, Mahatma Gandhi University, Kottayam, India

*Corresponding author. E-mail: arungowda9738@gmail.com

ABSTRACT

Cancer is one of the most deadly diseases in Western nations compared to infectious diseases of developing nations. There is an urgent need for new anticancer drugs with novel modes of action despite remarkable developments in cancer therapy in the past three decades. The large diversity of the marine environments offers a variety of secondary metabolites. New drugs from the marine environment act as an alternative source to meet the world population demand. In spite of vast diversity, the percentage of secondary metabolites screened for bioactivity is low in the marine environment. This chapter provides an insight into the unexplored area of marine anticancer compounds and anticancer research so far conducted in the area of marine anticancer drugs. In this review chapter, we summarized a class of marine anticancer agents from marine environment, their structure and the methods of isolation.

12.1 INTRODUCTION

Cancer is a frightful common class of disease in this era, rate of cancer-affected patients increases with changes in lifestyle, food habits, and environmental problems. Cancer is the uncontrolled growth of tissues accomplished by the formation of a mass of tissue called a tumor; however, cancer in blood, called leukaemia does not form any tumor. Cancer cells are different from normal cells in many ways, cancer cells grow out of control and became invasive. Cancer is a genetic disorder, generally caused by the changes to the genes, which control our cells function, these genetic mutations can be either inherited from the parents or arises due to the changes in the person's lifestyle. It is very important to notice that genetic changes in each person's cancer are unique and even within the same tumor different cells may have the different gene mutation. Carcinoma, sarcoma, melanoma, leukaemia, and lymphoma are different types of cancers found in humans. Different treatments are available for this, and the treatment type will choose on the basis of which type of cancer and how advanced it is but most of the medical practices suggest a combination of treatments, such as surgery with chemotherapy/radiation therapy, both the side effects of these radiation therapies are more shocking. In this context, plant-derived natural anticancer drugs gained significant attention. According to the reports of the World Health Organization, about 70% of population from the developing countries primarily depends on plant-derived medicines for health care, interestingly 70% of drugs for cancer treatments are of natural origin although natural products are usually recognized as secondary metabolites because they are not essential for our life

Marine environment has vast biodiversity; hence, it is a potential source of various bioactive components. About 30,000 described species of plants and animals live in the ocean environment. There are numerous sources for extracting novel potentially active biomolecules, but the marine environment is quite different from the existing sources due to the difference in the adaptation ability and physiology of the organisms in it. In this chapter, we deeply discuss the anticancer drugs from the marine environment and their efficiency. Exploitations of the marine environment started by collecting large creatures, such as corals, algae, and sponges, they have the ability to produce a variety of products with unique chemical structures and exhibit a broad panel of properties such as antitumor, antimicrotubule, antiproliferative, photoprotective, antibiotic, and anti-infective. Marine Natural Products are high-value ended products to be useful in the pharmaceutical industry and other drug developing companies in the world, interestingly they are frequently used in cosmetics too [1–7].

12.2   MARINE BACTERIA FAMILY

Microorganisms present in the marine environment gained considerable attention toward drug discovery from them. About 99% of the bacteria found in the marine environment are noncultarable in-vivo. Salinosporamide A is an important anticancer agent obtained from marine *Salinispora tropica* and *Salinispora arenicola*, which are commonly found in marine sediments. Salinosporamide is a generic name for the class of chemical compounds produced by marine bacteria Salinispora. Figure 12.1 represents the structure of Salinosporamide A similarly Byrostatin is another class of macrolide lactones produced by *Bugula neritina*. The structure of Byrostatin is represented in Figure 12.2 pharmacological studies of bryostatin revels that they have the ability to prevent tumor growth [8–10].

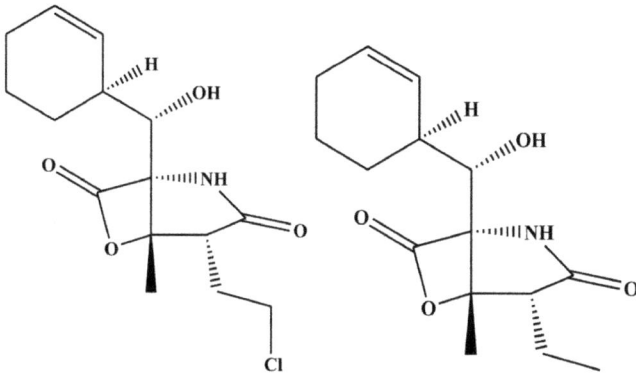

FIGURE 12.1 Salinosporamide A and B.

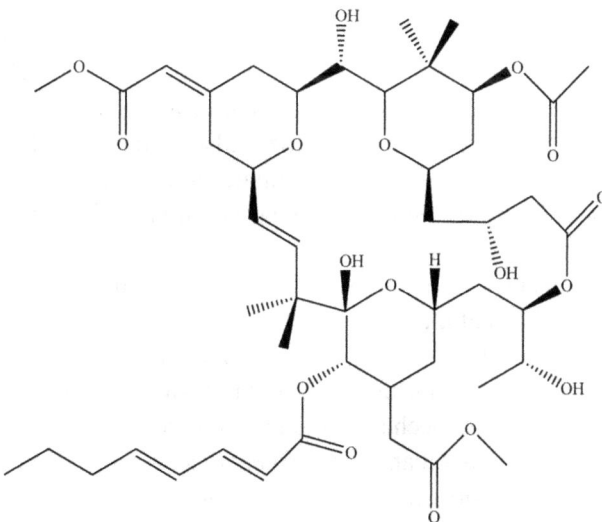

FIGURE 12.2 Structure of Bryostatin.

Marine cyano bacterias or blue-green bacterias are a class of bacterias of biological importance. These are gram-negative prokaryotes with the ability for O_2 photosynthesis, they are generally involved in the process of nitrogen fixation and global carbon flux. Cyanobacteria is an attractive source of anticancer drugs, curacin-A, dolastatin-10 are the two potential anticancer drugs of these bacterias. Curacin is isolated from cyano bacterium *Lyngbya majuscula*. Unique structure of curacin is represented in Figure 12.3. Curacin is characterized by the presence of a terminal alkene in its structure along with a thiazoline ring and a cyclopropyl moiety, they are responsible for its biological structures. The excellent anticancer activities of Curacin make a strong candidate for breast cancer and cancers on lines including colon and renal [11–14].

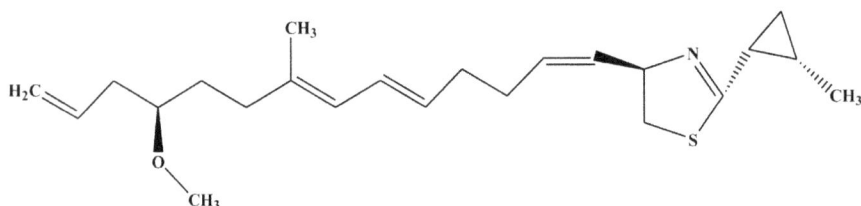

FIGURE 12.3   Structure of Curacin-A.

12.3   SEA WEED FAMILY

These are multicellular organisms (macroalgae) found in the shallow coastal waters greatly they grow in the deep sea. They may be *chlorophyceae, pheophyceae, or rhodophyceae.* Seaweeds have a variety of applications in foods, medicines, textiles, and as fertilizer also. Important phytochemicals such as agar–agar, carrageenan, and alginates are the algae products. Fatty acids, sterols, carotenoids, and polysaccharides are the bioactive compounds in seaweeds [14, 15].

Many biomolecules such as terpenoids, flavonoids, and various polyphenols have shown excellent antioxidant properties also. Brown seaweeds are characterized by its brown color due to the presence of photosynthesis pigment. Kelp, wracks, zonaria, dictyota are class of brown seaweeds. Fucodian is a class of sulfated complex polysaccharide found in brown seaweeds *Ecklonia cava* and *Costaria costata.* Fucodians show excellent anticancer properties in addition to their antiviral, antiadhesive, anti-inflammatory properties. Fucodian is a fucose-containing sulfated complex heteropolysaccharide and its structure highly depending on the species source of isolation, structure of fucodian is given in Figure 12.4. Fucodians are used as an additive in drinks, cosmetics, and health foods [16–18].

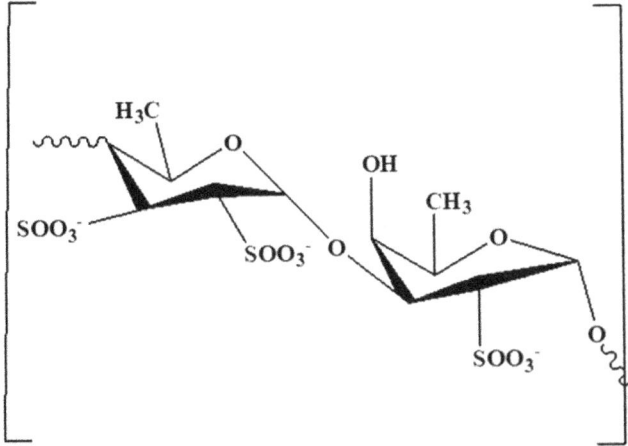

FIGURE 12.4   Structure of fucodian.

Similarly, laminarans are a useful anticancer product isolated from brown algae, namely *Laminaria species* Laminaran is a liner polysaccharide consists of $\beta(1\rightarrow3)$-glucan and $\beta(1\rightarrow6)$-branches. Figure 12.5 shows the structure of the laminarian.

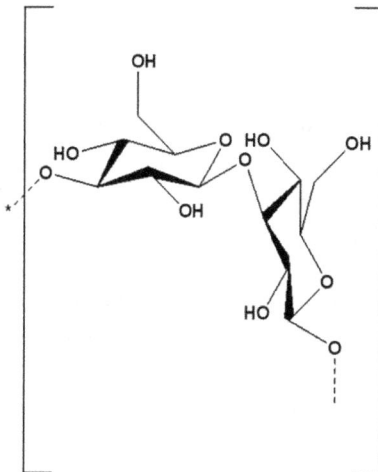

FIGURE 12.5   Structure of laminarian.

12.4   ANTICANCER AGENTS FROM CORAL REEFS

Coral reefs belong to the phylum *cinadria* and they provide habitat to a variety of marine organisms such as fishes, sponges, algae, and other crustaceans. Anticancer properties of corals are studied by various to explore them as potential aids for cancer therapy. Anticancer, anti-inflammatory, and antioxidant activities of corals have been reported already. The first anticancer drug isolated from corals was known under the trade name Cytosar-U*, it is chemically cytosine arabinoside consist of a cytosine base with an arabinose sugar. Cytarabine is mainly used for the treatment of leukaemia and lymphomas [19]. The structure of cytarabine is illustrated in Figure 12.6.

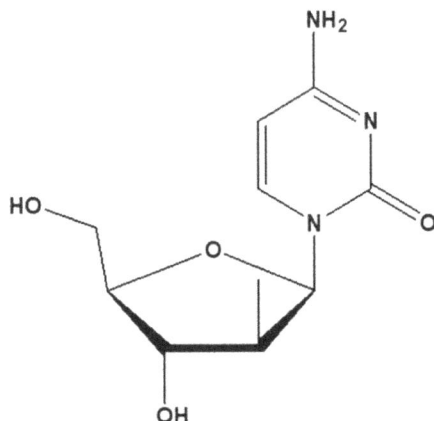

FIGURE 12.6   Structure of cytarabine.

Cytosine arabinoside interferes the synthesis of DNA. The sudden conversion of cytosine arabinoside into cytosine arabinoside triphosphate is an antimetabolic agent against deoxycytidine that prevents DNA synthesis. It is a Food and Drug Administration (FDA) approved anticancer drug from 1969. Halichrondin B is an important polyether macrolide isolated from *Halichondria okadai*. Various research studies report the anticancer properties of Halichrondin B against murine cancer cells. Eribulin is a complete analog Halichrondin B that was first chemically synthesized by Yoshito Kishi and his co-workers at Harvard University. Eribulin anticancer drug is marketed by Eisai.co under the trade name Halaven, it is generally used to treat breast cancer. It works by microtubule mechanism for blocking the growth of cancer cells [20, 21]. Figure 12.7 represents the structure of Eribulin and Halichrondin B.

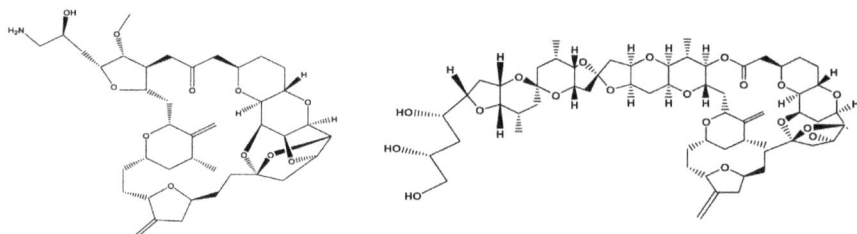

FIGURE 12.7 Structure of eribulin and halichrondin B.

Onnamide-A is a bioactive natural product isolated from marine spongaes and was isolated initially from the banks of Japan. The structure of onnamide-A is similar to pederin. Onnamide consists of a complex structure, as shown in Figure 12.8. Table 12.1 shows the clinical status and source of various anticancer agents.

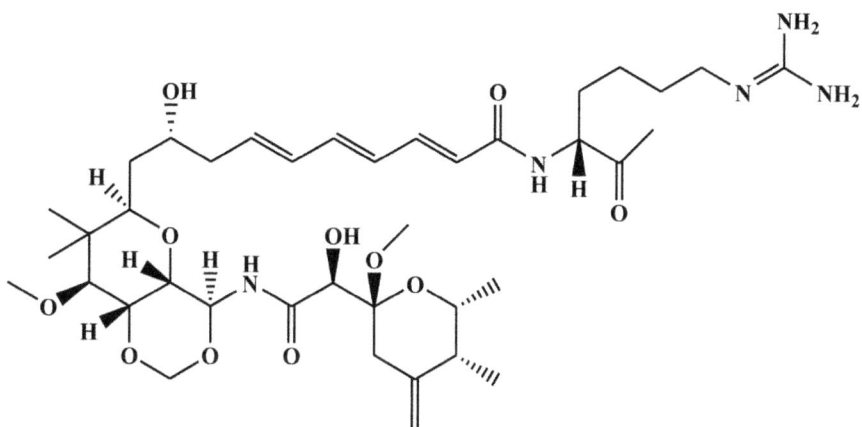

FIGURE 12.8 Structure of onnaminde-A.

12.5 MARINE ALKALOIDS

This term was initially introduced by the pharmacist Meissner in 1819, alkaloid means alkali-like material. Alkaloids are a class of naturally occurring organic nitrogen containing bases, they possess excellent pharmacological activities and are frequently used by mankind. Marine environment is a super source of a variety of alkaloids and chemistry of alkaloid has been studied well in terrestrial plants. Morphine was the first (1805) isolated alkaloid from a terrestrial plant by Kappelmayer, and Hordenine was the first (1969) alkaloid isolated from marine algae [22–25]. Alkaloids were found in the marine environment which is broadly classified into three classes:

1. Phenylethylamine alkaloids
2. Indole and halogenated indole alkaloids
3. Other alkaloids.

TABLE 12.1 Clinical Status and Source of Isolated Marine Drugs

S. No.	Compound Name	Source	Natural Product/ Derivative	Clinical Status
1	Cytarabine	Sponge	Derivative	FDA approved
2	Vidarabine	sponge	Derivative	FDA approved
3	Eribulin mesylate	sponge	Derivative	FDA approved
4	Trabectidin	Tunicate	Natural product	FDA approved
5	Brentuximab	Mollusk	Derivative	FDA approved
6	plitidepsin	Tunicate	Natural product	Phase III
7	Plinabulin	Fungus	Derivative	Phase II
8	Brentuximab vedotin	Mollusk	Derivative	FDA approved
9	Elisidepsin	Mollusk	Derivative	Phase II
10	Zalypsis	Nudibranch	Derivative	Phase II
11	Glembatumumab vedotin	Mollusk	Derivative	Phase II
12	Marizomib	Bacterium	Natural product	Phase II
13	Hemiasterlin	Sponge	Derivative	Phase II

12.5.1 PHENYLETHYLAMINE ALKALOIDS

It is the first class of marine alkaloid which is an aromatic monoamine alkaloid. Phenylethylamine alkaloids (PEA) consist of an ethylamine side chain on a benzene ring, structure is given in Figure 12.9. This is the main precursor of many natural and synthetic compounds. Several simple, as well as substituted phenylethylamines, are used by humans [27, 28]. Tyramine, hordenine, and catecholamine (dopamine) are examples of phenylethylamine. Generally, certain algae are the sources of phenylethylamine, *Desmerestia aculeate* and *Desmerestia viridis are the PEA containing brown algae, similarly Cystoclonium purpureum, Polysiphonia urceolata, Delesseria sanguine, Dumontia incrassate,* and *Ceramium rubrum* are the red algae used for the extraction of PEA. PEA can act as neurotransmitter and neuromodulator, it has been reported that deficiency of PEA can cause a depressive illness in humans. Substituted form of PEA is widely used in the medical area as stimulants, hormones, hallucinogens, and antidepressants, etc. [26, 29, 30].

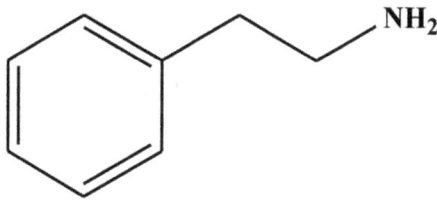

FIGURE 12.9 *Structure of* phenylethylamine.

Tyramine is chemically 4-hydroxyphenylethylamine, this is the mono-amine derivative of the amino acid tyrosine, structure of both tyrosine and Tyramine is given in Figure 12.10 [31]. It was found in red algae *Chondrus crispus &Polysiphonia urceolata and in* brown algae *Laminaria saccharina* Tyramine stimulates the central nervous system, causes vasoconstriction, increased heart rate, blood pressure.

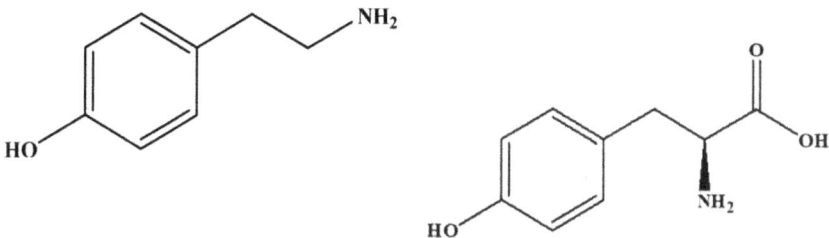

FIGURE 12.10 Structure of tyrosine structure of tyramine.

Dopamine is a type of catechol containing amine, structure of dopamine is represented in Figure 12.11, it is produced in the microorganism by decarboxylation of dihydroxyphenylalanine. Marine green algae *Monostroma fuscum* is the source of dopamine. Dopamine is mainly used as a neurotransmitter [33].

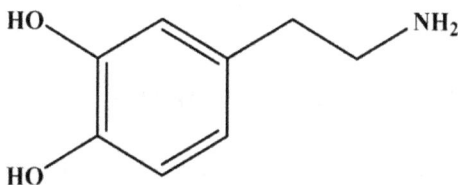

FIGURE 12.11 Structure of dopamine.

12.5.2   INDOLE AND HALOGENATED INDOLE ALKALOIDS

Indole alkaloids are the second class of marine alkaloids and are character-ized by the presence of an indole group or benzopyrrole in its structure, structure of indole is represented in Figure 12.12. Almazolone, martensine, martefragine, caulerpin, denticine, fragilamide, and caulersin are the main classes in this category [23, 34]. Figure 12.13 represents the structure of caulersin.

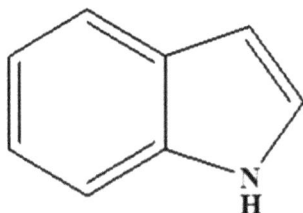

FIGURE 12.12   Structure of indole.

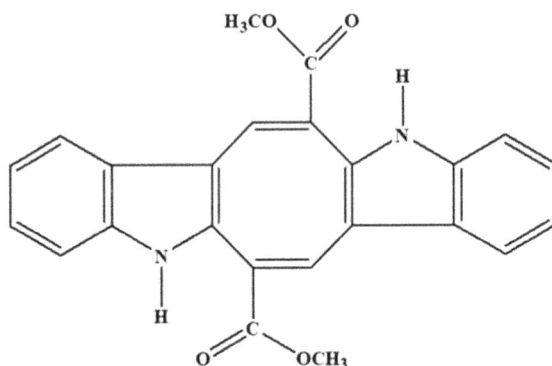

FIGURE 12.13   Structure of caulersin.

Almazolone was isolated from Haraldiophyllum species, it is a disub-stituted oxazolindole derivative. Almazolone has two stereoisomers and the structure of almazolone is represented in Figure 12.14.

12.5.3   HALOGENATED INDOLE ALKALOIDS

The halogenated metabolites from the marine environment are rich in bromine, whereas chlorinated compounds are preferably synthesized by terrestrial organisms. However, iodinated and fluorinated compounds are quite rare. About almost 4000 natural organohalogens were isolated from the marine world. Halogenated indole alkaloids contain an indole group substituted by bromine and chlorine atoms. They were isolated only from marine organisms, not from any terrestrial plants. Plakohypaphorine were first iodinated indoles isolated from Caribbean sponge *Plakortis simplex* and its structure is shown in Figure 12.15. Variolins, meriolins, aplysinopsins are the main classes in halogenated indole alkaloids [35–37].

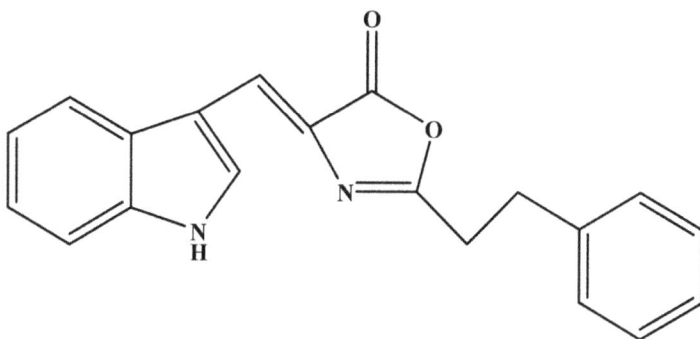

FIGURE 12.14   Structure of almazolone.

Psammopemmins, they are a class of halogenated indole alkaloids, isolated from Antarctic marine sponge *Psammopemma sp.* Psammopemmins consist of A–C, Figure 12.16 represents their structure. In general, 4-hydroxyindole moiety substituted at the 3-position by an unusual 2-bromopyrimidine system, presence of 4-oxygenated indole often exhibits potential pharmacological properties [35, 38, 39].

Aplicyanins are a new family of halogenated indeole alkaloids isolated from Antarctic tunicate *Aplidium cyaneum.* There are six types of aplicyanins, A–F, the structure of apicyanins consists of abromoindole nucleus and a 6-tetrahydropyrimidine substituent at third carbon, structure of aplicyanin is represented in Figure 12.17. They are cytotoxic to the human tumor cell lines such as colorectal carcinoma, lung carcinoma, and breast adenocarcinoma [40, 41].

Lophocladines belong to the third class of marine alkaloids, they are isolated from red algae *Lophocladia species* from New Zealand. Lophocladine A and B are the two types of lophocladines [42] and their chemical structure was given in Figure 12.18.

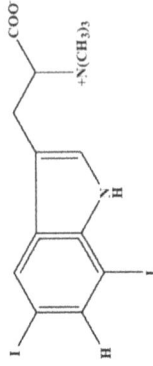

FIGURE 12.15 Structure of plakohypaphorine A, B, and C.

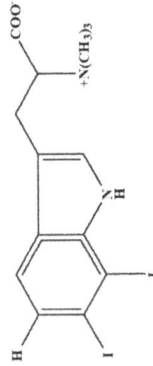

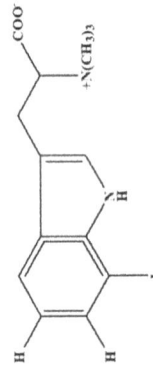

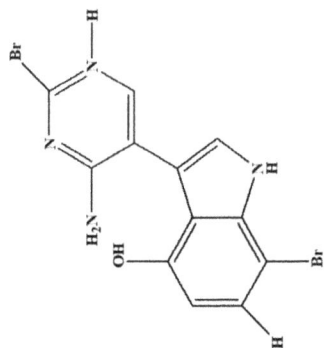

FIGURE 12.16 Psammopemmins A, B, and C.

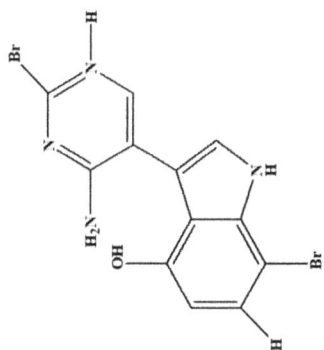

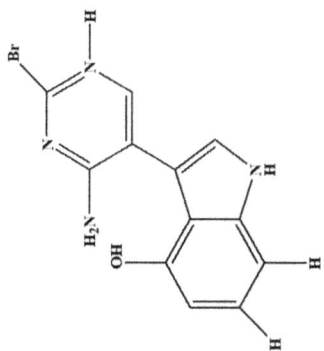

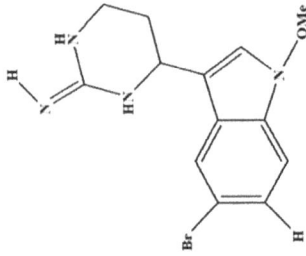

Aplicyanins C

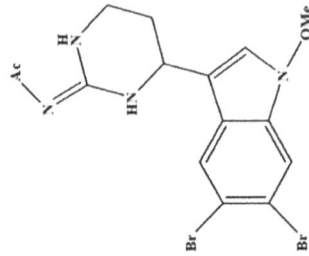

Aplicyanins A

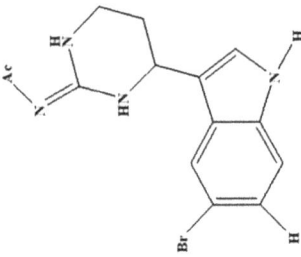

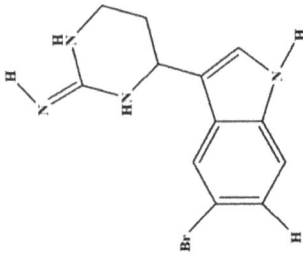

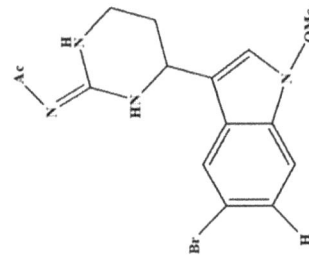

Aplicyanins B

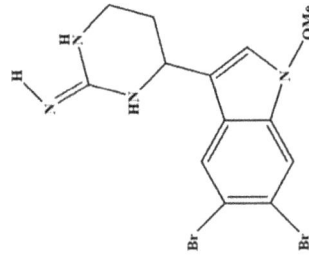

Aplicyanins A

Aplicyanins A

Aplicyanins D

FIGURE 12.17 Structure of aplicyanins.

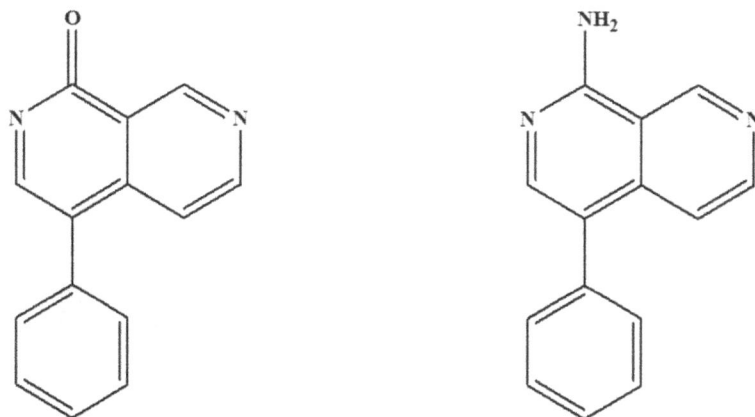

Lophocladines A Lophocladines B

FIGURE 12.18 Structure of lophocladines.

12.6 ISOLATION OF MARINE PRODUCTS

Nature has been a source of several compounds having excellent therapeutic effects on various diseases. There are several strategies used for the isolation of natural products from the source; however, the selection of extraction procedure depends on the nature of source and the type of compound, which is to be isolated. Figure 12.19 represents the typical isolation procedure employed. Isolation of marine products is somewhat more complicated [43, 44].

Marine products may contain extremely liable compounds, hence they are highly unstable and there is a chance to get decompose these products at any step during the purification process. To date, isolation and purification of marine products are time-consuming and costly. Collection and handling of marine organisms are extremely critical, hence several measures should be taken to avoid the decomposing of these unstable compounds also the information and place of collection should be recorded carefully for recollection and subsequent taxonomic identification. Voucher specimens for taxonomic purposes should be prepared by taking a small portion from the entire sample and preserved in formalin (10%)/seawater mixture and for algal samples 5% formalin solution is preferred, for the long-term storage formalin solution was replaced by 70% ethanol. To prevent the chemical degradation, collected samples are immediately lyophilized or kept at −20–0 °C if it is not possible then samples were kept in an ethanol/water mixture. Chromatographic processes are widely used for the isolation of individual

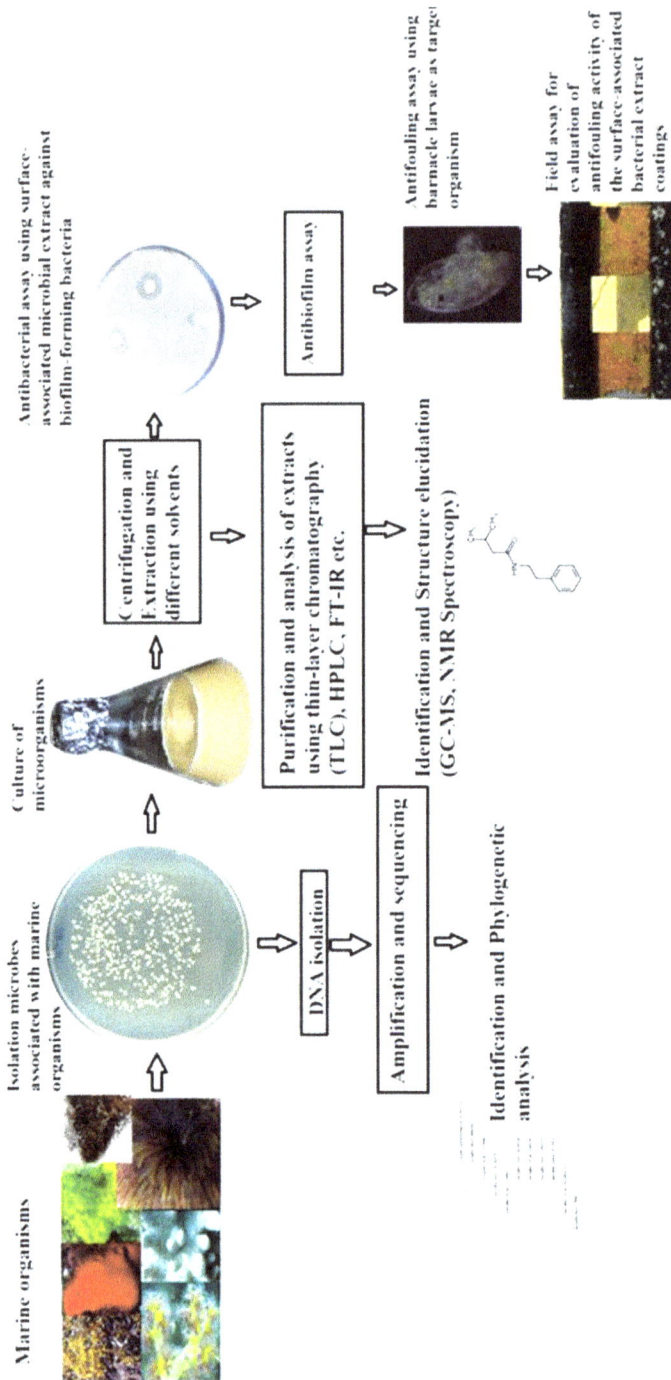

FIGURE 12.19 Flowchart for the isolation of marine product.

components from a mixture. In a chromatographic process, a mixture that is to be get separated is distributed between two phases, mobile phase, and stationary phase. Separation of individual components in a mixture is based on the difference in affinity of the compounds toward stationary and mobile phase. Chromatography can be classified into gas chromatography, liquid chromatography, and supercritical liquid chromatography, according to the nature of the mobile phase [45–49]

Extraction of marine products from the source can be done by three methods, most common method for the extraction is "maceration" with solvent [47]. Here samples are ground into fine particles to ensure the solvent penetration, sometimes enhanced penetration of solvent is carried out using stirring and sonication. Methanol and ethanol are the most preferred solvents for maceration. Filtration or centrifugation of the samples was continued until no extractive yield is obtained and solvent completely removed by rotary evaporation at a temperature <35 °C to avoid the degradation of compounds. The second method was the most efficient method, developed by National Cancer Institute. This method uses the frozen samples, grounded with dry ice and extracted with water at 4 °C. The remaining aqueous extract was removed by centrifugation and the sample was lyophilized. The final product was further successfully extracted with methanol and dichloromethane. The advantage of this method involves the lyophilization of the sample that eliminates the risk of thermal degradation and bumping. The third extraction process is based on the idea of supercritical fluid/supercritical point. The highest temperature and pressure above which there is no difference in between the liquid and this point is refereed as the critical point. Above the critical point, homogenous supercritical fluid is formed. This is the most efficient, fast, and widely used method for extraction [43, 50]

Marine extracts are complex, consist of acidic, basic, neutral lyophilic, and amphiphilic components in them, therefore the fractionation step is divided into four steps, as shown in Figure 12.20.

The first stage in the fractionation step is more important, it deals with the chemistry of material to be isolated as well as the probable impurities. Various sophisticated techniques such as NMR, TLC, and MS were employed for getting well knowledge about the compound. The second stage of fractionation is dereplication, it refers to an attempt to remove duplicate compounds and the third step is the crude fractionation, in this step compounds having similar physicochemical characteristics are separated; simply the unwanted materials are removed by this step, solvent partitioning, desalting, and defatting are the common procedures used for the removal of impurities. Solvent portioning is the most commonly employed method, here the organic extract

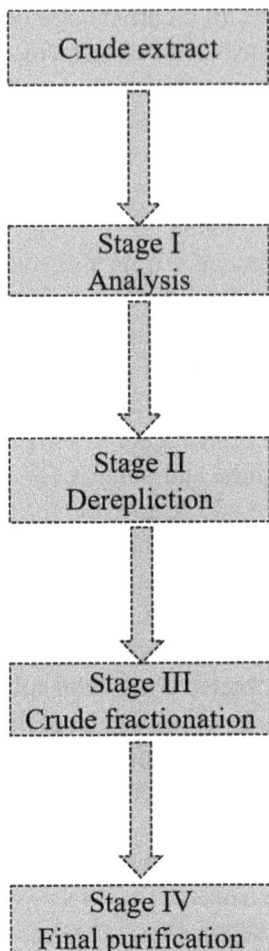

FIGURE 12.20 Fractionation step for marine product isolation.

is suspended in water followed by extraction using dicholromethane, aqueous layer formed was again extracted using secondary butanol, and organic layer was again extracted with hexane [43, 54].

Defatting is used for the removal of unwanted fatty components from the sample, this is usually done by employing sephadex LH-20 and methanol/dichloromethane mixture as solvent generally fats and other nonpolar compounds are eluted first [51, 52]. Desalting is the third method of fractionation, according to the method introduced by West et al., methanolic extract of the sample is passed through a column filled with styrenedivinyl benzene polymer, the resulting eluents are washed frequently with water and again passed to the column until all the hydrophobic components are adsorbed on the resin. The final and last stage in the fractionation step is purification, which is generally carried out using more sophisticated techniques, such as UV-diode array detector [53], evaporative light scattering detector [54], LC-MS [56], LC-NMR [57, 58], and so on.

12.7 CONCLUSIONS

Several anticancer are isolated from the marine world. The bioactive secondary metabolites obtained from the marine environment have outstanding commercial importance. In this chapter, we summarized the various marine anticancer agents that are isolated from various phylum as well as their way of isolation of marine bioactive compounds. We discussed in detail the chemical structure and pharmaceutical prospectus of these drugs, which provided crucial insights and valuable knowledge on the largely unexplored marine anticancer leads. Similarly, various classes of marine alkaloids have been discussed in this chapter; however, most of the alkaloids isolated from marine algae belongs to phenylethylamine and indole groups based on their structure.

KEYWORDS

- **cancer**
- **marine environment**
- **anticancer**
- **drugs**

REFERENCES

1. Simmons, T. L., Andrianasolo, E., McPhail, K., Flatt, P., & Gerwick, W. H. (2005). Marine natural products as anticancer drugs. *Molecular Cancer Therapeutics*, 4(2), 333–342.
2. Venter, J. C., Remington, K., Heidelberg, J. F., Halpern, A. L., Rusch, D., Eisen, J. A., et al. (2004). Environmental genome shotgun sequencing of the Sargasso Sea. *Science*, 304 (5667), 66–74.
3. Gorin, S. S. (2010). Theory, measurement, and controversy in positive psychology, health psychology, and cancer: basics and next steps. *Annals of Behavioral Medicine*, 39(1), 43–47.

4. Williams, D. H., Stone, M. J., Hauck, P. R., & Rahman, S. K. (1989). Why are secondary metabolites (natural products) biosynthesized? *Journal of Natural Products*, 52(6), 1189–1208.

5. Newman, D. J., Cragg, G. M., & Snader, K. M. (2003). Natural products as sources of new drugs over the period 1981–2002. *Journal of Natural Products*, 66(7), 1022–1037.

6. Sithranga Boopathy, N., & Kathiresan, K. (2010). Anticancer drugs from marine flora: an overview. *Journal of Oncology*, 2010, 1–17.

7. Kathiresan, K., & Duraisamy, A. (2005). Current issue of microbiology. *ENVIS Centre Newsletters*, 4, 3–5.

8. Hugenholtz, P., & Pace, N. R. (1996). Identifying microbial diversity in the natural environment: a molecular phylogenetic approach. *Trends in Biotechnology*, 14(6), 190–197.

9. Fenical, W. (1993). Chemical studies of marine bacteria: developing a new resource. *Chemical Reviews*, 93(5), 1673–1683.

10. Uzair, B., Tabassum, S., Rasheed, M., & Rehman, S. F. (2012). Exploring marine cyano-bacteria for lead compounds of pharmaceutical importance. *The Scientific World Journal*, 2012, 1–10

11. Jensen, P. R., & Fenical, W. (2000). Marine microorganisms and drug discovery: current status and future potential. In: Drugs from the Sea, 6–29.

12. Williams, P. G. (2009). Panning for chemical gold: marine bacteria as a source of new therapeutics. *Trends in Biotechnology*, 27(1), 45–52.

13. Fenical, W., Jensen, P. R., Palladino, M. A., Lam, K. S., Lloyd, G. K., & Potts, B. C. (2009). Discovery and development of the anticancer agent salinosporamide A (NPI-0052). *Bioorganic & Medicinal Chemistry*, 17(6), 2175–2180.

14. Gerwick, W. H., & Fenner, A. M. (2013). Drug discovery from marine microbes. *Microbial Ecology*, 65(4), 800–806.

15. Pal, A., Kamthania, M. C., & Kumar, A. (2014). Bioactive compounds and properties of seaweeds—a review. *Open Access Library Journal*, 1(4), 1–17.

16. Blunt, J. W., Copp, B. R., Munro, M. H., Northcote, P. T., & Prinsep, M. R. (2003). Marine natural products. *Natural Product Reports*, 20(1), 1–48.

17. Tang, H. F., Yi, Y. H., Yao, X. S., Xu, Q. Z., Zhang, S. Y., & Lin, H. W. (2002). Bioactive steroids from the brown alga Sargassum carpophyllum. *Journal of Asian Natural Products Research*, 4(2), 95–101.

18. Lins, K. O., Bezerra, D. P., Alves, A. P. N., Alencar, N. M., Lima, M. W., Torres, V. M., et al. (2009). Antitumor properties of a sulfated polysaccharide from the red seaweed Champia feldmannii (Diaz-Pifferer). *Journal of Applied Toxicology*, 29(1), 20–26.

19. Lindel, T., Jensen, P. R., Fenical, W., Long, B. H., Casazza, A. M., Carboni, J., & Fairchild, C. R. (1997). Eleutherobin, a new cytotoxin that mimics paclitaxel (Taxol) by stabilizing microtubules. *Journal of the American Chemical Society*, 119(37), 8744–8745.

20. Berman, E., Heller, G., Santorsa, J., McKenzie, S., Gee, T., Kempin, S., ... & Gabrilove, J. (1991). Results of a randomized trial comparing idarubicin and cytosine arabinoside with daunorubicin and cytosine arabinoside in adult patients with newly diagnosed acute myelogenous leukemia. *Blood,* 77(8), 1666–1674.

21. Chu, M. Y., & Fischer, G. A. (1965). Comparative studies of leukemic cells sensitive and resistant to cytosine arabinoside. *Biochemical Pharmacology*, 14(3), 333–341.

22. Bergmann, W., & Feeney, R. J. (1950). The isolation of a new thymine pentoside from sponges1. *Journal of the American Chemical Society*, 72(6), 2809–2810.

23. França, P. H., Barbosa, D. P., da Silva, D. L., Ribeiro, Ê. A., Santana, A. E., Santos, B. V., et al. (2014). Indole alkaloids from marine sources as potential leads against infectious diseases. *BioMed Research International*, 2014, 1–12.

24. Ang, K. K., Holmes, M. J., Higa, T., Hamann, M. T., & Kara, U. A. (2000). In vivo antimalarial activity of the beta-carboline alkaloid manzamine A. *Antimicrobial Agents and Chemotherapy*, 44(6), 1645–1649.

25. Güven, K. C., Percot, A., & Sezik, E. (2010). Alkaloids in marine algae. *Marine Drugs*, 8(2), 269–284.

26. Pelletier, S. W. (1970). Chemistry of the alkaloids. Van Nostrand Reinhold.

27. Güven, K. C., Percot, A., & Sezik, E. (2010). Alkaloids in marine algae. *Marine Drugs*, 8(2), 269–284.

28. Guven, K. C., Bora, A., & Sunam, G. (1969). Alkaloid content of marine algae. I. Hordenine from Phyllophora nervosa. *Eczacılık Bul*, 11, 177–184.

29. Guven, K. C., Bora, A., & Sunam, G. (1970). Hordenine from the alga Phyllophora nervosa. *Acta Pharmaceutica Sciencia*, 49(2), 127–132.

30. Barroso, N., & Rodriguez, M. (1996). Action of β-phenylethylamine and related amines on nigrostriatal dopamine neurotransmission. *European Journal of Pharmacology*, 297(3), 195–203.

31. Kneifel, H., Meinicke, M., & Soeder, Ç. J. (1977). Analysis of amines in algae by high-performance liquid-chromatography. *Journal of Phycology*, 13, 36–36.

32. Tocher, R. D., & Tocher, C. A. (1969). Biosynthesis of 3-hdroxy tyramine in plants Enz. Dopa decarboxylaze XI. *Photochemistry*, 9, 1893.

33. Liu, H., Mishima, Y., Fujiwara, T., Nagai, H., Kitazawa, A., Mine, Y., et al. (2004). Isolation of araguspongine M, a new stereoisomer of an araguspongine/xestospongin alkaloid, and dopamine from the marine sponge Neopetrosia exigua collected in Palau. *Marine Drugs*, 2(4), 154–163.

34. Chen, Y. F., Kuo, P. C., Chan, H. H., Kuo, I. J., Lin, F. W., Su, C. R., et al. (2010). β-carboline alkaloids from Stellaria dichotoma var. lanceolata and their anti-inflammatory activity. *Journal of Natural Products*, 73(12), 1993–1998.

35. Pauletti, P. M., Cintra, L. S., Braguine, C. G., Cunha, W. R., & Januário, A. H. (2010). Halogenated indole alkaloids from marine invertebrates. *Marine Drugs*, 8(5), 1526–1549.

36. Gribble, G. W. (2004). Natural organohalogens: a new frontier for medicinal agents? *Journal of Chemical Education*, 81(10), 1441.

37. Campagnuolo, C., Fattorusso, E., & Taglialatela-Scafati, O. (2003). Plakohypaphorines A−C, iodine-containing alkaloids from the caribbean sponge plakortis simplex. *European Journal of Organic Chemistry*, 2003(2), 284–287.

38. Walker, S. R., Carter, E. J., Huff, B. C., & Morris, J. C. (2009). Variolins and related alkaloids. *Chemical Reviews*, 109(7), 3080–3098.

39. Butler, M. S., Capon, R. J., & Lu, C. C. (1992). Psammopemmins (AC), novel brominated 4-hydroxyindole alkaloids from an Antarctic sponge, Psammopemma sp. *Australian Journal of Chemistry*, 45(11), 1871–1877.

40. Reyes, F., Fernandez, R., Rodriguez, A., Francesch, A., Taboada, S., Avila, C., & Cuevas, C. (2008). Aplicyanins A–F, new cytotoxic bromoindole derivatives from the marine tunicate Aplidium cyaneum. *Tetrahedron*, 64(22), 5119–5123.

41. Šíša, M., Pla, D., Altuna, M., Francesch, A., Cuevas, C., Albericio, F., & Álvarez, M. (2009). Total synthesis and antiproliferative activity screening of (±)-Aplicyanins A, B and E and related analogues. *Journal of Medicinal Chemistry*, 52(20), 6217–6223.

42. Gross, H., Goeger, D. E., Hills, P., Mooberry, S. L., Ballantine, D. L., Murray, T. F., et al. (2006). Lophocladines, bioactive alkaloids from the red alga Lophocladia sp. *Journal of Natural Products*, 69(4), 640–644.
43. Cannell, R. J. (1998). How to approach the isolation of a natural product. In: Natural Products Isolation. Humana Press, 1–51.
44. Rodríguez, J., Nieto, R. M., & Crews, P. (1993). New structures and bioactivity patterns of bengazole alkaloids from a Choristid marine sponge. *Journal of Natural Products*, 56(12), 2034–2040.
45. Rashid, M. A., Gustafson, K. R., Cartner, L. K., Pannell, L. K., & Boyd, M. R. (2001). New nitrogenous constituents from the South African marine Ascidian Pseudodistoma sp. *Tetrahedron*, 57(27), 5751–5755.
46. Chang, L. C., Otero-Quintero, S., Nicholas, G. M., & Bewley, C. A. (2001). Phyllolactones A–E: new bishomoscalarane sesterterpenes from the marine sponge Phyllospongia lamellosa. *Tetrahedron*, 57(27), 5731–5738.
47. Cannell, R. J. (Ed.). (1998). Natural products isolation (Vol. 4). Springer Science & Business Media.
48. Zhou, S., & Hamburger, M. (1996). Application of liquid chromatography-atmospheric pressure ionization mass spectrometry in natural product analysis evaluation and optimization of electrospray and heated nebulizer interfaces. *Journal of Chromatography A*, 755(2), 189–204.
49. Silva, G. L., Lee, I. S., & Kinghorn, A. D. (1998). Special problems with the extraction of plants. In: Natural Products Isolation. Humana press, 343–363.
50. Kupchan, S. M., Britton, R. W., Ziegler, M. F., & Sigel, C. W. (1973). Bruceantin, a new potent antileukemic simaroubolide from Brucea antidysenterica. *The Journal of Organic Chemistry*, 38(1), 178–179.
51. West, L. M., Northcote, P. T., & Battershill, C. N. (2000). Peloruside A: a potent cytotoxic macrolide isolated from the New Zealand marine sponge Mycale sp. *The Journal of Organic Chemistry*, 65(2), 445–449.
52. West, L. M., Northcote, P. T., Hood, K. A., Miller, J. H., & Page, M. J. (2000). Mycalamide D, a new cytotoxic amide from the New Zealand marine sponge Mycale species. *Journal of Natural Products*, 63(5), 707–709.
53. Stead, P. (1998). Isolation by preparative HPLC. In: Natural Products Isolation. Humana Press, 165–208.
54. Allgeier, M. C., Nussbaum, M. A., & Risley, D. S. (2003). Comparison of an evaporative light-scattering detector and a chemiluminescent nitrogen detector for analyzing compounds lacking a sufficient UV chromophore. *Lc Gc North America*, 21(4), 376–381.
55. Bobzin, S. C., Yang, S., & Kasten, T. P. (2000). LC-NMR: a new tool to expedite the dereplication and identification of natural products. *Journal of Industrial Microbiology and Biotechnology*, 25(6), 342–345.
56. Pannell, L. K., & Shigematsu, N. (1998). Increased speed and accuracy of structural determination of biologically active natural products using LC-MS. *American laboratory (Fairfield)*, 30(7), 28–30.
57. Pullen, F. S., Swanson, A. G., Newman, M. J., & Richards, D. S. (1995). 'On-line' liquid chromatography/nuclear magnetic resonance mass spectrometry—a powerful spectroscopic tool for the analysis of mixtures of pharmaceutical interest. *Rapid Communications in Mass Spectrometry*, 9(11), 1003–1006.

CHAPTER 13

Recent Advances in Scaffold Fabrication Techniques for Tissue Engineering

B. SWATHY KRISHNA[1*], and K. VANDANA[2]

[1]Central Institute of Plastic Engineering and Technology, Institute of Plastic Technology, Kochi, Kerala, India

[2]Quality Department, Quess Group of Companies, Bengaluru, India

*Corresponding author. E-mail: swathybhaskaran94@gmail.com

ABSTRACT

Tissue engineering is a boon to medical science as an alternative for organ transplantation and related problems. Human stem cells are allowed to grow in an artificial support, which can provide nutrients for the growth of cells to produce new tissues; these mechanical support/scaffolds are the backbone of tissue engineering. Scaffolds are preparing using various biocompatible polymers and ceramics. Several features of scaffolds are considered while the preparation for obtaining excellent cell adhesion and proliferation such as biocompatibility of the material, mechanical strength, and structural integrity of scaffolds. Most of the structural features depend upon the mechanism of preparation. In general, the techniques employed for scaffold preparation are classified into two classes such as conventional methods and rapid prototyping (RP) techniques. Several conventional techniques such as solvent casting and melt molding do not need any complex machinery whereas RP techniques are sophisticated techniques using complex machineries; stereolithography and 3D bioprinting are some of the efficient RP techniques, which are capable of scaffolds with high structural properties than conventional techniques. In this chapter, we deeply discuss the recent advances in conventional and RP techniques for scaffold preparation.

13.1 INTRODUCTION

Tissue engineering is an interesting field of science that promises a wonderful future to medical science. A few years ago, autografts and allografts were the important tissue or organ repair methods, but there are some adverse effects such as immune rejection, cell morbidity, unavailability of donors, and pathogen transfer behind these surgical procedures. Tissue engineering is the only efficient alternative for these methods and problems related to organ transplantation. It is the culture of cells in an in-vitro environment with the aid of interdisciplinary sciences such as chemistry, biological sciences, material science, and engineering. Here, stem cells are allowed to grow inside a mechanical support by feeding growth factors to produce functional tissues to repair the damaged organ. Enormous developments had been taken place in this field for the last two decades [1–5].

WT Green, an orthopedic surgeon, first proposed in the early 1970s that it would be possible to culture cells in predesigned biocompatible scaffolds. Later on, in 1988, Dr Vacanti at the Massachusetts Institute of Technology and Dr Langer at Boston Children's Hospital in Boston reported for the first time about culture of functional tissue equivalents by using branching network of synthetic biodegradable polymer scaffold and the journey of advanced tissue engineering started from here [6–8].

Scaffolds are artificial support for cells to grow using the signaling molecules, which are the essential proteins for cell growth [5]. Biocompatible polymers and ceramics are using for scaffold preparation. The common biomaterials include natural polymers such as collagen, fibrin, alginates, hyaluronic acid, and ceramics such as hydroxyapatite and bioglass. Materials property and scaffold parameters are crucial factor for determining the proper growth of cells. A scaffold degrades gradually inside the body with growth of cells. So, it should be biocompatible and should not make any toxins. Scaffold architecture also plays an important role in growth of cells, which, in turn, depends on the fabrication method of scaffold and parameters [9]. Scaffolds can be prepared through two different ways, which are known as conventional techniques and rapid prototyping (RP) techniques. Conventional techniques such as solvent casting, gas foaming, and phase separation have been using from the birth of tissue engineering concept. RP techniques began to use in tissue engineering from late 1980s. Both techniques have acquired potential developments in recent years.

13.2 BIOMATERIALS

"Any substance, other than a drug, or a combination of substances, synthetic or a natural in origin, which can be used for any period of time, as a whole or as a part of a system, which treats, augments, or replaces any tissue, organ, or function of the body" is the definition given by Chester in a conference held at UK in 1982. Biomaterials can be both natural and synthetic materials, which can be used inside the biological system for a therapeutic effect. Biocompatibility is the main property of a biomaterial should have and it defines the ability to sink with cellular environment to promote cell adhesion. Same like biocompatibility, bioactivity is another important property of the biomaterial which is the ability of a biomaterial to mimic the extracellular matrix or to recognize the cellular environment and activities related to correspondent cellular region. Biodegradability is another inevitable property that a biomaterial should have to successfully implant in biological system. Materials should degrade in accordance with the cell proliferation without making any toxic byproducts. Biomaterials are being used for drug delivery, biosensors, medical implants, and tissue engineering for decades. Polymers, ceramics, glasses, and living tissues itself can be used as biomaterials. Protein-based biomaterials such as silk, collagen, fibrin, gelatin, and polysaccharides such as alginate, hyaluronan, and chitosan (CS) are the naturally-derived biomaterials. Synthetic polymers such as polyvinyl alcohol, polyethylene glycol (PEG), and poly(lactic-*co*-glycolic acid) Poly- lactic- co- glycolic acid (PLGA) are some of the common materials used for tissue engineering. Alumina, zirconia, hydroxyapatite, and bioglass are some of the bioceramics for tissue engineering [9–11].

13.3 SCAFFOLDS

Properties and parameters of scaffold fabrication techniques are also crucial as properties of biomaterials. Properties, such as porosity, which is essential for good cell proliferation and mechanical strength, and surface modifications, depend upon the fabrication methods and parameters. Scaffolds are of three types of bioinert and such kinds of materials have minimal interaction with body such as bone replacement with steel. Bioactive scaffolds are opposite to bioinert scaffolds, having an interaction with surroundings such as hydroxyapatite. Next class is bioresorbable scaffolds, which are using for tissue engineering having interaction with surroundings and gradually degrade inside the biological environment without any toxic residues. Another classification is on the basis of structures, which are 3D porous scaffolds, nanofibers, and hydrogel scaffolds. Nanofibers are usually preparing by electrospinning. Polycaprolactone (PCL), CS, and polyvinyl alcohol are the most suitable materials for electrospinning. Nanofibers can have better mechanical strength than a glass/metal composite and good surface volume ratio with good homogeneous porosity compared to other kind of scaffolds. Hydrogel scaffolds are highly water absorbable mainly prepared by the materials such as gelatin, collagen, fibrin, polyacrylic acid, and polyvinyl alcohol. Low mechanical strength limits their utility in scaffold preparation for tissue engineering and normally it is used for encapsulation growth factors for drug delivery [12, 13].

13.3.1   DESIGN PARAMETERS FOR SCAFFOLD DEVELOPMENTS

Biocompatibility is not a point to discuss here as everyone knows that it is the inevitable part of scaffold whether it is polymer or ceramic; it should be capable to gradually degrade with the growth of cells in in-vivo environment and should mimic the natural extracellular matrix without any immune rejection.

Porosity of the prepared scaffold determines the strength of the scaffold depending upon the material. Even though porosity is essential for the adhesion and proliferation of cells, proper vascularization, and passage of signaling molecules, highly porous structure will probably reduce mechanical strength of the scaffold. Macropores having size more than 50 nm are usually preparing according to the required mechanical strength and host tissue. Generally, a pore size of 20 μm is needed for fibroblast growth, 200–400 μm for bone tissue formation, 20 μm for hepatocyte cells, 5 μm for neovascularization, 20–125 μm for mammalian tissue formation, etc. Mechanical support to the growing cells by the scaffold is as important as pore size that scaffold should be capable of bearing external stress such as new tissues will bear. Mechanical properties such as tensile modulus, compressive strength, and flexural modulus should match the extracellular matrix. Mechanical properties are inversely proportional to pore density as shown in Figure 13.1. Increase in porosity decreases mechanical strength.

Mechanical modulus for hard tissue ranges between 10 and 1500 MPa and for soft tissue, it is between 0.4 and 350 MPa. Biomaterial can be functionalized to increase the adhesion, biocompatibility, and mechanical modulus. Cell adhesion can be achieved through processing techniques such as electrospinning and 3D bioprinting. High surface volume ratio fibers are possible to spin through electrospinning that can increase the cell adhesion without any compromise in mechanical properties. Research is going onto modify the factors such as hydrophilicity/hydrophobicity, surface charge, surface roughness of the polymer material along with grafting of external moieties, or surface coatings including conducting polymers [12–18].

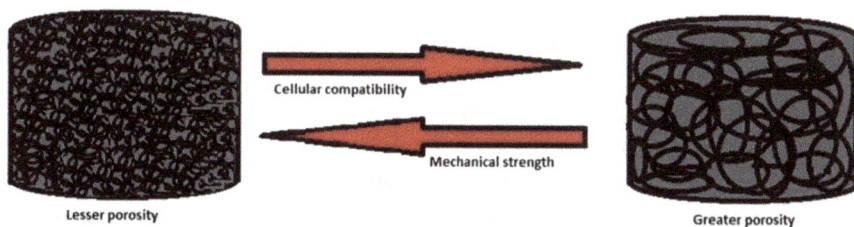

FIGURE 13.1 Schematic representation of the relation between scaffold and mechanical strength (reprinted from [1], copyright (2020), with permission from Elsevier).

Conducting polymers such as polyaniline, polypyrrole, and polythiophene and derivatives can effectively transform to biomaterials due to tunable physical and chemical properties including biocompatibility and response of tissues in brain, heart, and neural tissues toward electrical stimulation that can help in the proliferation of cells. Recently, Sanjairaj et al. fabricated conductive and bioprintable hydrogels based on collagen and block copolymer of polypyrrole and PCL for neural tissue scaffolds, which have shown better biocompatibility and bioprintability [19].

Solid freeform techniques and conventional methods are two kinds of fabrication methods, which have been using for decades to prepare scaffolds in which conventional methods are simple methods which are suitable to prepare highly porous scaffolds but better mechanical properties are difficult to achieve and solid freeform techniques or RP techniques work based on predesigned computer-aided design (CAD) and sophisticated machines such as bioprinter [20, 21].

13.4 CONVENTIONAL TECHNIQUES

Comparatively easy method for preparing highly porous interconnects but minimum mechanical properties, use of toxic solvents, and difficulty to control the design parameters reduced the utilization to soft-tissue repairs and other suitable scaffolds. Solid freeform techniques or RP techniques deposit the biomaterial that can be polymerized by photopolymerization or temperature on a platform through layer-by-layer to mold a complete design. Control of design and high porosity without any compromise in mechanical properties are the better characteristics of solid freeform techniques. Limited availability of suitable material is a big issue facing by the modern techniques.

13.4.1   SOLVENT CASTING/PARTICULATE LEACHING

Simplest method for preparing highly porous scaffold material in which selected salt solution contains predetermined salt particle with specific diameter in a suitable solvent is mixed with a polymer solution and allows the solvent to evaporate leaving a salt polymer mixture. Leaching of salt particle can give a highly interconnected porous scaffold.

Sola et al. utilized solvent casting/particulate leaching technique to prepare scaffolds, which can mimic bone marrow niche. They have used rigid polymethyl methacrylate and flexible polyurethane as polymers and sodium chloride as porogen. Prepared scaffolds have shown 82%–91% porosity (as shown in Figure 13.2) and better mechanical property. HS-5 cells cultured along with leukemic cells have shown better proliferation than leukemic cells, which are due to protective or prosurvival action of HS-5 cells [22]. Recently, Jamshidi et al. fabricated nanoclay reinforced starch-PCL scaffolds through solvent casting–salt leaching method for bone tissue engineering. Resulted scaffold material has high mechanical modulus of about 5.8 MPa and a porosity of 70%. Inclusion of montmorillonite nano-clays decreased the contact angle from 133° to 122° and, thus, increased the hydrophilicity [23].

However, the technique is easy and cheap to carry out without any complex equipment; it is difficult to control the shape of pores and inner connectivity. Even if solvents are evaporating, traces of some of the toxic solvents can affect the cell growth and denature the proteins. Difficulty in salt leaching is also problem related to this technique.

Chia et al. found an enhanced solvent casting/particulate leaching technique to develop the homogeneous distribution of porogens to get equal density of pores and good interconnectivity. They produced bioglass incorporated polyurethane scaffolds by particle leaching followed by centrifugation at different rpm ranged from 1500 to 3000. The centrifugation caused homogeneous distribution of porogens. The estimated porosity was about 88%–90%, which is about 8% higher than scaffolds prepared by normal SCPL method [24].

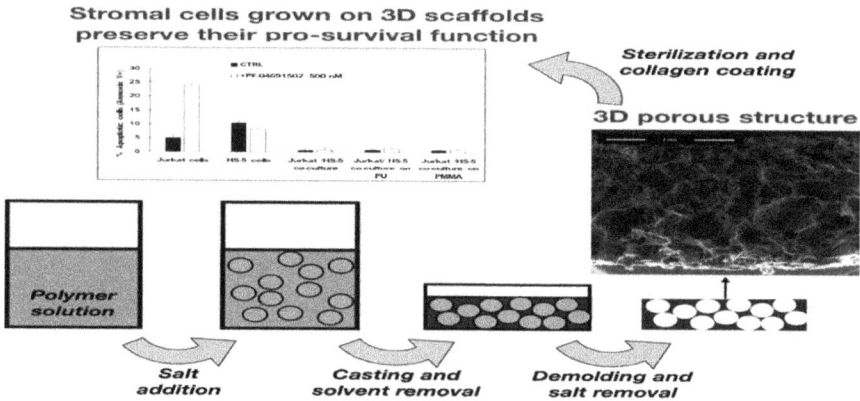

FIGURE 13.2 Schematic representation of solvent casting technique (reprinted from [22], copyright (2019), with permission from Elsevier).

13.4.2 MELT MOLDING

Thermoplastic biomaterials can be easily molded to a scaffold material by melting it above the glass transition temperature. The molten material then poured into an appropriate mold that can produce good porous scaffold without the use of toxic solvents. It can be used in tandem with particle leaching to prepare suitable porosity. Injection molding, compression molding, and extrusion molding are the main approaches using for melt molding as shown in Figure 13.3 which represents the melt molding using compression mold [25]. Highly porous structure can produce with melt molding. A combination of melt molding with solvent particulate leaching or phase separation can favor the better pore formation. Most of the biomaterials are susceptible to thermal degradation, so materials having high melting temperature are more suitable than materials having low melting temperature. D mao et al. recently fabricated PCL/58s bioactive glass-sodium alginate/gelatin hybrid scaffold for bone tissue engineering through a modified melt molding technology. PCL–bioglass composite was prepared by solvent casting and sodium/gelatin composite microspheres were prepared by a syringe dropping method that was used as a porogen while melt molding process. Scaffold showed good porosity and cell adhesion. This simple modified two-step process could be potential technique for bone tissue engineering [26].Oh et al. evaluated the biodegradability of polydioxanone-*b*-PCL scaffolds using melt molding particulate leaching technology. Scaffolds with higher polydioxanone content have shown much more degradation kinetics than other scaffolds. Scaffaro et al. investigated on solvent less melt molding selective leaching technology for preparing PCL/PEG scaffolds. Three-layered scaffolds were prepared by compression molding and porogens leached out with water. Scaffolds showed good biocompatibility with 70% porosity [27]. These are found to be useful in bone-cartilage interface tissue engineering.

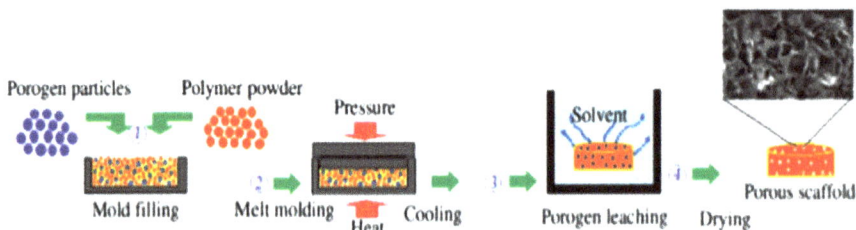

FIGURE 13.3   Melt molding using compression mold (reprinted from [25], copyright (2019), with permission from Elsevier).

13.4.3   GAS FOAMING

An effective method to reduce the use of toxic solvents and high temperature was first proposed by Nam et al. in 2000. Carbon dioxide dissolves under high pressure about 5.5 MPa in polymer solution at room temperature. Pore nucleation can be done by reducing the pressure of carbon dioxide, which can make a phase separation of carbon dioxide from polymer solution and leaving it as a porous scaffold. The supercritical fluid can act as a plasticizer to reduce the glass transition temperature or crystallization temperature to initiate pore formation inside it. Porogens can add to modify the pore size and shape. Porosities as high as 90% with pore sizes from 200 to 500 μm are attained using this technique. Pore interconnectivity and low mechanical strength are still remains to be solved. Crystalline materials are not suitable for gas foaming, as it is difficult to decrease the glass transition temperature. So, mostly semicrystalline or amorphous materials are suitable for this technique.

Iman et al. recently used gas foaming technique to synthesize scaffolds of polypropylene blended with starch and bioglass as supplement particles to improve the mechanical strength. Porosity was around 100–500 μm. The optimized parameters such as temperature and pressure resulted in a material having good mechanical property and in-vitro cell proliferation assays have shown the materials suitability for cell proliferation and nontoxicity. Figure 13.4 represents the screw for bone fixation prepared by polypropylene carbonate (PPC)-starch-bioglass blend [26].

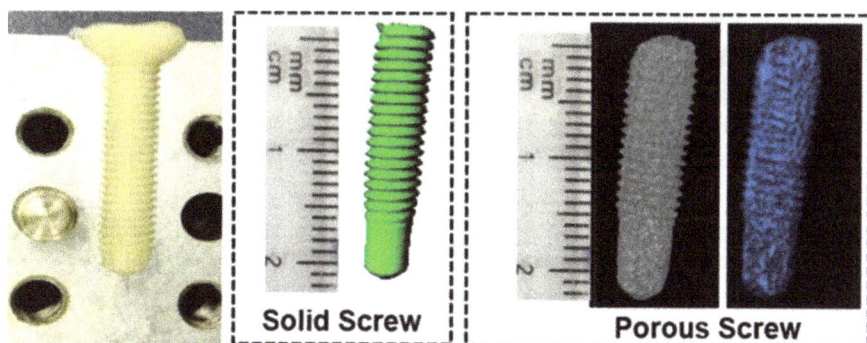

FIGURE 13.4 (A) Melt molded PPC-starch-bioglass screw, (B) the constructed image of the solid screw, and (C) the reconstructed images of porous implant scanned with micro-CT (reprinted from [28], copyright (2018), with permission from Elsevier).

Poursamar et al. fabricated gelatin scaffolds stabilized by glutaraldehyde using modified gas foaming technology. Gelatin has a superior foaming capacity. Stabilization with glutaraldehyde formed cross-linking between gelatin molecules, which have increased the mechanical properties and porosity of the scaffolds. Cytotoxicity assays showed that glutaraldehyde is nontoxic to cells. So, this modified gas foaming technique is suitable to prepare better scaffolds for tissue engineering than normal gas foaming [29].

13.4.4 PHASE SEPARATION

Mikos et al. proposed phase separation technique in which polymer is dissolved in phenol or naphthalene-like suitable solvents followed by dispersion of bioactive molecules. A phase separation or two phases of polymer solution containing high concentration and low concentration of polymer are created by lowering the temperature. Three-dimensional nanofibers can be created by quenching the separated liquid phase to solid phase and evaporation or extraction of solvents. Two kinds of phase separation are there such as solid–liquid phase separation and liquid–liquid phase separation. In solid–liquid phase separation, polymer-rich part acts as a matrix and polymer-less part acts as pores after solvent evaporation while in liquid–liquid phase separation, polymer-less part dissolves in solvent and becomes like a tunnel after evaporation of solvent. Homogeneous pores can be prepared from solvent to liquid phase separation but liquid–liquid separation method cannot provide homogeneous and good interconnected pores [30]. Selection of solvents and temperature is of great importance to create phase separation because it is not possible with all solvents. A phase inversion can be done by precipitating polymer solution in water too. Water-soluble polymers such as collagen and polysaccharides have proven their efficiency to use with phase separation.

Salehi et al. prepared poly-L-lactic acid (PLLA)/CS scaffolds for neural tissue repair through solid–liquid phase separation. The prepared PLLA/CS scaffolds had shown 87.55% porosity and better cell proliferation, which could be due to the hydrophilicity of PLLA and cationic charge of CS with high mechanical properties [31].

Wang et al. proposed a dual-phase separation method for better biodegradation of PLLA. PLLA is miscible with PLGA but not with PCL. So, PCL acts as a porogen while phase separation. Mechanical properties, porosity, and degradation increased as compared to previous work due to the addition of PLGA. Such kind of ternary or multinary systems are useful for modifying the properties of scaffolds [32].

13.4.5 FREEZE DRYING

Freeze drying is an industrial process for removing water content of industrial products. It is also known as lyophilization or cryodesiccation. In this method (shown in Figure 13.5), surrounding pressure of the material reduced after freezing the polymer material under 0 °C and then water sublimed directly using enough heat or vacuum distillation. Thus, we can prepare satisfactory porous scaffold without use of any porogens because ice crystals formed during freezing itself act as porogens. Surfactants such as water-soluble polyurethane are needed for stabilize the emulsion.

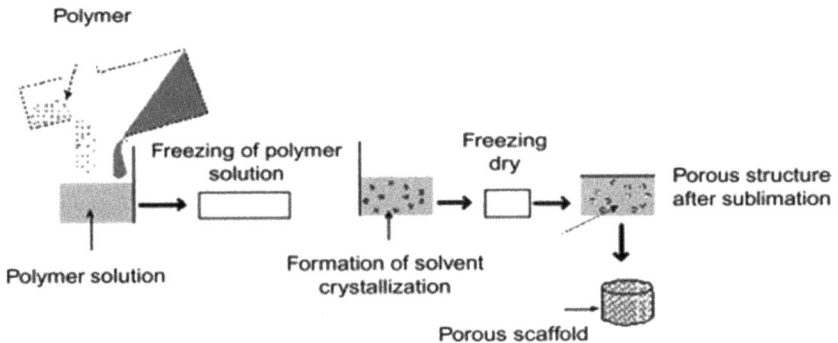

FIGURE 13.5 Schematic representation of freeze drying process (reprinted from [68], copyright (2019), with permission from Elsevier).

Recently, Khan et al. fabricated grafted beta-glucan/hydroxyapatite scaffolds coated with silver through freeze drying method. Prepared scaffold has shown good mechanical strength as a cancellous bone and better porosity [33]. Shahbazarab et al. fabricated highly porous scaffold for bone tissue engineering with more than two compounds. They have incorporated zein, a vegetable protein with CS and hydroxyapatite. Zein scaffolds have good porosity and cell adhesion like CS. Addition of hydroxyapatite increased the mechanical properties of the prepared scaffolds and it has shown better adhesion of MG-63 cells [34]. Govindan et al. investigated the effect of incorporating phosphate glass in gelatin and preparation of scaffold material for bone tissue engineering. They have found 70% porosity with a pore diameter of 100–500 nm. Proliferation of cells was found to be high in scaffold containing more PG content than gelatin scaffold. PG/gelatin scaffolds were found to be good for bone tissue engineering [35].

13.4.6 FIBER BONDING

Technique utilizing the unique properties of fiber such as high surface area to volume ratio is proposed by Mikas et al. in 2003. Mikas and his coworkers prepared polyglycolic acid (PGA) mesh by immersing PGA mesh in PLLA solution. Upon heating, PGA fiber cross-linked and formed an interconnected fiber mesh. Due to the immiscibility of PLLA with PGA, it is easy to remove PLLA from PGA solution by dissolving in methylene chloride. The obtained porosity was about 81% [36].

High surface area to volume ratio of fibers can improve the cell adhesion of scaffold material and simple manufacturing technique making them a better option to prepare biocompatible scaffolds. Immiscibility of the polymer material and lack of control on porosity are main drawbacks of this technique. Although limitations are serious, still works are going on in this technique.

Svobodova et al. investigated the fibrous scaffold formation of poly (γ-benzyl-L-glutamate) through solvent-assisted fiber bonding technique. The fibers bonded by dissolving in isopropyl alcohol and toluene further modified with N5-hydroxyethyl-L-glutamine units through aminolysis followed by addition of a peptide chain. The prepared scaffolds have a pore size of 20–400 μm and scaffold remained intact during the modification times. Modified scaffold having concentration of peptide chains between 90 and 3000 fm/cm^2 showed better growth of chondrogenic cells [37].

13.4.7 ELECTROSPINNING

It is the most effective and widely used conventional technique for preparation of nonwoven nanofibers with sufficient surface area and pore volume. Electrospinning attained its fame in the last decades of 20th century and still persisting and developing in both scientific and industrial areas. More than 200 natural polymers as well as synthetic polymers can spin to nanofibers using this technique.

Basic needle spinners can be setup in vertical or horizontal manner. Spinner has three main parts, which are collector screen, syringe, and a high voltage source. Feeding of polymer solution from the fed system can make one droplet at the tip of syringe. Given high voltage induces high charge difference between syringe and collector along with the formation of electric charge at the surface of polymer solution, which can disturb the surface tension of liquid surface due to mutual charge repulsion. When electric field increases the liquid, it attains the shape of a cone which is known as Taylor cone at the tip of syringe. Polymer solution flows like a jet to the collector when the repulsive electric force increases than the surface tension of the liquid. The thin jet travels toward the collector due to the accelerative Coulombic force from the external electric field and gets collected as thin fibers in collector while solvent gets evaporated [38–40].

Multiaxial spinning, triaxial spinning, bicomponent electrospinning, and magnetic field electrospinning are different varieties of electrospinning. Bicomponent electrospinning uses two vertically joined compartments in syringe having two polymer solutions and one needle. The spinneret system can prepare fibers having properties of both polymer solutions. Multineedle eletrospinning uses different needles attached to a single voltage supply and polymer reservoir. Bubble electrospinning is one of the simple methods that uses bubbles without needle to create fiber jet. Polymer solution aerates in the absence of electric field to produce bubbles. Presence of electric field produces a tangential stress on the surface of bubble due to the combined effect of electric charge and surface tension, which, in turn, makes a protuberance in the smallest bubble to create upward jet-like motion. When electric charge overcomes, the surface tension solution emerges out like a jet fiber [38, 39].

Recently, Sadeghi et al. synthesized polyvinyl alcohol/gelatin/chondroitin sulfate scaffolds using electrospinning technique (Figure 13.6). Solvent selection is the main problem related with electrospinning.

They have used water and acetic acid mixture as a nontoxic solvent, which helped them to prepare nontoxic scaffolds. Gelatin usually forms gel while mixing with water. Aqueous solution of acetic acid can dissolve gelatin in room temperature. So, electrospinning using water and acetic acid can give nontoxic scaffolds and can reduce the problem of solvent selection [42].

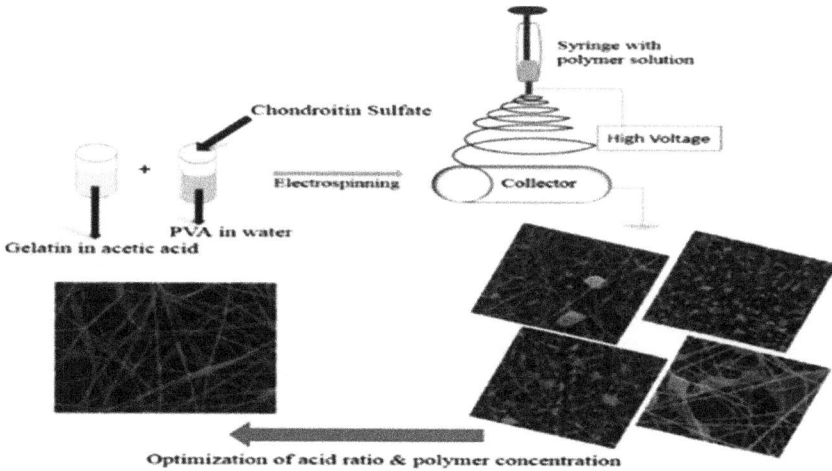

FIGURE 13.6 Schematic representation of electrospinning technique and SEM images of prepared scaffold materials (reprinted from [42], copyright (2019), with permission from Elsevier).

Scaffolds having porosities ranging from few microns to hundred microns and better mechanical strength are possible to prepare by changing the parameters such as strength of electric field, length and radius of spinneret, and viscosity and ionic strength of the solution. In-situ modifications of fibers, composite spinning, spinning of hydrogels, and easy delivery of growth factors by varying the concentrations of polymer solutions made electrospinning more relevant than other fabrication techniques.

Composite electrospinning is trending for few years, as it is possible to eliminate several issues related to a single material. Jiang et al. recently fabricated a scaffold with a blend of polyglycerol sebacate (PGS) and thermoplastic polyurethane (TPU) for vocal fold tissue engineering. PGS is a biocompatible material using for the first time for preparing scaffold due to the elastic modulus as of vocal fold. TPU can give mechanical properties of extracellular matrix of vocal fold tissue. Different structures were prepared through electrospinning including a leaf-like structure. Scaffold with a 6:4 ratio of PGS and TPU has shown good proliferation of fibroblast cells due to a better amount of PGS which has shown a good contact angle of 65.4° which is suitable for cell adhesion. The electrospuned PGS/TPU is a successful material for using soft tissues such as vocal fold [43].

Tan et al. fabricated cellulose acetate butyrate/PEG composite fibers through electrospinning (as shown in Figure 13.7). The nanofiber found to be having good hydrophilicity than normal cellulose acetate butyrate fiber.

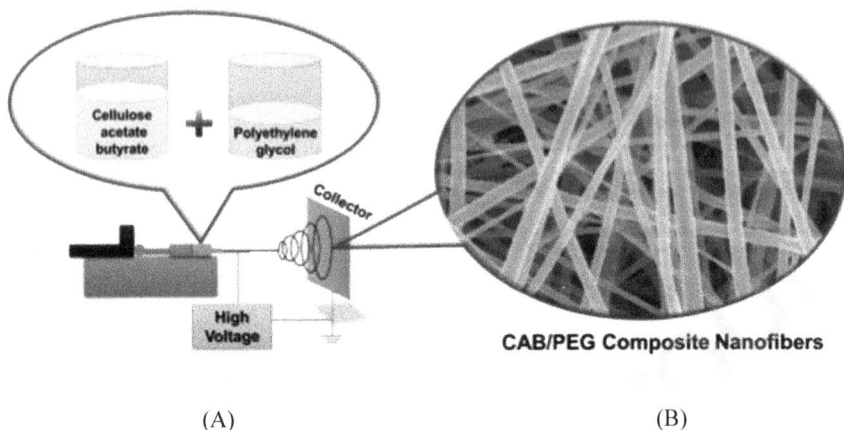

(A)	(B)

FIGURE 13.7 (A) Schematic representation of electrospinning and (B) SEM image of nanofibers (reprinted from [44], copyright (2018), with permission from Elsevier).

CAB fibers are normally hydrophobic and incorporation of PEG reduced the hydrophobicity, so that the adhesion of dermal fibroblast cells increased as well as good mechanical properties. Recently, nanofibrous hydrogels have been started to use in electrospinning. Hasanzadeh et al. investigated on 3D nanofibrous scaffolds made up of fibrin/polyurethane and multiwall carbon nanotube (MWCNT) for applications in neural tissue engineering. MWCNT could enhance the conductivity of neural tissues and polyurethane increased the mechanical property and decreased the degradation time of fibrin gel [44].

Although all the conventional techniques are reliable and easy to prepare, it is difficult to control the pore size and interconnectivity of pores. Strong care and skill are needed to prepare scaffolds having sufficient mechanical properties and also most of the techniques are not suitable for making big membranes. Solid freeform techniques are the current alternate and efficient method for makeup all the limitations of conventional techniques.

13.5 RAPID PROTOTYPING TECHNOLOGIES

Rapid prototyping technologies, also known as solid freeform techniques or layer-by-layer techniques, works on the base of predesigned CAD. RP techniques are efficient to create three-dimensional structures with vey minute features, which make it suitable to prepare minute pore structures than conventional techniques. CAD data stored in stereolithography (STL) [from stereolithography (SLA)] format is seen as two-dimensional layers, which is used by computers to print two-dimensional layers. The movement of printer head from bottom to top or according to the design can generate a complete three-dimensional solid. The use of these techniques started in 1980s and it proved the ability to use in biomedical field by 1990s. SLA is the oldest RP techniques, which had been used for industries. SLA, fused deposition modeling, selective laser sintering, and 3D bioprinting are the four main techniques used for tissue engineering. All these techniques are capable of producing very minute and complex architectures for tissue engineering having distinguishable properties such as pore size, volume, interconnectivity, geometry, mechanical properties, and even to control the biodegradation of material.

Currently, advancements in RP techniques lead to production of patient-specific implantable according to the need of a repair along with the incorporation of stem cells during processing. Using computed tomography or MRI scan details, personalized implantable can prepare in situ by adding stem cells to it with high accuracy. Polymers and ceramics both are suitable for processing through these techniques. Even soft hydrogels can be processed easily through RP techniques. Multimaterial additive manufacturing techniques are another significant development in RP technology in which more than one material can be used to manufacture a scaffold. All these qualities made it superior than conventional techniques, but still certain drawbacks are there to be solved [45, 46].

13.5.1 STEREOLITHOGRAPHY

It is the oldest 3D modeling system based on photopolymerization of polymers under ultraviolet rays. It is also known as Hull SLA and invented by Charles Hull in 1986. Accurate small features less than 5 μm can be easily molded by this technique.

Mastuda et al. reported fabrication of biodegradable scaffolds using copolymers of trimethylene carbonate and PCL for the first time using SLA. Two kinds of SLA techniques are there which are based on technology (SLA) and they have been using which are laser-based SLA and digital light projection (DLP) SLA. In laser-based SLA, UV light from the source polymerizes the resin in the tank according to the data of sliced 2D layers of actual design from CAD file. Once the layer is polymerized, the platform lowers to build the next layer. The process continues up to preparing the whole object. DLP is comparatively faster than laser-based technique. DLP uses lamp light rather than UV light. In DLP technique, an image of the layer to be produced flashes on the bottom of the tank, so that it can produce the entire layer at once whereas SLA needs more time to polymerize from point to point of the resin. Elevator moves downward after the formation of one layer for the printing of next layer. After the formation of whole object, it should have undergone some post curing methods for complete curing. Usually, gaited solvent bath is using for draining extra solvent and subsequent curing according to the material structure. The minimum thickness of the layers or the cure depth is 25–50 μm. Liquid crystal displays digital micromirror devices (DMDs) that are using to control the irradiation pattern. DMDs can control the irradiation by reflecting it in specific pattern to give rise to more accurate models than SLA. DLP has several advantages over SLA as the illuminating surface should not smoothen again. Material required is less than SLA and the surface being protected from surroundings can prevent oxygen inhibition of the polymerization reaction. Polypropylene fumarate, trimethylene carbonate, poly(ε-caprolactone), poly-L-lactide, and hydroxyapatite are some of the materials suitable for SLA [45–47].

Schmidleithner et al. experiment the utility of high-resolution DLP SLA for preparing tricalcium phosphate scaffolds for bone tissue engineering. β-tricalcium phosphates have excellent biodegradation kinetics than other ceramics. β-tricalcium phosphates have mixed with a solvent containing acrylates and methacrylates with a photoinitiator. They have designed scaffolds in four geometries such as rectilinear grid, a hexagonal kagome, Schwarz primitive, and a hollow Schwarz with a porosity of 75% and pore diameter of 400 μm. Rectilinear grid and hexagonal kagome structures have shown good mechanical properties with a compressive strength of 44.7 MPa, which is around the strength of a cortical bone. Cell growth was good up to 14 days with confirmed osteogenesis and collagen deposition. So, high-resolution-based DLP can produce biocompatible scaffolds with both ceramics and polymers with good mechanical properties and cell proliferation [48].

Xiangquan Wu et al. utilized multimaterial mask projection stereolithography (MMSL) to fabricate a biphasic osteochondral scaffold. Scaffolds were fabricated using PEG, diacrylate hydrogel, and β-tricalcium phosphate. MMSL is useful to prepare layer of one material over another layer or mixture of two materials on a layer of single material or mixture of materials. These scaffolds made up by the multimaterial algorithm/CAD format prepared by the team that could successfully create the product with good interfacial adhesion. Multimaterial additive manufacturing has an important place in the near future of RP techniques [49].

13.5.1.1 TWO-PHOTON POLYMERIZATION

Two-photon polymerization is an important class of SLA, which uses energy from two packets of radiation for photopolymerization. Fabrication of a complete three-dimensional object without moving the platform and with minute features is the significance of this method. Two-photon polymerization method polymerizes a small three-dimensional volume of the resin called voxel. Two mechanisms proposed behind two-photon excitation. In the first mechanism, the first photon excites the initiator molecules to a definite intermediate time of 10^{-9} s. The second photon arriving within this time excites the molecule to original excited state followed by releasing of energy to form free radicals for polymerization. In the second method, there is no real intermediate state and time. So, high-frequency radiation is needed to completely excite the molecule after first incident ray within 10^{-15}s. Titanium-sapphire lasers or femtosecond lasers are widely using for this technique to produce high-frequency radiation. These kinds of radiation can penetrate deep into the vat column, which can create nanoscale structures. The maximum resolution possible is 100–200 nm [29] and the minimum possible is 52 nm [30]. Moreover, it can prevent the overheating and, thus, allowing the transportation of molecules such as proteins or cells [50, 51]. Felfel et al. studied the degradation rate of scaffolds prepared from poly(DL-lactide-co-ε-caprolactone) copolymer with lactic acid by 2PP polymerization. The scaffolds made in different concentrations of lactic acid have a maximum size of $2 \times 4 \times 2$ mm^3 and 300 μm pore size. The prepared concentrations of 16:4, 18:2, and 9:1 were undergone degradation test for several days at different temperature. Rate of mass loss for 16:4 was lower at all temperatures compared to other, which is attributed to the high degradation time of caprolactone. Mechanical strength also showed proportionality with amount of caprolactone during degradation. The obtained values for activation energy (EA) were 87.9, 82.7, and 94.7 kJ/mol for 16:4, 18:2, and 9:1 lactic acid – caprolactone copolymer (LC) ratios. All of them exhibited fast degradation kinetics around 60 °C [52]. Demina et al. have used two-photon-induced microstereolithography for the preparation of CS-g-oligolactide copolymer scaffolds. They have evaluated the mechanism of cross-linking through two-photon SLA and optimized the processing conditions for good mechanical properties [53]. The potential of two-photon polymerization is still need to be evaluated and explored for more medical applications. Less availability of photopolymerizable resins which are biodegradable and difficulty to fabricate multimaterial scaffolds are the main issues related to SLA.

13.5.2   *FUSED DEPOSITION MODELING (FDM)*

Fused deposition modeling is an extrusion-based printing technology emerged in 1990s but gained more significance since 2010. FDM is highly material-specific, which is suitable to process semicrystalline or amorphous thermoplastics and less complicated than other techniques. The desired material is fed into the machine in the form of a filament having 1.75 mm diameter and passed through a liquefier to melt the material and extruded through the head to create a layer of the specified product. Extruder head moves in *x–y* plane while platform moves downward in z direction to a definite distance (as shown in Figure 13.8). The process repeated to produce a complete product. This is a highly effective method like other methods to print various fine structures with integral mechanical properties. Unlike other methods, variety of thermoplastics can be used for this technique and material wastage is very less [54]. PCL, poly(D,L-lactide-co-glycolide) (PDLGA), polyamides, polylactides, polyetheramides, and hydroxyapatite composites of polymers and ceramics such as PCL-hydroxyapatite and PDLGA-tricalcium phosphate are the main materials, which are stable for FDM process. Polymer–ceramic composites are the new trend in printing technology, which can be easily done by using FDM. Zein et al. fabricated honeycomb-like PCL scaffold using FDM in 2002. Mechanical properties were found to be good for prepared scaffolds with a compressive strength of 77 MPa and porosity in the range of 48%–77% after that FDM acquired lots of importance in tissue engineering [55]. Recently, Nevado et al. fabricated polylactic acid (PLA) and biphasic calcium phosphate composite scaffolds using FDM. Composites of polymers with hydroxyapatite and β-tricalcium phosphate are very common, but composite with biphasic calcium phosphate is for the first time in literature. Prepared scaffolds have shown good mechanical strength and better cell proliferation. Corcione et al. evaluated the properties of highly loaded hydroxyapatite microsphere in PLA matrix through FDM. 50 wt% of hydroxyapatite particles increased the roughness of the PLA matrix. Similarity toward bone matrix and high porosity due to the mesoporous structure of hydroxyapatite increased the cell proliferation of scaffolds [56].

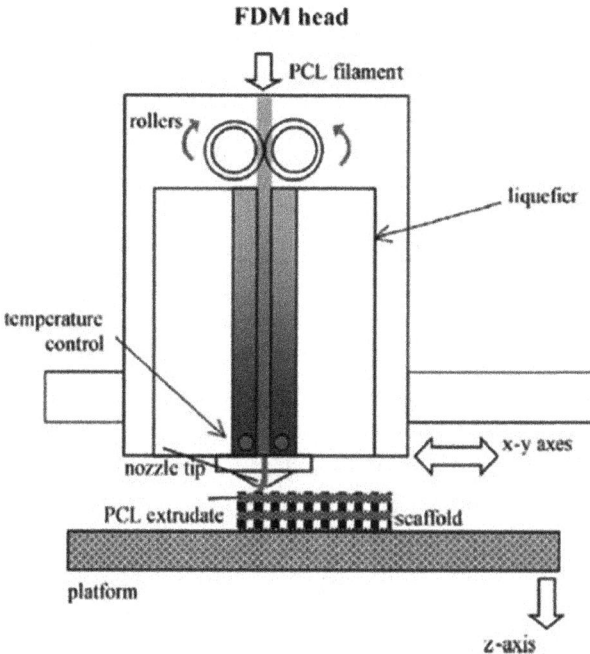

FIGURE 13.8 Schematic representation of FDM (reprinted from [11], copyright (2019), with permission from Elsevier).

Time-consuming handwork for polishing surface and support for hangings are main downsides of FDM. High material temperature is not suitable to seed cells and growth factors along with material because temperature could destroy the properties of cell. Liquid frozen deposition was emerged as a solution for seeding cells with a lower temperature cooling platform.

Liquid frozen deposition system or low temperature manufacturing system uses a low temperature platform for cooling the molten material from the extruder nozzle. Solvent evaporates using freeze drying or direct evaporation after the formation of one layer. The process repeats to get the whole object.

Yen et al. investigated the utility of liquid frozen deposition in preparing scaffolds for cartilage tissue engineering. They have prepared scaffolds using different concentrations of PDLGA. Scaffolds with high concentration of PDLGA exhibited high compression modulus around 1.17 MPa which is near to the articular bone compression modulus of 1.42 MPa but less than scaffolds fabricated by the FDM. High compression modulus is attributed to the high pore volume in the surface. Cell proliferation was found to be high in scaffolds with 15% and 20% of PLGA, respectively. Chondrocytes proliferation increased up to 1.7% after 7 days of growth from first day. Sufficient collagen deposit was found after 14 days. Fine porosity of scaffolds with 15% and 20% increased the cell proliferation than other scaffolds. FDM proved its ability to grow cells for cartilage bones [58].

13.5.3 SELECTIVE LASER SINTERING (SLS)

Polymeric scaffold fabrication technology was developed by Carl Deckard at University of Texas in 1989. High-power laser such as carbon dioxide laser system is using for melting a thin layer of a polymer material of around 100–200 μm thickness. The laser system controlled by a cad program can locally and selectively melt the powdered material and to produce bonds through sintering in required shape. After the formation of first layer, the process repeated to get the complete structure. Excess unsintered material can support the system while processing. Good sphericity or density is essential to control the flow of material under high temperature. Flow can be controlled by adding some flow ability additives also.

Bin Duan et al. fabricated three-dimensional nanocomposite microspheres using SLS from calcium phosphate/poly(3-hydroxybutyrate-*co*-3-hydroxyvalerate) (PHBV) and carbonated hydroxyapatite/PLA. The sintered scaffold exhibited complete interconnected porous structure and high porosity in which the incorporation of osteoconductive calcium particles helped to improve the cell proliferation. These scaffold material showed a good biomimetic environment for both cell growth and differentiation [59].

Shaun Eshraghi et al. have found that the mechanical properties of PCL-based one-, two-, and three-dimensional and orthogonally oriented scaffolds synthesized through SLS are high than other layer manufacturing technology. Diermann et al. studied the hydrolytic degradation of poly (3-hydroxybutyrate-*co*-3-hydroxyvalerate) (PHBV) scaffolds prepared through SLS. The predesigned architectures made by SLS had larger surface area for high intake of water. These structures increased the hydrolytic degradation. The estimated pore size was 80 nm. These scaffolds made through SLS showed high porosity, high relative density, high molecular weight, and high degradation rate after incubation of 6 weeks in lead sulfate solution compared to PHBV scaffolds prepared through conventional techniques. The rough powder adhesion makes SLA a good candidate for bone tissue engineering. Cells adhesion is high compared to other techniques [60].

13.5.4   3D BIOPRINTING

It is one of the most promising technologies, which prints cells along with biomaterial directly to get scaffold in which cells proliferate and biomaterial degrades gradually to repair the tissue. The combination of cells and biomaterial is known as bioink. The concept was proposed by Mironov et al., which is working according to the same STL file format of other printing techniques. The printing technique can make pores of micrometer scale ranging from 10 to 10,000 μm. Three kinds of bioprinting are there such as extrusion-based, jetting-based, and SLA-based 3D bioprinting. One of the major challenges of 3D bioprinting is multiple cell printing. Research is going on this area. Possibility of 4D printing is another major feature of 3D bioprinting, which is also in earlier stage of research.

13.5.4.1   INKJET PRINTING

3D bioprinting, also known as inkjet printing or drop-on-demand printing, is invented in Massachusetts Institute of Technology. Wide range of materials can be printed in less time with minute features. It had been became a common printer everywhere, but differences are there for biomaterial printing. Three kinds of inkjet bioprinting are there named according to the heating source, which are thermal, piezoelectric, and electrostatic bioprinting. In thermal inkjet printing, the heater attached to the binding head produces heat energy using electric pulses, which, in turn, produces bubbles in the ink. These bubbles force the binder through the nozzle as droplets. In the second method, an actuator placed in head deformed by applying voltage pulses. During this time, the binder squeezes out of the nozzle. In the third one, a solenoid valve, which is controlled by a microcontroller, is attached at the end of head. The valve controls the shape of droplets [61, 62].

Saijo et al. fabricated maxillofacial implants of hydroxyapatite using inkjet printing. Addition of water to calcium phosphate can convert it to hydroxyapatite during the inkjet printing. Prepared scaffolds have shown good biocompatibility and osteoconductivity [63]. The method is highly inexpensive compared to other RP techniques. Several biomaterials such as fibrin, collagen, alginates, PCL, PLA, and living cells can be used for printing. Printing density or cell volume can be adjusted by varying the concentration of binder solution, but viscosity below 18 MPa is only possible to print up-to-date. Formation of uniform microchannel inside the scaffold could increase the cells seeding and proliferation. Different nozzles can be used for preparing different size pores, but the maximum pore size prepared is below 300 μm for 3D structures. One of the main features of this technology is multicolor printing on specific positions. Printability of living cells or decellularized extracellular matrix is another important feature of inkjet printing.

Two kinds of cell printing are there among which one is cell scaffold-based approach and other is scaffold-free cell-based approach. In first method, biomaterial and cell together are using for printing and in second approach, living cells are printing directly. Decellularized extracellular matrix is another category of bioinks, which is preparing by removing the living cells through definite steps. High biocompatibility of decellularized extracellular matrix gained more attention than other materials. Limitation in material viscosity, mechanical stress, difficulty in bioink dispensing, and nozzle clogging are the main disadvantages of inkjet printing.

Chaofan et al. investigated the properties of inkjet printing and get the optimal solution. Sodium alginate is used as bioink [64]. A jet of sodium alginate printed to the solution of calcium chloride was gelatinized by the solution. Scaffolds achieved a porosity of 75% with good interconnectivity and degraded 90% over 16 weeks.

Tao et al. invented a hybrid technology for making cartilage tissues having good mechanical property. They have combined electrospinning and inkjet printing in which PCL was electrospuned and a composite of fibrin-alginate suspended with elastic chondrocyte cells was added to electrospuned fibers using inkjet printing. Scaffold consists of five layers and is prepared by alternative electrospinning and jet printing. Cell viability was more than 80% with high mechanical properties. So, this hybrid technique is a good candidate for tissue engineering [65].

13.5.4.2   MICROEXTRUSION

Microextrusion-based printing is the cheapest bioprinting method, which forces bioink through a nozzle to the platform. It can be divided into two categories, which are pneumatic and mechanical extrusion systems. Pneumatic system uses the air pressure to push the material out of nozzle. Compressed gas pressure can cause discrete flow of material inside nozzle, which can affect the printing resolution. Even though cell viability is less than inkjet printing due to the forces inside nozzle, it is better technology to print viscous material and high cell density than inkjet printing. Mechanical-based systems use a piston or screw to extrude material. Spatial resolution is high and extrusion of high viscous material is possible due to high shear forces than jetting method. It can print material having viscosity in the range of 30,000–50,000 MPa [61, 62]. Mendibil et al. fabricated tubular poly(L-lactide-co-ε-caprolactone) scaffolds for soft-tissue regeneration. Microextrusion is proved to be a high throughput method for preparing long porous scaffolds with similar mechanical properties of human soft tissues. Tensile modulus of the prepared scaffold was about 15 MPa, which is equal to human nerve tissue. Control over concentration gradient of nanoparticles in a scaffold material is difficult during manufacturing process. Trachtenberg et al. created polypropylene fumarate scaffolds with hydroxyapatite nanoparticles using extrusion-based printing [66].

13.6 ELECTROHYDRODYNAMIC (EHD) JET PRINTING

Electrohydrodynamic jet printing is latest derivative of electrospinning and a noncontact jet printing technology. It can be used to print very fine structures with large resolution without any problems related to nozzle diameter. It produces mobile ions in the polarizable liquid by an electric field. The columbic repulsion of ions alters the shape of meniscus to a Taylor cone. At certain electric field, the repulsion forces increase the surface tension of the droplet and material emitted toward the substrate.

Liu et al. used EHD jet printing (E-jet) to investigate on the control of cell proliferation on PLGA scaffolds. In this project, various structures were fabricated by varying the electric field [67]. MTT assay confirmed the cell proliferation after the first day of seeding. At 3 days, the cells were grown in a spindle-like structure. From the third day, they have started to grow in the direction of fiber alignment. E-jet printing can provide an environment for aligned growth of cells in in-vivo and in-vitro conditions. Wei et al. investigated the resolution of scaffolds prepared using EHD technique. They have prepared 3D and 2D porous PCL scaffolds from hot melt PCL. The 3D scaffolds with layered pattern and high pore interconnectivity have shown a pore diameter less than 10 μm. Experiment has proven the ability of EHD to print high-resolution scaffolds using a stable jet than electrospinning and other traditional printing techniques.

13.7 CONCLUSION

Scaffolds are the backbone of tissue engineering and these scaffold preparation techniques play an important role in tissue engineering. Scaffold preparation techniques have acquired prominent developments in recent years. Conventional techniques have started in the early 1950s, which are still used for scaffold preparation due to its simplicity and effectiveness. Solvent casting/particulate leaching, phase separation, and freeze drying can be used to prepare highly porous structures with simple equipment. Electrospinning is the superior conventional method, which is using most widely for biomedical research. Even though conventional techniques can prepare good scaffolds, control on porosity and mechanical strength is very difficult. These issues related with conventional techniques that lead to the emergence of RP techniques over conventional techniques. RP techniques such as SLA, FDM, and 3D bioprinting can produce scaffolds with better porosity and mechanical strength. Possibility to process composite materials more than one material together and different kinds of modification on polymer chains during processing make RP techniques more advantageous than conventional techniques. Emergence of 3D bioprinting increased the possibility of printing organs successfully with biomaterials. 4D printing of organs and tissues using RP techniques is also started in different forms, which is not so far from humankind.

Scaffold preparation techniques need to be developed more for solving current problems related with processing. Limited biomaterials for each techniques and fine inner architecture are the main hurdles for RP and conventional techniques. Currently, the plethora of works is going on processing techniques and biomaterials, which have the potential to turn mankind to a new era of science and technology.

KEYWORDS

- **scaffolds**
- **biomaterials**
- **RP techniques**
- **3D bioprinting.**

REFERENCES

1. Stratton, S., Shelke, N. B., Hoshino, K., Rudraiah, S. and Kumbar, S. G. (2016). Bioactive polymeric scaffolds for tissue engineering. *Bioactive Materials*, *1*(2), 93–108.

2. Howard, D., Buttery, L. D., Shakesheff, K. M. and Roberts, S. J. (2008). Tissue engineering: strategies, stem cells and scaffolds. *Journal of Anatomy, 213*(1), 66–72.

3. Vacanti, J. P. and Langer, R. (1999). Tissue engineering: the design and fabrication of living replacement devices for surgical reconstruction and transplantation. *The Lancet, 354*, S32–S34.

4. Wu, G. H. and Hsu, S. H. (2015). Polymeric-based 3D printing for tissue engineering. *Journal of Medical and Biological Engineering, 35*(3), 285–292.

5. Subia, B., Kundu, J. and Kundu, S. C. (2010). Biomaterial scaffold fabrication techniques for potential tissue engineering applications. *Tissue Engineering, 141*, 13–18.

6. Chaignaud, B. E., Langer, R. and Vacanti, J. P. (1997). The history of tissue engineering using synthetic biodegradable polymer scaffolds and cells. In: Atala, A and Mooney, J. (Eds) *Synthetic Biodegradable Polymer Scaffolds* (pp. 1–14). Birkhäuser, Boston.

7. Meyer, U. (2009). The history of tissue engineering and regenerative medicine in perspective. In: Meyer, U., Meyer, T., Handschel, J. and Wiesmann, H. P. (Eds) *Fundamentals of Tissue Engineering and Regenerative Medicine* (pp. 5–12). Springer, Berlin, Heidelberg.

8. Berthiaume, F., Maguire, T. J. and Yarmush, M. L. (2011). Tissue engineering and regenerative medicine: history, progress, and challenges. *Annual Review of Chemical and Biomolecular Engineering, 2*, 403–430.

9. Hubbell, J. A. (1995). Biomaterials in tissue engineering. *Biotechnology, 13*(6), 565–576.

10. Kim, B. S., Baez, C. E. and Atala, A. (2000). Biomaterials for tissue engineering. *World Journal of Urology, 18*(1), 2–9.

11. Singh, R., Singh, S. and Hashmi, M. S. J. (2016). Implant materials and their processing technologies. In: *Reference Module in Materials Science and Materials Engineering,* pp. 1–31. *In book; Reference Module In Material Science And Materials Engineering.*

12. Dhandayuthapani, B., Yoshida, Y., Maekawa, T. and Kumar, D. S. (2011). Polymeric scaffolds in tissue engineering application: a review. *International Journal of Polymer Science, 2011,* 29062.

13. Stratton, S., Shelke, N. B., Hoshino, K., Rudraiah, S. and Kumbar, S. G. (2016). Bioactive polymeric scaffolds for tissue engineering. *Bioactive Materials, 1*(2), 93–108.

14. Weigel, T., Schinkel, G. and Lendlein, A. (2006). Design and preparation of polymeric scaffolds for tissue engineering. *Expert Review of Medical Devices, 3*(6), 835–851.

15. Abdelaal, O. A. and Darwish, S. M. (2011). Fabrication of tissue engineering scaffolds using rapid prototyping techniques. *International Journal of Industrial and Manufacturing Engineering, 5*(11), 2310–2318.

16. Hutmacher, D. W. and Cool, S. (2007). Concepts of scaffold-based tissue engineering—the rationale to use solid freeform fabrication techniques. *Journal of Cellular and Molecular Medicine, 11*(4), 654–669.

17. Hutmacher, D. W. (2001). Scaffold design and fabrication technologies for engineering tissues—state of the art and future perspectives. *Journal of Biomaterials Science, Polymer Edition, 12*(1), 107–124.

18. Murphy, M. B. and Mikos, A. G. (2007). Polymer scaffold fabrication. In: Lanza, R., Langer, R. and Vacanti, J. (Eds) *Principles of Tissue Engineering* (pp. 309–321). Academic Press, United States.

19. Vijayavenkataraman, S., Vialli, N., Fuh, J. Y. and Lu, W. F. (2019). Conductive collagen/polypyrrole-b-polycaprolactone hydrogel for bioprinting of neural tissue constructs. *International Journal of Bioprinting, 5*(2.1), 229.

20. Zhang, Y., Tse, C., Rouholamin, D. and Smith, P. (2012). Scaffolds for tissue engineering produced by inkjet printing. *Open Engineering, 2*(3), 325–335.
21. Leong, K. F., Cheah, C. M. and Chua, C. K. (2003). Solid freeform fabrication of three-dimensional scaffolds for engineering replacement tissues and organs. *Biomaterials, 24*(13), 2363–2378.
22. Sola, A., Bertacchini, J., D'Avella, D., Anselmi, L., Maraldi, T., Marmiroli, S. and Messori, M. (2019). Development of solvent-casting particulate leaching (SCPL) polymer scaffolds as improved three-dimensional supports to mimic the bone marrow niche. *Materials Science and Engineering C, 96,* 153–165.
23. Jamshidi, M., Akbari, B. and Nourmohammadi, J. (2019). Nanoclay reinforced starch-polycaprolactone scaffolds for bone tissue engineering. *Journal of Tissues and Materials, 2*(1), 55–63.
24. Chia, O. C., Suhaimin, I. S., Kassim, S. A., Zubir, S. A. and Abdullah, T. K. (2019). Effect of modified solvent casting/particulate leaching (SCPL) technique on the properties of bioactive glass reinforced polyurethane scaffold for biomedical applications. *Journal of Physical Science, 30,* 115–126.
25. Allaf, R. M. (2018). Melt-molding technologies for 3D scaffold engineering. In: Deng, Y. and Kuiper, J. (Eds). *Functional 3D Tissue Engineering Scaffolds: Materials, Technologies, and Applications* (pp. 75–100). Woodhead Publishing, United Kingdom.
26. Mao, D., Li, Q., Li, D., Tan, Y. and Che, Q. (2018). 3D porous poly(ε-caprolactone)/58S bioactive glass–sodium alginate/gelatin hybrid scaffolds prepared by a modified melt molding method for bone tissue engineering. *Materials and Design, 160,* 1–8.
27. Oh, S. H., Park, S. C., Kim, H. K., Koh, Y. J., Lee, J. H., Lee, M. C. and Lee, J. H. (2011). Degradation behavior of 3D porous polydioxanone-b-polycaprolactone scaffolds fabricated using the melt-molding particulate-leaching method. *Journal of Biomaterials Science, Polymer Edition, 22*(1–3), 225–237.
28. Manavitehrani, I., Le, T. Y., Daly, S., Wang, Y., Maitz, P. K., Schindeler, A. and Dehghani, F. (2019). Formation of porous biodegradable scaffolds based on poly(propylene carbonate) using gas foaming technology. *Materials Science and Engineering C, 96,* 824–830.
29. Poursamar, S. A., Hatami, J., Lehner, A. N., da Silva, C. L., Ferreira, F. C. and Antunes, A. P. M. (2015). Gelatin porous scaffolds fabricated using a modified gas foaming technique: characterisation and cytotoxicity assessment. *Materials Science and Engineering C, 48,* 63–70.
30. Martínez-Pérez, C. A., Olivas-Armendariz, I., Castro-Carmona, J. S. and García-Casillas, P. E. (2011). Scaffolds for tissue engineering via thermally-induced phase separation. *Advances in Regenerative Medicine, 35,* 275–294.
31. Salehi, M., Farzamfar, S., Bozorgzadeh, S. and Bastami, F. (2019). Fabrication of poly(L-lactic acid)/chitosan scaffolds by solid–liquid phase separation method for nerve tissue engineering: an in vitro study on human neuroblasts. *Journal of Craniofacial Surgery, 30*(3), 784–789.
32. Wang, S. D., Ma, Q., Wang, K. and Ma, P. B. (2018). Strong and biocompatible three-dimensional porous silk fibroin/graphene oxide scaffold prepared by phase separation. *International Journal of Biological Macromolecules, 111,* 237–246.
33. Khan, M. U. A., Al-Thebaiti, M. A., Hashmi, M. U., Aftab, S., Abd Razak, S. I., Abu Hassan, S. and Amin, R. (2020). Synthesis of silver-coated bioactive nanocomposite scaffolds based on grafted beta-glucan/hydroxyapatite via freeze-drying method: anti-microbial and biocompatibility evaluation for bone tissue engineering. *Materials, 13*(4), 971.

34. Shahbazarab, Z., Teimouri, A., Chermahini, A. N. and Azadi, M. (2018). Fabrication and characterization of nanobiocomposite scaffold of zein/chitosan/nanohydroxyapatite prepared by freeze-drying method for bone tissue engineering. *International Journal of Biological Macromolecules*, *108*, 1017–1027.
35. Govindan, R., Gu, F. L., Karthi, S. and Girija, E. K. (2020). Effect of phosphate glass reinforcement on the mechanical and biological properties of freeze-dried gelatin composite scaffolds for bone tissue engineering applications. *Materials Today Communications*, *22*, 100765.
36. Mikos, A. G. and Temenoff, J. S. (2000). Formation of highly porous biodegradable scaffolds for tissue engineering. *Electronic Journal of Biotechnology*, *3*(2), 23–24.
37. Svobodová, J., Proks, V., Karabiyik, Ö., Çalıkoğlu Koyuncu, A. C., Torun Köse, G., Rypáček, F. and Studenovská, H. (2017). Poly(amino acid)-based fibrous scaffolds modified with surface-pendant peptides for cartilage tissue engineering. *Journal of Tissue Engineering and Regenerative Medicine*, *11*(3), 831–842.
38. Begum, H. A. and Khan, K. R. (2017). Study on the various types of needle based and needleless electrospinning system for nanofiber production. *International Journal of Textile Science*, *6*, 110–117.
39. Li, Y. and Bou-Akl, T. (2016). Electrospinning in tissue engineering. *Electrospinning-Material, Techniques, and Biomedical Applications*, *3*, 117–139.
40. Lin, W., Chen, M., Qu, T., Li, J. and Man, Y. (2020). Three-dimensional electrospun nanofibrous scaffolds for bone tissue engineering. *Journal of Biomedical Materials Research Part B: Applied Biomaterials*, *108*(4), 1311–1321.
41. Vong, M., Speirs, E., Klomkliang, C., Akinwumi, I., Nuansing, W. and Radacsi, N. (2018). Controlled three-dimensional polystyrene micro- and nano-structures fabricated by three-dimensional electrospinning. *RSC Advances*, *8*, 15501. DOI: 10.1039/C7RA13278.
42. Sadeghi, A., Pezeshki-Modaress, M. and Zandi, M. (2018). Electrospun polyvinyl alcohol/gelatin/chondroitin sulfate nanofibrous scaffold: fabrication and in vitro evaluation. *International Journal of Biological Macromolecules*, *114*, 1248–1256.
43. Jiang, L., Jiang, Y., Stiadle, J., Wang, X., Wang, L., Li, Q. and Turng, L. S. (2019). Electrospun nanofibrous thermoplastic polyurethane/poly(glycerol sebacate) hybrid scaffolds for vocal fold tissue engineering applications. *Materials Science and Engineering C*, *94*, 740–749.
44. Tan, H. L., Kai, D., Pasbakhsh, P., Teow, S. Y., Lim, Y. Y. and Pushpamalar, J. (2020). Electrospun cellulose acetate butyrate/polyethylene glycol (CAB/PEG) composite nanofibers: a potential scaffold for tissue engineering. *Colloids and Surfaces B: Biointerfaces*, *188*, 110713.
45. Yuan, B., Zhou, S. Y. and Chen, X. S. (2017). Rapid prototyping technology and its application in bone tissue engineering. *Journal of Zhejiang University-Science B*, *18*(4), 303–315.
46. Yeong, W. Y., Chua, C. K., Leong, K. F. and Chandrasekaran, M. (2004). Rapid prototyping in tissue engineering: challenges and potential. *Trends in Biotechnology*, *22*(12), 643–652.
47. Ronca, A. and Ambrosio, L. (2017). Polymer-based scaffolds for tissue regeneration by stereolithography. *Advanced Biomaterials and Devices in Medicine*, *4*(1), 300–317.
48. Schmidleithner, C., Malferrari, S., Palgrave, R., Bomze, D., Schwentenwein, M. and Kalaskar, D. M. (2019). Application of high resolution DLP stereolithography for fabrication of tricalcium phosphate scaffolds for bone regeneration. *Biomedical Materials*, *14*(4), 045018.

49. Wu, X., Lian, Q., Li, D. and Jin, Z. (2019). Biphasic osteochondral scaffold fabrication using multi-material mask projection stereolithography. *Rapid Prototyping Journal*, *25*, 355–546.

50. Bourdon, L., Maurin, J. C., Gritsch, K., Brioude, A. and Salles, V. (2018). Improvements in resolution of additive manufacturing: advances in two-photon polymerization and direct-writing electrospinning techniques. *ACS Biomaterials Science and Engineering*, *4*(12), 3927–3938.

51. Miwa, M., Juodkazis, S., Kawakami, T., Matsuo, S. and Misawa, H. (2001). Femtosecond two-photon stereolithography. *Applied Physics A*, *73*(5), 561–566.

52. Felfel, R. M., Poocza, L., Gimeno-Fabra, M., Milde, T., Hildebrand, G., Ahmed, I. and Liefeith, K. (2016). In vitro degradation and mechanical properties of PLA-PCL copolymer unit cell scaffolds generated by two-photon polymerization. *Biomedical Materials*, *11*(1), 015011.

53. Demina, T. S., Bardakova, K. N., Minaev, N. V., Svidchenko, E. A., Istomin, A. V., Goncharuk, G. P. and Akopova, T. A. (2017). Two-photon-induced microstereolithography of chitosan-g-oligolactides as a function of their stereochemical composition. *Polymers*, *9*(7), 302.

54. Wugh, H. S. (2015). Review: polymeric-based 3D printing for tissue engineering. *Journal of Medical and Biological Engineering*, *35*, 285–292.

55. Zein, I., Hutmacher, D. W., Tan, K. C. and Teoh, S. H. (2002). Fused deposition modeling of novel scaffold architectures for tissue engineering applications. *Biomaterials*, *23*(4), 1169–1185.

56. Nevado, P., Lopera, A., Bezzon, V., Fulla, M. R., Palacio, J., Zaghete, M. A., Biasotto, G., Montoya, A., Rivera, J., Robledo, S. M., Estupiñan, H., Paucer, C. and Garcia, C. (2020). Preparation and in vitro evaluation of PLA/biphasic calcium phosphate filaments used for fused deposition modelling of scaffolds. *Materials Science and Engineering C*, *114*, 111013.

57. Wu, G. H. and Hsu, S. H. (2015). Polymeric-based 3D printing for tissue engineering. *Journal of Medical and Biological Engineering*, *35*(3), 285–292.

58. Yen, H. J., Hsu, S. H., Tseng, C. S., Huang, J. P. and Tsai, C. L. (2009). Fabrication of precision scaffolds using liquid-frozen deposition manufacturing for cartilage tissue engineering. *Tissue Engineering Part A*, *15*(5), 965–975.

59. Duan, B., Wang, M., Zhou, W. Y., Cheung, W. L., Li, Z. Y. and Lu, W. W. (2010). Three-dimensional nanocomposite scaffolds fabricated via selective laser sintering for bone tissue engineering. *Acta Biomaterialia*, *6*(12), 4495–4505.

60. Eshraghi, S. and Das, S. (2010). Mechanical and microstructural properties of poly-caprolactone scaffolds with one-dimensional, two-dimensional, and three-dimensional orthogonally oriented porous architectures produced by selective laser sintering. *Acta Biomaterialia*, *6*(7), 2467–2476.

61. Dababneh, A. B. and Ozbolat, I. T. (2014). Bioprinting technology: a current state-of-the-art review. *Journal of Manufacturing Science and Engineering*, *136*(6), 610–616.

62. Noh, S., Myung, N., Park, M., Kim, S., Zhang, S. U. and Kang, H. W. (2018). 3D bioprinting for tissue engineering. In: Kim, B. W. (Ed). *Clinical Regenerative Medicine in Urology* (pp. 105–123). Springer, Singapore.

63. Saijo, H., Igawa, K., Kanno, Y., Mori, Y., Kondo, K., Shimizu, K. and Sasaki, N. (2009). Maxillofacial reconstruction using custom-made artificial bones fabricated by inkjet printing technology. *Journal of Artificial Organs*, *12*(3), 200–205.

64. Lv, C. F., Zhu, L. Y., Shi, J. P., Li, Z. A., Tang, W. L., Liu, T. T. and Yang, J. Q. (2018). The fabrication of tissue engineering scaffolds by inkjet printing technology. In: *Materials Science Forum* (Vol. 934, pp. 129–133). Trans Tech Publications Ltd., Switzerland.

65. Xu, T., Binder, K. W., Albanna, M. Z., Dice, D., Zhao, W., Yoo, J. J. and Atala, A. (2012). Hybrid printing of mechanically and biologically improved constructs for cartilage tissue engineering applications. *Biofabrication*, 5(1), 015001.

66. Mendibil, X., Ortiz, R., Sáenz de Viteri, V., Ugartemendia, J. M., Sarasua, J. R. and Quintana, I. (2020). High throughput manufacturing of bio-resorbable micro-porous scaffolds made of poly(L-lactide-co-ε-caprolactone) by micro-extrusion for soft tissue engineering applications. *Polymers*, 12(1), 34.

67. Liu, T., Huang, R., Zhong, J., Yang, Y., Tan, Z. and Tan, W. (2017). Control of cell proliferation in E-jet 3D-printed scaffolds for tissue engineering applications: the influence of the cell alignment angle. *Journal of Materials Chemistry B*, 5(20), 3728–3738.

68. Ghalia, M. A. and Dahman, Y. (2016). Advanced nanobiomaterials in tissue engineering: synthesis, properties, and applications. In: Grumezescu, A. (Ed). *Nanobiomaterials in Soft Tissue Engineering* (pp. 141–172). William Andrew Publishing, United States.

CHAPTER 14

An Overview of Polymeric Hydrogels for Drug Delivery Applications

NEETHA JOHN

CIPET: IPT-Kochi, HIL Colony, Edyar Road, Udyogamandal PO, Eloor, Cochin 683501, India

*Corresponding author. E-mail: neethajob@gmail.com

ABSTRACT

Hydrogels are three-dimensional polymeric materials with a network structure designed for various medical applications. It has the porous structure and can be able to swollen to a greater extent and to absorb large amounts of medicinal compounds and other types of molecules. They are biocompatible and biodegradable with a controlled-release mechanism. The hydrogels are, therefore, an effective drug delivery system. Various studies have been conducted and found that hydrogels are giving greater efficiency in curing various diseases and infections compared to the conventional drug delivery systems. Therefore, polymeric hydrogels are having a greater future prospective not only in medicinal fields but also in allied areas.

14.1 INTRODUCTION

Hydrogels are basically polymers having network structure with controlled cross-links and they are water soluble. It can be made from water-soluble polymer and can have a wide range of chemical and physical properties. It is available in various physical forms such as slabs, even microparticles, nanoparticles, coatings, and films. Hydrogels are used for various applications other than direct clinical processes in tissue engineering, regenerative medicine, diagnostics, immobilization of cells and biomolecules separation and act as barrier materials for the controlling of adhesion between biological components. Hydrogels have very peculiar and unique physical properties that lead to the wide range of usage in drug delivery applications [1–7].

The physical structure of hydrogels is based on the density of cross-links formed, which can lead to a highly porous structure. These hydrogels have a gel matrix with greater affinity toward aqueous environment and it can be easily swollen in aqueous medium. The porosity of hydrogels leads to higher loading of drugs into the gel matrix. These drugs can be released at a specified rate. The drug release rate will be dependent on the diffusion coefficient of the small molecule or macromolecule through the hydrogel network. There are several conditions created for the successful delivery of drugs from the hydrogels. The hydrogels created with a formulation in which the drugs slowly elute out. It should maintain a high local concentration of drug in the surrounding tissues over an extended period of time. The delivery of drug should be a systemic delivery with the proper rate. Hydrogels are highly biocompatible in nature and, therefore, successful to use in the peritoneum and in vivo sites [8].

Hydrogels contain higher water content that is one of the reasons for biocompatibility. There are many similarities of hydrogels to the native extracellular matrix. It can be both physical and chemical in nature. Hydrogels can be designed to get biodegradability or dissolution. There are enzymatic, hydrolytic, or environmental methods available and they are pH, temperature, or electrical field. The degradation of hydrogels is designed based on the time requirements and the location of the delivery systems. Hydrogels are easily deformable and can attain the shape of the applied surface. They have very good adhesive properties also by which it can be used for complex surfaces also.

Hydrogels are polymer matrices that can swell in water with a tendency to assimilate into water when placed in aqueous environment. The swelling characteristics make it the best material under biological conditions. It can be easily and very well used in drug delivery and immobilization of proteins, peptides, and other biological compounds. It has the similarity of natural living tissue due to its higher water content. The cross-links in hydrogels make it three-dimensional structures suitable for the immobilization of biologically active agents. It holds the compounds by the physical entanglements and forming the crystallites. These types of entanglement can release the compounds in a controlled manner. In totality, the cross-linked and biocompatible structure of the hydrogels makes it useful for various diverse applications.

14.2 CHARACTERISTICS OF HYDROGELS

Hydrogels can be characterized for its morphology, swelling property, and elasticity. Porous structure can be explained by the morphology studies. The release mechanism of the drug from the swollen polymeric mass is determined by cross-linking, elasticity effects, and the mechanical strength [9]. There are several methods to characterize the hydrogels.

Cross-linking Ratio: The factor that control swelling of hydrogels is its cross-linking ratio. It can be termed as the ratio between moles in the cross-linking agents and total moles of the polymer. If more cross-linking agents are present, cross-linking ratio will be higher. Those hydrogels with more cross-links will swell lesser. It can affect the mobility of the polymer chain and lower the swelling ratio. The hydrogels with water loving chemical groups will swell more compared to water hating or hydrophobic group. There will be collapsing of hydrophobic groups that leads to the lower contact between water molecules and swelling will be lesser. There are various stimulating mechanisms also to control swelling. Swelling will be controlled by various environmental factors. Hydrogels can be sensitive toward temperature and can be affected by temperature during the swelling process. Similarly, pH and presence of ions can also influence the swelling. Various other stimulating parameters can change the swelling of hydrogels.

Mechanical Properties: One of the very important characteristics of hydrogels is the mechanical properties. It should satisfy the mechanical integrity to work as a drug carrier in a biological environment. The hydrogels should satisfy the properties during the lifespan to get the approvals from concerned authorities. Hydrogels are used to protect the drug until it is released in the controlled fashion. The drug may contain sensitive components such as proteins and lipids that should give the correct level of protection until they are released into the medium it is set. Mechanical properties are highly influenced by the cross-linking given to the gel. A stronger gel can be formed, if more cross-linking is given. But, in order to maintain the elastic nature of the hydrogels, the amount of cross-links is to be controlled to the desired level only. There are several modifications done for the polymer molecules, so that the mechanical strength is controlled. Addition of a comonomer and making a copolymer are one of the methods tried in this respect. Comonomers can function in many ways to increase the mechanical strength by the addition of polar bonds in addition to the cross-links given.

Toxicity: Hydrogels toxicity is very important aspect to be evaluated, as it is to be applied in living organisms. They can be toxic to the environment due to many reasons. For example, unreacted monomers, half reacted polymers, and other additives such as initiators that come out to the system which are unwanted may create the toxicity. Cytotoxicity measurements have to be satisfied by the hydrogels. This is done by the extraction method in which the components leaching to an agar solutions are analyzed. Hydrogels made up of acrylate and methacrylates are studied in many systems. Cytotoxicity of the components is related to the chemical structure. Polymerization reactions are modified to get better and more conversions, so that it can reduce the unreacted monomers. As initiators are making the system toxic, polymer formation without initiators is also studied like using high-energy radiations. Polyvinyl alcohol-based hydrogels are made by thermal methods without the use of initiators. The structure is made with more crystals, so that it can act as cross-links in the hydrogels [8, 10–15].

In-vivo Biocompatibility and Biodegradability: It is very necessary to evaluate its biocompatibility in order to compare and investigate the effects of hydrogels in vivo. The living organisms are subjected to develop inflammatory reactions when come in contact by the degradation of the synthetic polymers [16, 17]. Hydrogel toxicity and biocompatibility are highly dependent on the breakdown of the polymer into monomers or oligomers, the cross-linking agents, or trace polymerization agents [18]. From the use of hydrogel formulations, drug delivery has changed to a favorable condition. It also performs without toxicity screening [19], maintaining long-term stability, and getting proper control over the release properties of the therapeutic agents. It also gives long life. When it is derived from natural materials such as collagen, chitosan, fibrin, and hyaluronic acid [20], it produces the minimum toxic and biocompatible material. In-vitro studies are showing promising results with hydrogels in case of biodegradability and biocompatibility and in-vivo studies are also promising [21].

Bioadhesion: The bioadhesive properties of hydrogels are predominant factors in the selection of their drug delivery routes. Biological systems such as intestinal epithelium and mucosa are generally in wet condition, mobile, and slippery. Adhesion of hydrogels is difficult or limiting. In nasal and oral delivery [22, 23], hydrogel that adheres to the epithelium gives prolong effects and can give higher the retention of the system at a target site that gives better therapeutic effect. Large efforts are made to develop bioadhesive hydrogels to get improved drug delivery [22, 24]. Polymers such as chitosan and poly(acrylic acid) are found to be mucoadhesive [25–27]. Hydrogen bonds with the mucosa in poly(acrylic acid). Positively-charged chitosan can form electrostatic interactions with negatively charged surfaces of tissues and cells [27]. Hydrogels having mucoadhesive polymers have longer retention for oral and nasal drug delivery [28–31].

By incorporating a catechol compound such as 3,4-dihydroxy-L-phenyl-alanine (DOPA) in hydrogels to promote bioadhesion, it is the strategy inspired by marine mussels. Hydrogel-based poly(ethylene glycol) (PEG) containing a DOPA ingredients has shown greater adhesion on epididymal fat pad and external liver surfaces for over year [32–34].

Toughness: The toughness of a hydrogel is very important aspects to maintain its structure and to avoid fracture during the usage on tissue adhesion. Hydrogel matrices should have enough toughness to resist rupture and to prevent the escape of cells [35]. Hydrogels are working as immune isolating membranes and it is needed to ensure that the hydrogel matrix is modulating with the proper cross-link density [36]. One can use interpenetrating networks to form hydrogels [37] for such applications. Alginate and polyacrylamide interpenetrating network of hydrogel possess very high toughness [38, 39] and they are mechanically identical to soft tissues such as cartilage and tendon [40].

Mesh Size Controls on Diffusion and Release: Hydrogels consist of a cross-linked polymer network and have open spaces between polymer chains. It allows the liquid and small solute diffusion. Generally, mesh sizes [41, 42] obtained are in the range from 5 to 100 nm and a number of methods to determine the mesh size. The mesh size depends on polymer, cross-linking, and external stimuli such as temperature and pH. Hydrogels are having wide range of mesh size and having network of heterogeneity and polymer polydispersity. Hydrogels also have nonideal network structures such as dangling chains and closed loops that come from gelation mechanisms, for example, free radical polymerization [43]. Homogeneous mesh size network can be obtained when gelation of symmetrical tetrahedron-like macromeres of the same size [44–46] are used.

Other Related Characteristics: Morphology characteristics of the hydrogels are analyzed by equipment called stereomicroscope. The texture is analyzed by SEM for the hydrogels to know about the granular structures [47]. The polymers are characterized by the X-ray methods to know whether they maintain their crystalline structure. The materials may get deformed during the processing and loose its crystalline structures [47–49]. IR absorption spectra due to stretching and O–H vibration can cause change in the morphology of hydrogels. There can be changes in the formation of coil or helix that indicates cross-linking appearance of bands near 1648 cm^{-1} [48, 49]. The hydrogels are immersed in aqueous medium or medium of specific pH to know the swellability of these polymeric networks. Hydrogels polymers will increase its dimensions due to swelling [47–51]. Hydrogels are also studied for its viscosity at constant temperature by using cone plate type viscometer [52].

14.3   TYPES OF HYDROGELS

Smart Hydrogels: The word smart is associated with hydrogels as they are very different from inert hydrogels. They can sense changes in environmental properties and they will respond by increasing or decreasing their degree of swelling. These hydrogels have wide range of applications in various fields as it can change with respect to the environment. It can change the volume and particularly used for drug delivery applications and controlled drug release. These intelligent hydrogels can sense and deliver the drug in the required intervals. The hydrogels will be responding to various stimuli such as temperature, pH, and ions. According to the stimuli, it may undergo phase transitions. Gelrite® is an example of a Gellan gum. It can undergo anionic polysaccharide in in-situ manner and gelling takes place in the presence of mono- and divalent cations, including Ca^{2+}, Mg^{2+}, K^+, and Na^+ [1, 53].

pH-sensitive or Ion-sensitive Hydrogels: Hydrogels, which respond to changes in pH of the external environment, are called pH-sensitive hydrogels. Ionic groups are attached in those hydrogels and produce special characteristics. pH-sensitive polymers used in hydrogels' preparations are polymethyl methacrylate (PMMA), polyacrylamide, polyacrylic acid, polydiethylaminoethyl methacrylate (PDEAEMA), and polyethylene glycol. These polymers are hydrophobic in nature and can swell in water. The swelling will be dependent on its pH of the external environment. If there is a pH change of the biological environment, it can cause changes in the swelling pattern. In case of hydrogel of caffeine, it is prepared with polymer PDEAEMA at pH below 6.6. This polymer has very high swellability. If the pH of the system increases, drug release will occur and the polymer will shrink. PMMA and polyhydroxyethyl methacrylate (PHEMA) are pH-sensitive hydrogels made up of a copolymer. It swells very high in neutral or high pH, but does not swell in acidic medium. PHEMA and guar gum swelling depend on pH and ionic strength [54, 55]. To encapsulate proteins in acrylamide, polymer cross-linked with bisacrylamide acetal cross-linkers pH-sensitive hydrogels has been used. When the pH is 5, protein is released as the pore size of the acetal cross-linked hydrogels increases. At neutral pH, protein does not diffuse and the acetal groups remain unaffected [56, 57].

Temperature-sensitive Hydrogels: The hydrogels are temperature sensitive as it contains cross-links. There are large numbers of temperature-sensitive drugs made by hydrogels, which are temperature sensitive. These drugs are accepted by pharmaceuticals. Due to this, a large number of drugs are being used. The change in the temperature of external environment can change the release mechanisms and mechanical characteristics of the hydrogels [58]. There are hydrogels, which contract upon heating and are called negative thermosensitive hydrogels. These hydrogels work below their low critical solution temperature of the system. During cooling above their upper critical solution temperature, positive thermosensitive hydrogels contract [59]. Hydrogels are mainly polymers with hydrophobic nature that have varying network structure and the response to temperature is controlling release of the drug. Thermosensitive hydrogels are biodegradable, specific to a particular system, can be controllable by various parameters, and biocompatible drug delivery devices.

There are in situ gel-forming hydrogels which could be in sol state before administration but converts into nonflowing gels after administration [60–62]. These hydrogels are formed by chemical cross-linking or covalent bonds or physical junctions or hydrophobic interactions or electrostatic interactions or chain entanglements [60, 62]. In the in situ gel-forming hydrogels, permanent networks are formed by chemical cross-linking or physical junctions. As environmental conditions change the materials, it can show reversible phase transition behavior [63]. Such hydrogels have no cross-linking agents, no photoirradiation, no organic solvents, and no heat released during polymerization. Due to this, the thermosensitive physical cross-linked in situ gel-forming hydrogels with sol–gel transition are studied to a greater extent. It gains wide applications in biomedical fields, which include controlled drug delivery, cell encapsulation, and tissue engineering [60–73].

The drugs for anticancer, antidiabetic, hormones, or proteins and peptides are widely been used with such thermosensitive devices. The hydrogels can be formed within the system and beneficial for the inflamed or diseased tissue areas [74–76]. Such hydrogels can deliver drugs such as insulin, heparin, and indomethacin. A thermosensitive hydrogels made up of poly-isopropylacrylamide was developed by Tanaka (1978) [77]. Temperature-dependent swelling was shown by the cross-linked polymers containing 75% N-isopropylacrylamide and rest of methacrylic acid.

There will be combined effect of temperature and pH on the drug release when the hydrogel is in a swollen state [78, 79]. Ethylcellulose polymer being coated with thermosensitive membrane was prepared by cross-linking polyisopropylacrylamide hydrogel. This is a thermosensitive macrocapsules of nanoparticles developed in which matrix consists of temperature-sensitive hydrogel. In such hydrogels, the drug release is very high as the high temperature causes large void formation due to collapsing of membrane. At the lower critical solution temperature of about 32 °C, these polymers exhibit phase separation in aqueous solution [80, 81] and synthesized thermosensitive hydrogel of poly(*N*-isopropyl-3-butenamide). The hydrogel was with smaller pore size and when the concentration of cross-linker increases, the same material showed high swelling ratio with a gel containing low concentration of cross-linker. There are more thermosensitive hydrogel of polyorganophosphazene polymers containing alpha-amino-omega-methyl-poly(ethylene glycol) and hydrophobic L-isoleucine ethyl ester side groups. This material showed varying physical appearance such as transparent sol to translucent gel when the temperature was used to entrap natural insulin source for prolonged release [82]. Anticancer drug—doxorubicin was added to it for the controlled release. The drug was performing very well and has no effect on gel properties such as viscosity and gel strength. It was observed successfully for 20 days. This was used for the depot therapy [83].

Glucose-sensitive Hydrogels: The hydrogels response depending upon the presence of glucose or sugar is called glucose-sensitive hydrogels. The cross-linked poly(methacrylamidophenylboronic acid-co-acylamide) hydrogel is a pharmaceutical hydrogel system and is also a glucose-sensitive hydrogel. When the concentration of glucose is high in the surrounding environment, the hydrogel will swell and can liberate the drug in a controlled manner [84, 85]. Glucose-sensitive hydrogels contain an implantable sensor, which can sensitize the glucose concentration from 0 to 20 mM [86]. Partitioning the insulin concentration is possible by insulin-loaded hydrogels of cross-linked copolymers of PEG and methacrylic acid. The microparticles of hydrogels showed the release highest at pH 7.4 and no leakage under acidic conditions [87]. Photopolymerization of 2-hydroxyethyl methacrylate and 3-acrylamidophenylboronic acid can create glucose-sensitive hydrogel. The liberation of insulin will be based on the glucose concentration [88]. There can be an enzymatic reaction in the hydrogels based on sulfonamide where the hydrogel is showing maximum swelling at pH 7.4 in a local glucose environment of 0–300 mg/dL [83] for the controlled delivery of insulin.

Another hydrogel made of poly(2-hydroxyethyl methacrylate-co-*N,N*-dimethylaminoethyl methacrylate) or poly(HEMA-co-DMAEMA) polymer containing insulin in which the glucose oxidase acts as catalyst for the enzymes. In the presence of glucose, swelling of the hydrogel causes by the raise in the pH due to the glucose diffuses in the hydrogel from blood and gets converted to gluconic acid. When hydrogels swell in the presence of glucose, liberation of insulin starts and this can control the glucose level in the blood. Such devices can release insulin in a controlled manner. The morphology of the hydrogel also regulated by oxygen uptake [89].

Depending on the concentration of glucose in the external environment, stimuli-sensitive hydrogels can show reversible gel to sol phases. For example, a conjugated polymer of monomethoxypoly(ethylene glycol) with glucose-containing polymer. When glucose is added, viscosity of hydrogels decreases [90]. Glucose-sensitive hydrogels can bind insulin to concanavalin A. It is a lectin protein that reacts with specific sugar residues present at terminals. In this case insulin, it is displaced in the presence of glucose [91, 92]. Immobilization of glucose oxidase enzyme catalyzes beta-D-glucose to gluconic acid and hydrogen peroxide and glucose-sensitive hydrogels are formed. There will be decrease in swelling when the release of gluconic acid decreases pH of the external environment.

In the polymer chain, enzyme can be in the bound form or it could be attached form [93]. Hydrogels have the conducting behavior that lead to the swelling and ions liberation. There will be formation of gluconic acid or ionization of amines in the polymer, which could be made use for preparation of hydrogels. Smart biomaterials can show controlled delivery of solute proteins such as insulin, lysozyme, or bovine serum albumin (BSA) in response to external environment [94]. There are many other parameters such as temperature, pH, light, electric field, chemicals, and ions in formulation of glucose-responsive hydrogels [95–98].

Nanohydrogels: Hydrogels prepared in water by self-aggregation of polymers of natural origin such as dextran are called nanohydrogels. Natural polysaccharides such as dextran, pullulan, or cholesterol-containing polysaccharide are the sources for these types of hydrogels. Such hydrogels can be prepared from cholesterol-containing polysaccharide. It is the reaction in which swelling of the cholesterol-containing polysaccharide takes place and leads to the formation of hydrogel nanoparticles. The properties of hydrogel can be controlled by changing the degree of substitution of cholesterol polysaccharides. The properties are size and density of nanoparticles [99, 100]. The hydrogels formed by these methods are nanoparticles with dimensions 20–30 nm. These hydrogels can be used for and releasing the entrapped drug by swelling. The swelling may occur due to the pH change of the surrounding environment. Study has been conducted on adriamycin-like drugs and found delivering to infected tumor cells. Here, the release of the drug occurred due to the pH change. When the pH was below 6.8, the release was found to be the highest for Na [101]. Proteins named lysozyme, albumin, and immunoglobulin are also released in controlled manner by such hydrogels nanoparticles.

Protein released amount is dependent on the square root of time. Dextran-type hydrogels are encapsulated with enzyme dextranase and made biodegradable [102]. Pullulan nanoparticles hydrogels are used for targeting a cell by encapsulating active drug in aqueous score of aerosol OT in n-hexane solvent [103]. Linoleic acid modified with chitosan also can be made into hydrogels by self-assembling nanoparticles that can be used for targeting tissues and are biocompatible and biodegradable [104]. Polysaccharide mannose from *Saccharomyces cerevisiae* has been prepared or encapsulating insulin or BSA is another nanohydrogel that can be used for controlled drug delivery [105].

14.4   DRUG DELIVERY SYSTEMS (DDSS)

One of the very fast developing areas is the DDSs, which are connected to the fields of pharmacology, chemistry, chemical, and biotechnology [106–108]. There are a lot of shortcomings for the conventional drug administrations, which have been overcome by the controlled DDS. The controlled rates of delivery in this system are giving much better treatment effects compared to the conventional treatment methods [109]. There are a lot of experiments and researches are already progressed in this areas; still lot more are expected in the future.

The role of hydrogels is very predominant in this field [110–112]. It has gained much more attention in the years due to their excellent response in the systems. They are smart in their action and they have various properties that support the controlled release of drugs to the system. There are many special properties that it can contribute such as the special response to the particular environment and changes as per the parameters such as light, pressure, temperature, pH, and electric fields [113–115].

More attentions are given to the application of hydrogels, which can provide stable and economical DDSs. It helps in the advanced drug delivery formulations and can reduce problems of conventional drugs and its dosages. Hydrogels form the novel DDSs with variety of special features. They are stable and biocompatible and very convenient to use for both big and small molecules. Drugs such as nonsteroidal anti-inflammatory drugs are easily administrated using the hydrogels. It can be very well suitable for large proteins and peptides [116, 117]. Hydrogels can constantly provide drugs in the controlled rate, which is not possible by the conventional drug administration. A diabetic patient needs insulin in the blood at a controlled rate throughout the time, which can be provided by a hydrogel-based DDS.

The design of controlled DDSs is in such a way that the drug release will occur for a long time at a controlled rate. This mechanism is designed as zero-order release kinetics where the release rate is constant. Here, biocompatible polymers containing the drugs are used. These polymers will contain the required drug and the drug will be targeted to those infected cells. The advantage is that it will not be targeting the normal cells. There will be a protection for the normal cells by this system [118, 119]. The basic requirement for this system is a carrier. The carrier should be biocompatible and biosensitive. This can be materialized by the use of hydrogels containing hydrophobic polymeric network with three-dimensional structures. These polymers are cross-linked to the optimum levels for maintaining insolubility in water [120]. The hydrogels will be swollen many times to their molecular structure in water or biological fluids [121] at the same time maintaining the mechanical strength due to the cross-links.

The injectable-type thermosensitive hydrogels are very important [122–124] in the advanced DDSs. Thermosensitive hydrogels are free flowing sol at or below ambient temperature. These hydrogels convert into nonflowing gel at body temperature, if injected by in vivo. This system could release the drug when it is loaded with pharmaceutical agents [123–127]. Such drug incorporation has many advantages. They are injectable, with greater solubility of hydrophobic drugs, greater safety, as it does not use solvent, initiators, and make lesser toxicity. It is also beneficial as the formulation and administration are simpler, not surgery procedure, prolonged releasing pattern, and specifically adhere to the sites. This became a convenient administration route by in situ for the local drug delivery and can administrate hydrophilic drugs, hydrophobic drugs, peptides, proteins, and nucleic acids.

Xerogels are formed when water is removed from the hydrogels. The hydrogels after drying can absorb water to a greater extent and form superabsorbent [128]. Aerogels are dehydrated hydrogels in which water is removed without change in structure. Small particles with a diameter of 100 nm are called microgels and also swell in water. The structure of hydrogels is further termed as macroporous, microporous, or nonporous that depends on the porosity. The pore size of macroporous hydrogels is 0.1–1 μm having comparatively larger pores. The drug released from the pore by the value of drug diffusion coefficient. Small-sized pores are microporous hydrogels of 100–1000 A° range. In microporous hydrogels, the drug release will be based on molecular diffusion and convection. There will be partitioning of the drug through the hydrogel walls when the drug and polymer are compatible to each other. There are hydrogels in nonporous nature containing cross-linking of monomers of size 10–100 A°. In such cases, drug releases by diffusion [129–131].

14.5   HYDROGEL ADMINISTRATION

It becomes very complex problem when various biomaterials are administrated in vivo to a biological environment. The material should be biologically safe environment for the subjected animals. The testing in vivo is challenging because there should be an established and reliable animal model to achieve the biomechanical restoration. There are various injectable hydrogels protocols developed by following all the standards and optimizations. If the body could tolerate them, it becomes an ideal system for performing in vivo testing on rodents [132]. Figure 14.1 represents all types of administration methods.

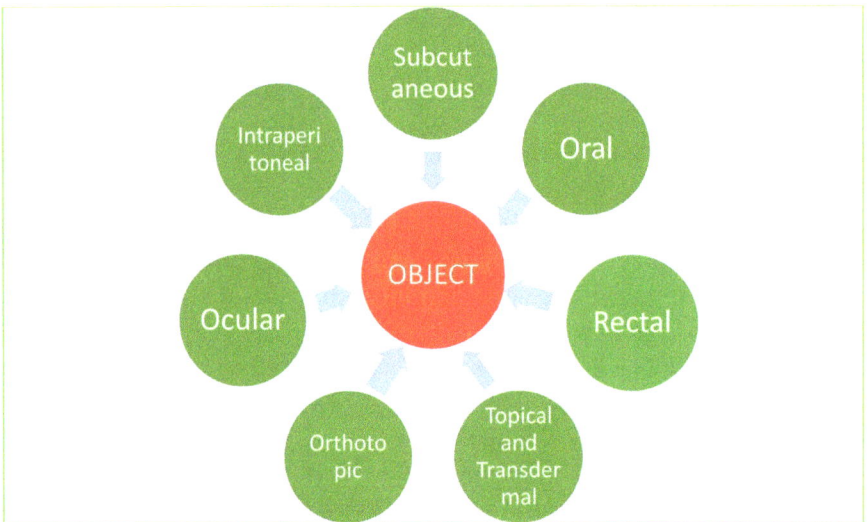

FIGURE 14.1   Various types of drug administration systems.

Subcutaneous Hydrogel Delivery System: To analyze the response of the therapy or medicine, toxicity response can be conducted more effectively by the use of a subcutaneous injection. The area where the injection is given gets vascularized and there can be a very mild amount of reaction that can be observed [132]. Polyethylene-based hydrogels have proven without cytotoxicity in murine models even after 60 days are injected subcutaneously [133]. There are many other examples were the hydrogels are working effectively. They are ellagic acid-based hydrogels [134], nanosized polyacrylamide hydrogels [135], chitosan and gelatin hydrogels [136, 137], alginate [138], and pectin [139]. Mild inflammatory responses are observed in the majority of the studies.

Oral Delivery: One of the very convenient methods is oral delivery of drugs [140]. These hydrogels should give bioavailability, which depend on medium parameters such as pH variations along the line of intestinal tract [141]. There is acute oral toxicity for mono polyethylene glycol (MPEG), caprolactone, and itaconic acid by such pH-sensitive hydrogels in BALB/c mice and showed no signs of toxicity [142]. In oral ingestion, most significant aspect is the metabolic effect of monomers on the organism. Very healthy metabolism is observed on polyglycolic and poly(lactic-*co*-glycolic) acid hydrogel degradation [131]. This can lead to some limitations in terms of hydrogel such as digestive enzymes that could make denaturation, lower permeability through the epithelial membrane into the bloodstream, and superior or inferior digestive systems can convert into potential therapeutic targets [143].

Rectal Delivery: There are several advantages for rectal administration. This can give very rapid absorption of the compound, gastrointestinal tract can be avoided, very minimum adverse reactions, and provides stable environmental conditions and controlled release of the compound. This gives very good biocompatibility on the digestive tract [144]. When rectally administrated these hydrogels such as catechol-chitosan, tests conducted on mucoadhesive properties in murine models give no toxic effects even for 10 days [145]. Afaf et al. developed a hydrogel-based product that can work in vitro and in vivo with promising results [138].

Topical and Transdermal Delivery: Topical and transdermal hydrogel therapy is another suitable approach. The skin may act as barrier, which restricts the delivery via epidermis and dermis is the general concept. The skin will act as macroscale mesh-like structure that would prohibit penetration in the case of collagen hydrogels [146]. Hydrogel-based formulations are developed with no discernable side effects compared to other gel-based used in hospital conditions [147]. This system depends on nanoparticles diameter, charge penetration rate, and structure. Drug delivery using nanoparticles found very effective as per the studies. It is found that peptide-layered nanocarriers are much more efficient than pegylated ones. Skin samples collected from mouse and human through surgical resection and ex-vivo studies were carried out [148].

Orthotopic Injections: It is a practical approach of administration of hydrogels via intratumoral injection. This will result in release of the nanostructure system loaded in a hydrogel matrix. These hydrogel structures are macroscopic gels coming needed to decrease the damage of tissues while taking the injection [149]. A smart hydrogel, which is responsive to temperature and preventing the formation of peritoneal adhesion on a damaged abdominal wall, was synthesized by Qinjie Wu et al. in 2015 [150]. Hydrogel-based orthotopic treatment postresection cavity gives slow release that will improve the long-term survival [151].

Intraperitoneal Delivery: The medicine injection directly into the body gives very good results. This method is called intraperitoneal administration. Hydrogel systems are administrated in such a manner that give excellent results and it is a noninvasive option and can use optimum formulation of various pharmaceutical agents. There are dual actions such as drug delivery and postoperative antiadhesiveness. It is developed by Chih-Hao Chen et al. in 2018 that could incorporated in mouse [152].

Intraperitoneal hydrogels such as mostly gelatin-based gels do not show cytotoxicity and have high degrees of biocompatibility [153]. Hydrogels have the greater capacity to absorb water, so that it can be used for the injection-based formulations [141].

Ocular Delivery: This is the delivery of drugs through the eye of the patients. It is very complicated to develop formulations for ocular delivery; there are several implications that may create limitations of inferior bioavailability and absorption [142]. There can be eye topical applications to be performed but will address the diseases in minimum levels only. When delivering therapeutic agents to a higher concentrations to the posterior segments, failure observed in many situations [154]. In posterior segment, intraocular injections are tried giving primary concern to ocular complications. There are other approaches such as intravitreal, intracameral, or periocular injections, but have high side effects possible [155]. Hydrogels are used for contact lenses made of silicone and polymethylmethacrylate and are highly biocompatible [156]. Silicone hydrogels causing eye inflammation have been reported [157].

14.6   DESIGN OF HYDROGELS

Hydrogels are of various size, architecture, and function. As per these features, the hydrogels are utilized for drug delivery. They are available in various dimensions such as centimeters from subnanometers. Hydrogel delivery to human body will depend on the design aspects. It can form any size and shape. Presence of micropores will be affecting the overall physical properties such as deformability. This can allow convective drug transport to the system. Water absorbed will be surrounded by the cross-links network formed in the hydrogels. The open spaces in the network are termed as mesh size and they are characterized as per the mesh size value. Depends on the mesh size, the drug diffuses through it. There is the possibility of various chemical reactions between the drug and the polymer chains. Depends on the physical and chemical structure designed, there can be large number of binding points for the drug and the polymer. For the controlled release of the drug, there should be suitable conditions at the molecules even at the atomic scale. Therefore, hydrogels are to be designed in macroscopic level with the desirable features which may vary from one system to other system. Hydrogel possesses a multiscale pattern in their structure, hence it is, thus, enabling to design it based on the applications [158].

Some of the design aspects are common to many types of hydrogel systems. There are also specific cases depending on the therapeutic application. There are several conditions to be satisfied for the DDSs based on hydrogels. It should maintain the drug activity during the packaging, transport, and storage. The drug and hydrogel need to maintain its stability both chemically and physically. The delivery of hydrogels can be done by various methods. It can be done by implantation done using surgery, needle injection given locally, or through intravenous infusion method. Depending on the overall efficacy and patient compliance, delivery methods can be chosen. The pattern by the drug releases to get the required results is very important. The availability of the drug and the profile of drug release need to be analyzed and accordingly the system is designed. The release pattern can be short term, long term, continuous, or pulsatile types. There should be proper disposal mechanism when the drug amount finishes and design should include self-degradation of the polymer and no need of a surgery to remove it. Cases are there in which the hydrogel carrier polymer can be used again for another application.

Macroscopic Design: Hydrogels have the peculiarity that it can be made into any size or shape according to the human body requirements during the delivery methods and procedures. There are mainly three hydrogel categories based on the size: macroscopic hydrogels, microgels, and nanogels. Microgels and nanogels are hydrogels with dimensions of micrometers and nanometers, but macroscopic hydrogels are typically in the order of millimeters to centimeters. These hydrogels are surgically implanted into the body or kept so that it is contact with body to get the delivery of drug [159]. A type I collagen gel that releases recombinant human bone morphogenetic protein-2 achieved success with surgically implanted hydrogels for drug delivery in the clinical trials. This was implanted for the treatment of long bone fracture and spinal fusion [160].

The skin, intestinal epithelium, and mucosa are epithelial barriers for drug delivery. These cannot allow the penetration of macroscopic hydrogels and can permit the drugs come out from the hydrogels. Such hydrogels are widely used in wound dressing. Examples are poly(vinyl alcohol) and poly(hydroxyalkyl methacrylate) [161] and biopolymers such as alginate [162], collagen [163], and chitosan [158] that are made from synthetic polymers. These hydrogels can adapt to the skin very easily and widely used in protein delivery for insulin and calcitonin [164]. Wounds are treated nicely by alginate-based hydrogels from long back [165, 166]. Many new materials are coming up in clinical trials. For the healing of deep, second-degree burn wounds [167], recent clinical trials are found effective and safer using a hydrogel delivering recombinant human granulocyte-macrophage colony-stimulating factor.

In Situ-gelling Hydrogels: The hydrogels are subjected to liquid to solid transition after injected into human body in normal liquid form. The gel formed can take up the shape as the space available. Here, a slow gelling process takes place and while injection, the solution will be in the liquid form and the gelation starts slowly. The ideal system kinetics are designed not to clot while injection inside the needle. At the same time, as the solution enters into the body, it should get gelled and should not get mixed up and diluted further with body fluids. There are various standards of gelation mechanism such as charge interaction [168, 169], stereocomplexation [170], and Michael addition [171].

The cross-linking mechanism includes electrostatic charges. Peptides can be cross-linked using cationic lysine and anionic organophosphorus [172]. There are noncovalent interactions also possible between heparin and heparin-binding peptides and proteins. These cross-linkings are helpful to form hydrogels for growth factor delivery [173, 174]. There are another types of gelling of hydrogels in situ. It was formed with a complex polyelectrolyte that can release the proteins, insulin, and avidin within 2 weeks [175]. Some of the cross-linking systems are toxic and damage the cells and tissues. It is, therefore, necessary to develop biobased cross-linking reactants such as copper free for the purpose of gelation [176–178].

Shear-thinning Hydrogels: There are hydrogels, which are pregelled outside of the body. It is then injected by the application of shear stress. They are shear-thinning type hydrogels that can flow like low-viscosity fluids under applied shear stress during injection. It can easily recover their original stiffness after the removal of shear stress happens inside the body. Shear thinning means a reversible cross-links occur physically. Physical cross-links are reversible not like covalent bonding. It occurs because of lot of interactions between many types of forces such as hydrophobic interactions, electrostatic interactions, and hydrogen bonding. There are also antiassembly forces such as solvation and electrostatic repulsion [179]. There are peptides having self-assembling properties studied to a greater extent for making shear-thinning hydrogels. It is available in variety with many types of amino acids that are very easy in modification [180–182] with sequence-specific peptide. For making injectable hydrogels for drug delivery [183, 184], a group of β-hairpin peptides such as Max peptides are developed. The solution to gel transition facilitated by the peptides which having long fibrils up to 200 nm containing two blocks of hydrophobic and charged amino acids.

The peptide self-assembly can occur between metal cations and amino acid and it is illustrated by the gelation of a β-containing sheet of fibrillar hydrogel with zinc ions [185]. Another materials with shear-thinning behaviors are alginate hydrogels. Using electrostatic interactions between alginate and multivalent cations, hydrogels are formed with calcium and zinc. These hydrogels are very well accepted and used to get permanent local delivery with a bioactive vascular endothelial growth factor (VEGF). It was found successful in ischemic murine hindlimbs for 15 days by local drug delivery. It is effective than bolus injection [186, 187], which takes to complete VEGF deprivation after 72 h.

Microgels and Nanogels: A very effective method in invasive delivery of hydrogels is by the use of microgels and nanogels. It got advantages over macrosized gels. It got very small size even smaller than the needle diameter and give larger effective surface area. It can be more convenient to penetrate through the tissue barriers. Hydrogel transport and their adhesion to the blood vessels, airways, or intestinal tract all depend on the size of the particles. Microgels and nanogels can do intraperitoneal and intrabony injection in addition to other normal methods of transport. In case of oral or pulmonary delivery, microgels smaller than 5 μm are used. It has a rapid circulation, therefore not suitable for intravascular injection. The nanogels of size 10–100 nm can leave small blood vessels through fenestrations in the endothelial lining suitable for systemic drug administration, facilitate extravasation into tissues. Hydrogels having size below 10 nm in diameter can be passed by the kidney filtration, but gels of 0.5–10 μm can be phagocytized by macrophages [188].

Designing of the DDSs [189, 190] is influenced by the size and size distribution, deformability, shape, and surface chemistry. Nanogels of positive zeta potential or with high aspect ratios have cellular internalization that is faster especially with a rod-like shape [191]. Biodistribution and circulation persistence of microgels in mice [192] are influenced by the size and deformability. Drugs that are used in gene therapy such as delivery of nucleotide-based drugs such as plasmid DNA, nanogels are very effective. Treatment of cancers, hemophilia, and viral infections [193] is effective with gene therapy. Cellular uptake and prolong circulation time can be improved by nanogels containing DNA compared to nonencapsu-lated DNA.

Leaky tumors are treated with such drugs were vasculature enhances nanoparticle accumulation; in such cases, ineffective lymphatic drainage limits nanoparticle clearance and it can have enhanced permeability and retention effect [194]. PEO- and poly(ethylenimine)-based cationic nano-gels can increase the transport of oligonucleotides across the gastrointestinal epithelium and even the blood–brain barrier [195]. The plasma half-life and protein stability [196] can be enhanced by nanogels consisting of polymer–protein conjugates. DNA nanogels and DNA enzymes-based hydrogels can integrate multiple modular elements that can be used for targeting specific cancer cells [197].

To produce hydrogels of different sizes, various techniques are devel-oped. The size can be also controlled by gelation conditions. The parameters such as polymer and surfactant concentrations or the fabrication parameters, nozzle size, and flow rate can also influence the [198] size of hydrogels. Microfluidics and micromolding methods are used for the production of microgels emulsion and nanomolding techniques used by nanogels. Particle replication in nonwetting templates (PRINT) is a molding technique to produce monodisperse hydrogel particles [6, 199–202] ranging from below 200 nm to 10 μm.

Oral Mucoadhesive DDSs: When there is an adhesion between biological components with other material, it is called mucoadhesion. It will be held by the interfacial forces. The bond formed here is between mucosal surfaces. The attachment of the drug with a carrier to the mucous membrane is a complex phenomenon called mucoadhesion. It is occurring by wetting, adsorption, and interpenetration of polymer chains. The mucoadhesion requires intimate contact between a bioadhesive and a membrane along with wetting and swelling. It requires penetration of the bioadhesive into the tissue or into the surface of the mucous membrane termed as interpenetration. Time for mucosal is very less in minutes and can be increased by the addition of adhesives agents; thus, contact time can be more [203–209]. The theory states that there is a close contact occurs between the mucoadhesive polymer and mucin and interpenetration of polymer and mucin. There can be van der Waals forces, hydrogen bonds, and electrostatic bonds [1].

14.7 DRUG RELEASE MECHANISMS FROM HYDROGELS

Hydrogels have special unique combination of characteristics that make them useful in drug delivery applications. Due to their hydrophilicity, hydrogels can intake large amounts of water. The hydrogels have a very different molecule release mechanisms from hydrophobic polymers. There are simple as well as sophisticated models developed to predict the release of an active agent from a hydrogel device as a function of time. These models are based on diffusion, swelling, and chemically controlled mechanisms that can predict the rate of controlled release.

Network Degradation: There should be a regulated network degradation for the control release of drugs present in the hydrogels. Drugs will be diffusing out when network degrades and mesh size increases. Degradation occurs basically by hydrolysis [210–212] or enzyme activity [213–215] onto the backbone of the polymer. Biodegradable PEG hydrogels can protein release with a half-live period up to 17 days as it contain ester bonds which can hydrolyze slowly. Hydrogel with matrix metalloproteinases (MMPs) has cleavable oligopeptide bonds. MMP-cleavable peptide (GGRMSMPV) into a hyaluronic acid hydrogel can be used to release an inhibitor of MMPs in myocardial infarction [216]. There are hydrogel responds to glucose for insulin delivery [217, 218] and thrombin-responsive hydrogels which can control blood coagulation [219, 220].

There can be triggered degradation in the system for time control that can be provided like getting hydrolysis [221] by giving acidic conditions. Degradation of microgels containing *o*-nitrobenzyl ether (NBE) moieties due to cleavage of the NBE can be triggered by high-energy ultraviolet (UV) light. It can then release the encapsulated transforming growth factor beta-1 (TGF-β1) [222]. Degradation of a hydrogel by a conversion nanoparticles to convert two or more near-infrared (NIR) photons into a UV photon [223] can be triggered by low-energy NIR light.

Swelling: Another important method of drug release is by controlled swelling of hydrogels. As when hydrogel is swelling, the mesh size increases automatically. There should be balance between network deformation and osmosis, as these parameters control the swelling of hydrogels and that lead to water absorption [224, 225]. There are various other external parameters such as temperature [226], glucose [227, 228], pH [229], ionic strength [230], light [231], and electric fields [232]. All these conditions are to be selectively used in the drug delivery.

In case of oral and cancer delivery systems, pH-responsive swelling is widely used. Hydrogels swelling in the acidic stomach will be minimum; therefore, drug is entrapped inside and, hence, protected. When the hydrogel passes through a pH, neutral design is given so that it swells and drug diffusion takes place. Alginate is one of the more commonly hydrogels using a variety of polymers with acidic or basic groups. Alginate hydrogel can hold drugs tightly in acidic conditions, when the pH is neutral. The carboxylic acid groups on the alginate deprotonate and create large osmosis effects leading to swelling of network and drug release [233].

Solid tumors in which the extra- and intracellular environments are more acidic than in normal tissues [234] hence, pH triggered release of drug can be applicable. There are other stimuli-responsive swelling mechanisms used for drug release. Chemotherapy drug cisplatin for breast cancer cells was used to deliver in which the temperature was slightly higher than normal body temperature [235] as it is a temperature-responsive nanogel.

Mechanical Deformation: When the network mechanically deforms [236], it can both increase the mesh size by changing the network structure and trigger convective flow within the network. A pulsatile release patterns can be generated very fine control over the magnitude of the instantaneous release rate. There can be pulsatile release of insulin, which could be the actual pattern in the body for delivery of insulin following eating [237]. From mechanical deformation or using ultrasound and magnetic field-induced deformations, a network of the deformation can be obtained.

To enhance tissue vascularization [238], a direct mechanical deformation can be used to regulate growth factor. Magnetic fields are used to deform a hydrogel network that containing presence of magnetic nanoparticles [239, 240]. Macropores are included and cause a large and rapid deformation of the scaffold, which increase the release of drug molecules from the hydrogels [241]. The hydrogel structure can be transiently disrupted by ultrasound. This is very effective due to its very high resolution and deep penetration within body tissues. Insulin and interferon-gamma [242] can provide pulsatile drug delivery using ultrasound.

In the mechanical deformation, there is a greater damage to the hydrogels and finally results in mechanical failure. This can be solved by the use of self-healing hydrogels. Alginate hydrogels can be repeated in recovery. It can work with reversibly cross-linked divalent cations that can heal back under physiological conditions and ultrasound disruption. It will enable near digital-type release of small molecules, proteins, and condensed oligonucleotides.

Drug–polymer Interactions: Chemical bonds can be designed between the drug and the polymer chains are another approach to control drug release from hydrogels. These chemical bonds give high affinity interactions that can slow down reaction and sometime terminate drug diffusion through the network. This type of reactions is required in small drugs to control the fast release. There are variety of chemical and physical interactions such as covalent conjugation to secondary interactions and electrostatics and hydrophobic associations between the drug and hydrogels.

Covalent Conjugation: Covalent linkages may be stable or cleavable between drug and polymer can immobilize the drug. If the covalent linkage is highly stable, drug can retain in the polymer for a long time. The cleavable covalent linkages just like breaking of cross-links in degradable networks can be programmed. The breakage can be taking place over a time or in response to environmental conditions. The drugs are released rate can be programmed as per the requirements. Many types of covalent linkages are possible. To conjugate TGF-β1 to a PEG hydrogel via an amine-N-hydroxysuccinimide reaction [243], an amide bonds have been used. Steric hindrance on the tethered drugs was reduced by the hydrogel matrix [244] by a long-chain linkage of hetrobifunctional PEG.

Electrostatic Interactions: There is a strong affinity between drugs and the polymer chains; therefore, electrostatic interactions are widely used. It can work on controlled delivery of multiple drugs from a single system [245, 246] as the charge-based interaction is nonspecific in nature. The drugs can be released from the hydrogel when it is degraded or when the electrostatic interaction is stopped by mobile ions from the system environment. This is applicable to many types of drugs and polymers have charges. Alginate hydrogels carry negative charges used to deliver cationic heparin-binding growth factors such as VEGF to promote tissue regeneration [247, 248]. When the polymer–drug electrostatic interactions are not sufficiently strong for the controlled release, then it can be incorporated as a third agent for interactions [249]. Heparin has incorporated into hydrogels to control the delivery of heparin-binding proteins such as VEGF and basic fibroblast growth factor [250]. There are sulfonate functional groups, which can increase the electrostatic interactions between alginate and protein drugs to extend the release time [251]. The sulfation pattern of heparin has been modified to adjust the affinity of heparin to growth factors and thus control their release mechanism [252].

Hydrophobic Association: Hydrogels possess a large amount of water and having the hydrophilic nature. Due to this, the encapsulation and release of hydrophobic drugs can be a problem. Deterioration and stability and strength of the hydrogel may be affected by phase separation between encapsulated hydrophobic drugs and the hydrogel. Because of this, hydrogels contain hydrophobic polymers that are developed. It can give the components many binding sites for hydrophobic drugs [253].

Copolymerizing hydrophobic monomers and the incorporation of hydrophobic molecules to provide hydrophobic domains in hydrogels are tried. A hydrogel for the delivery of hydrophobic anticancer drugs [254, 255] was developed by hydrophobic aliphatic chains that were incorporated into peptides that can be self-assembled. For the delivery of hydrophobic drugs [256], thiocholesterol was incorporated into polyvinyl alcohol hydrogels. Incorporation of hydrophobic domains may reduce the water content of the hydrogels and can alter their biochemical and physical properties. The overall hydrophobicity of the hydrogels does not change by inclusion of cyclodextrins into hydrogels. These macrocyclic oligosaccharides contain an external hydrophilic character and internal hydrophobic character and in pockets hydrophobic drugs are attached. The drug release is controlled by the relative partitioning of solubilized drugs between the hydrogel and the release medium. which is independent of the mesh size of the hydrogel [257].

It is important to recognize that hydrogels often provide large number of sites for interactions with drugs. It also allows us to hybridize multiple interactions into a single hydrogel [258]. More degree of freedom is designed by modifying the drug release through the chemical interactions. This potential advantage must be considered against the hydrogel biocompatibility. Drug activity is reduced [259, 260] by chemical modifications, active site, or a region of a protein that causes a conformational change. Some types of enzymes lose its bioactivity when PEGylated via the ε-amino group of lysine resides [261].

14.8 FUTURE PERSPECTIVES

As a whole about the outcome, hydrogels are found to be feasible tools for the microfluidics, tissue regeneration engineering, biosensors, and a potential tissue scaffold for new organs.

Future prospects say about the tremendous improvement in their biomimetic capabilities to change the structural and morphological properties. In addition, hydrogel used in 3D multicell model complex generating gives promise in reducing the usage of the number of animals used for testing the activities. This will be giving the closest resemblance of the human body.

It is clear from the outcomes that there is tremendous acceleration in the formulation, development, and deployment in the pharmaceutical market. The uses and roles of hydrogels in biomedical research are not restricted to any particular level as it is gaining importance to a wide spectrum. Technology has improved to a greater extent and the growth of hydrogel also reached to greater level and their still scope of growing to a wider range. Hydrogel became a common material in medical field not only for medical professional but also for common people. The electronics field also proves the growth of hydrogels in various healthcare-oriented applications. The development of the concept "lab-on-a-chip" takes place in which hydrogels play a major role. Diagnostic and drug screening investigations and generation of wearable sensors in which microfluidic devices are more practical and compelling in the present's scenario. This is a strong platform to monitor pathological characteristics of the human. Such devices can also perform a controlled release of pharmaceutical formulations according to the monitored parameters. Hydrogel can act as scaffolds in biomedicine and biomedical research became very relevant material.

Novel hydrogels have greater reach in the coming era where very fine structures are made where it can solve practical applications in the real world such as contact lenses, wound dressing, and 3D culture scaffolds. It also was getting the hold in other potential areas such as robotics, aerospace engineering, solar cells and photoreactors, environmental research, and sports science.

14.9 CONCLUSION

Hydrogels are the polymer with cross-linked networks and can absorb very higher amounts of aqueous medium. Because of the water intake capacity, hydrogels resemble natural living tissue compared to any other types of synthetic material. In most of the drug delivery applications, hydrogels have being used as it has the unique combination of characteristics. Hydrogels, being hydrophilic in nature, can intake large amounts of water. The molecular release pattern from a hydrogel is different from hydrophobic polymers. Hydrogels-based creams are better than conventional creams with better results and biocompatibility. Scaling and dryness are not observed when hydrogels are used as it has moisturizing properties.

KEYWORDS

- **hydrogels**
- **biodegradable**
- **crosslinking**
- **swollen**
- **hydrophilic**

REFERENCES

1. Bindu SM, Ashok V, Chatterjee A. Review on hydrogels as drug delivery in the pharmaceutical field. Int J Pharm Chem Sci. 2012; 1(2):17–30.
2. Lee KY, Mooney DJ. Hydrogels for tissue engineering. Chem Rev. 2001; 101(7): 1869–1879.
3. van der Linden HJ, Herber S, Olthuis W, Bergveld P. Stimulus-sensitive hydrogels and their applications in chemical (micro)analysis. Analyst. 2003; 128:325–331.
4. Jen AC, Wake MC, Mikos AG. Review: hydrogels for cell immobilization. Biotechnol Bioeng. 1996; 50(4):357–364.
5. Wang KL, Burban JH, Cussler EL. Hydrogels as separation agents. In: Dušek K. (Ed). Responsive Gels: Volume Transitions II. Advances in Polymer Science, vol 110. Springer, Berlin, 1993. p. 67–79.
6. Bennett SL, Melanson DA Torchiana DF, Wiseman DM, Sawhney AS. Next-generation hydrogel films as tissue sealants and adhesion barriers. J Card Surg. 2003; 18 (6): 494–499.
7. Sutton C. Adhesions and their prevention. Obstet Gynecol. 2005; 7:168–176.
8. Peppas NA, Colombo P. Analysis of drug release behavior from swellable polymer carriers using the dimensionality index. J Control Release. 1997; 45:35–40.
9. Khare AR, Peppas NA. Swelling/deswelling of anionic copolymer gels. Biomaterials. 1995; 16:559–567.
10. Yoshii E. Cytotoxic effects of acrylates and methacrylates: relationships of monomer structures and cytotoxicity. J Biomed Mater Res. 1998; 37:517–524.
11. Peppas N, Huang Y. Nanoscale technology of mucoadhesive interactions. Adv Drug Deliv Rev. 2004; 56:1675–1687.
12. Nedkov E, Tsvetkova S. Structure of poly(ethylene glycol) hydrogels obtained by gamma irradiation. Radiat Phys Chem. 1994; 44:81–87.
13. Peppas NA, Keys KB, Torres-Lugo M, Lowman AM. Poly(ethylene glycol)-containing hydrogels in drug delivery. J Control Release. 1999; 62:81–87.
14. Allcock HA, Ambrosio AMA. Synthesis and characterization of pH-sensitively (organophosphazene) hydrogels. Biomaterials. 1996; 17:2295–2302.
15. Stringer JL, Peppas NA. Diffusion of small molecular weight drugs in radiation cross-linked poly(ethylene oxide) hydrogels. J Control Release. 1996; 42:195–202.

16. Akkas P, Sari M, Sen M, Guven O. The effect of external stimuli on bovine serum albumin adsorption capacity of poly(acrylamide/maleic acid) hydrogels prepared by gamma rays. Radiat Phys Chem. 1999; 55:717–721.

17. Han TS, Hur K, Choi B, Lee JY, Byeon SJ, Min J, Yu J, Cho JK, Hong J, Lee HJ, Kong SH, Kim WH, Yanagihara K, Song SC, Yang HK. Improvement of anti-cancer drug efficacy via thermosensitive hydrogel in peritoneal carcinomatosis in gastric cancer. Oncotarget. 2017; 8:108848–108858.

18. Naahidi S, Jafari M, Logan M, Wang Y, Yuan Y, Bae H, Dixon B, Chen P. Biocompatibility of hydrogel-based scaffolds for tissue engineering applications. Biotechnol Adv. 2017; 35:530–544.

19. Palmer BC, DeLouise LA. Nanoparticle-enabled transdermal drug delivery systems for enhanced dose control and tissue targeting. Molecules. 2016; 21:1719.

20. Gomes M, Azevedo H, Malafaya P, Silva S, Oliveira J, Silva G, Sousa R, Mano J, Re R. Natural polymers in tissue engineering applications. Tissue Eng. 2008; 5:145–192.

21. Ma X, Sun X, Hargrove D, Chen J, Song D, Dong Q, Lu X, Fan TH, Fu Y, Lei YA. Biocompatible and biodegradable protein hydrogel with green and red autofluorescence: preparation, characterization, and in vivo biodegradation tracking and modeling. Sci Rep. 2016; 6:19370.

22. Peppas NA, Sahlin JJ. Hydrogels as mucoadhesive and bioadhesive materials: A review. Biomaterials. 1996; 17:1553–1561.

23. Chaturvedi M, Kumar M, Pathak K. A review on mucoadhesive polymer used in nasal drug delivery system. J Adv Pharm Technol Res. 2011; 2:215.

24. Reece TB, Maxey TS, Kron IL. A prospectus on tissue adhesives. Am J Surg. 2001; 182: S40–S44.

25. Xu J, Strandman S, Zhu JX, Barralet J, Cerruti M. Genipin-crosslinked catechol-chitosan mucoadhesive hydrogels for buccal drug delivery. Biomaterials. 2015; 37: 395–404.

26. Nho YC, Park JS, Lim YM. Preparation of poly(acrylic acid) hydrogel by radiation crosslinking and its application for mucoadhesives. Polymers. 2014; 6:890–898.

27. Bhattarai N, Gunn J, Zhang M. Chitosan-based hydrogels for controlled, localized drug delivery. Adv Drug Deliv Rev. 2010; 62:83–99.

28. Ponchel G, Irache JM. Specific and non-specific bioadhesive particulate systems for oral delivery to the gastrointestinal tract. Adv Drug Deliv Rev. 1998; 34:191–219.

29. Shojaei AH, Paulson J, Honary S. Evaluation of poly(acrylic acid-co-ethylhexyl acrylate) films for mucoadhesive transbuccal drug delivery: Factors affecting the force of mucoadhesion. J Control Release. 2000; 67:223–232.

30. Neves JD, Bahia M. Gels as vaginal drug delivery systems. Int J Pharm. 2006; 318:1–14.

31. Luppi B, Bigucci F, Mercolini L, Musenga A, Sorrenti M, Catenacci L, Zecchi V. Novel mucoadhesive nasal inserts based on chitosan/hyaluronate polyelectrolyte complexes for peptide and protein delivery. J Pharm Pharmacol. 2009; 61:151–157.

32. Lee H, Dellatore SM, Miller WM, Messersmith PB. Mussel-inspired surface chemistry for multifunctional coatings. Science. 2007; 318:426–430.

33. Lee BP, Messersmith PB, Israelachvili JN, Waite JH. Mussel-inspired adhesives and coatings. Ann Rev Mater Res. 2011; 41:99.

34. Brubaker CE, Kissler H, Wang LJ, Kaufman DB, Messersmith PB. Biological performance of mussel-inspired adhesive in extrahepatic islet transplantation. Biomaterials. 2010; 31:420–427.

35. Nafea E, Marson A, Poole-Warren L, Martens P. Immunoisolating semi-permeable membranes for cell encapsulation: Focus on hydrogels. J Control Release. 2011; 154: 110–122.

36. Lake GJ, Thomas AG. Strength of highly elastic materials. Proc R Soc A. 1967; 300: 108–119.

37. Kong HJ, Wong E, Mooney DJ. Independent control of rigidity and toughness of polymeric hydrogels. Macromolecules. 2003; 36:4582–4588.

38. Gong JP, Katsuyama Y, Kurokawa T, Osada Y. Double-network hydrogels with extremely high mechanical strength. Adv Mater. 2003; 15:1155–1158.

39. Sun JY, Zhao X, Illeperuma WRK, Chaudhuri O, Oh KH, Mooney DJ, Vlassak JJ, Suo Z Highly stretchable and tough hydrogels. Nature. 2012; 489:133–136.

40. Li J, Illeperuma WR, Suo Z, Vlassak JJ. Hybrid hydrogels with extremely high stiffness and toughness. ACS MacroLett. 2014; 3:520–523.

41. Lin CC, Metters AT. Hydrogels in controlled release formulations: network design and mathematical modeling. Adv Drug Deliv Rev. 2006; 58:1379–1408.

42. Burczak K, Fujisato T, Hatada M, Ikada Y. Protein permeation through poly(vinyl alcohol) hydrogel membranes. Biomaterials. 1994; 15:231–238.

43. Dubrovskii SA, Rakova GV. Elastic and osmotic behavior and network imperfections of nonionic and weakly ionized acrylamide-based hydrogels. Macromolecules. 1997; 30:7478–7486.

44. Sakai T, Matsunaga T, Yamamoto Y, Ito C, Yoshida R, Suzuki S, Sasaki N, Shibayama M, Chung U. Design and fabrication of a high-strength hydrogel with ideally homogeneous network structure from tetrahedron-like macromonomers. Macromolecules. 2008; 41: 5379–5384.

45. Lee KY, Mooney DJ. Hydrogels for tissue engineering. Chem Rev. 2001; 101: 1869–1880.

46. Vermonden T, Censi R, Hennink WE. Hydrogels for protein delivery. Chem Rev. 2012; 112:2853–2888.

47. Szepes A, Makai Z, Blumer C, Mader K, Kasa P, Revesz PS. Characterization and drug delivery behavior of starch-based hydrogels prepared via isostatic ultrahigh pressure. Carbohyd Polym. 2008; 72:571–575.

48. Yu H, Xiao C. Synthesis and properties of novel hydrogels from oxidized Konjac glucomannan cross-linked gelation for in-vitro drug delivery. Carbohyd Polym. 2008; 72:479–489.

49. Pal K, Banthia AK, Majumdar DK. Effect of heat treatment of starch on the properties of the starch hydrogels. Mater Lett. 2008; 62:215–218.

50. Yin Y, Ji X, Dong H, Ying Y, Zhing H. Study of the swelling dynamics with overshooting effect of hydrogels based on sodium alginate-g-acrylic acid. Carbohyd Polym. 2008; 71: 682–689.

51. Kim SW, Bae YH, Okano T. Hydrogels: swelling, drug loading, and release. Pharm Res. 1992; 9(3):283–290.

52. Schuetz YB, Gurny R, Jordan O. A novel thermoresponsive hydrogel of chitosan. Eur J Pharm Biopharm. 2008; 68:19–25.

53. Xia LW, Xie R, Jiu XJ, Wang W, Chen Q, Chu LY. Nano-structured smart hydrogels with rapid response and high elasticity. Nat Commun. 2013; 4:2226.

54. Peppas LB, Peppas NA. Dynamic and equilibrium behavior of pH-sensitive hydrogels containing 2-hydroxyethyl methacrylates. Biomaterials. 1990; 11:635–644.

55. Das A, Wadhwa S, Srivastava AK. Cross-linked guar gum hydrogels discs for colon-specific delivery of ibuprofen: formulation and in vitro evaluation. Drug Deliv. 2006; 13:139–142.

56. Murthy N, Thng YX, Schuck S, Xu MC, Frecher JMJ. A novel strategy for encapsulation and release of proteins: hydrogels and microgels with acid-labile acetal cross-linkers. J Am Chem Soc. 2002; 124:12398–12399.

57. Gupta P, Vermani K, Garg S. Hydrogels: from controlled release to pH-responsive drug delivery. Drug Discov Today. 2002; 7:569–579.

58. Prabaharan M, Mano JF. Stimuli-responsive hydrogels based on polysaccharides incorporated with thermoresponsive polymers as novel biomaterials. Macromol Biosci. 2006; 6(12):991–1008.

59. Soppimath KS, Aminabhavi TM, Dave AM, Kumbar SG, Rudzinski WE. Stimulus-responsive smart hydrogels as novel drug delivery systems. Drug Deliv Ind Pharm. 2002; 28(8):957–974.

60. He C, Kim S, Lee D. In situ gelling stimuli-sensitive block copolymer hydrogels for drug delivery. J Control Release. 2008; 127(3):189–207.

61. Hatefi A, Amsden B. Biodegradable injectable in situ forming drug delivery systems. J Control Release. 2002; 80(1–3):9–28.

62. Yu L, Ding J. Injectable hydrogels as unique biomedical materials. Chem Soc Rev. 2008; 37(8):1473–1481.

63. Nguyen M, Lee D. Injectable biodegradable hydrogels. Macromol Biosci. 2010; 10(6): 563–579.

64. Jeong B, Bae YH, Lee DS, Kim SW. Biodegradable block copolymers as injectable drug-delivery systems. Nature. 1997; 388:860–862.

65. Kissel T, Li Y, Unger F. ABA-triblock copolymers from biodegradable polyester A-blocks and hydrophilic poly(ethylene oxide) B-blocks as a candidate for in situ forming hydrogel delivery systems for proteins. Adv Drug Deliv Rev. 2002; 54:99–134.

66. Lee JW, Hua FJ, Lee DS. Thermoreversible gelation of biodegradable poly(caprolactone) and poly(ethylene glycol) multiblock copolymers in aqueous solutions. J Control Release. 2001; 73(2–3):315–327.

67. Song MJ, Lee DS, Ahn JH, Kim DJ, Kim SW. Thermosensitive sol–gel transition behaviors of poly(ethylene oxide)/aliphatic polyester/poly(ethylene oxide) aqueous solutions. J Polyp Sci Pol Chem. 2004; 42:772–784.

68. Markland P, Zhang Y, Amidon GL, Yang VC. A pH- and ionic strength-responsive polypeptide hydrogel: synthesis, characterization, and preliminary protein release studies. J Biomed Mater Res. 1999; 47(4):595–602.

69. Torres-Lugo M, Peppas NA. Molecular design and in vitro studies of novel pH-sensitive hydrogels for the oral delivery of calcitonin. Macromolecules. 1999; 32(20):6646–6651.

70. Kim B, Flamme KL, Peppas NA. Dynamic swelling behavior of pH-sensitive anionic hydrogels used for protein delivery. J Appl Polym Sci. 2003; 89(6):1606–1613.

71. Ichikawa H, Peppas NA. Novel complexation hydrogels for oral peptide delivery: in vitro evaluation of their cytocompatibility and insulin-transport enhancing effects using Caco-2 cell monolayers. J Biomed Mater Res A. 2003; 67A(2):609–617.

72. Ruel-Gariépy E, Leroux J. In situ-forming hydrogels—review of temperature-sensitive systems. Eur J Pharm Biopharm. 2004; 58(2):409–426.

73. Jeong B, Kim SW, Bae YH. Thermosensitive sol-gel reversible hydrogels. Adv Drug Deliv Rev. 2002; 54(1):37–51.

74. Ramanan RM, Chellamuthu P, Tang L, Nguyen KT. Development of a temperature-sensitive composite hydrogel for drug delivery applications. Biotechnol Prog. 2006; 22(1):118–125.

75. Ruel GE, Leroux JC. In-situ forming hydrogels: a review of temperature-sensitive systems. Eur J Pharm Biopharm. 2004; 58(2):409–423.

76. Bae YH, Okano T, Kim SW. On-off thermocontrol of solute transport II: solute release from thermosensitive hydrogels. Pharm Res. 1991; 8(5):624–628.

77. Tanaka T. Collapse of gels and the critical endpoint. Phys Rev Lett. 1978; 40:820–823.

78. Peppas NA, Burer P, Leobandung W, Ichikawa H. Hydrogels in pharmaceutical formulations. Eur J Pharm Biopharm. 2000; 50:27–46.

79. Kim MR, Park TG. Temperature-responsive and degradable hyaluronic acid/pluronic composite hydrogels for controlled release of human growth hormone. J Control Release. 2002; 80(1–3):69–77.

80. Sershen SR, Westcott SL, Halas NJ, West JL. Temperature-sensitive polymer nanoshells composite for photothermally modulated drug delivery. J Biomed Mater Res. 2000; 51(3):293–298.

81. Xu X, Zhang X, Wang B, Cheng S, Zhuo R, Wang Z. Fabrication of a novel temperature sensitive poly(n-isopropyl-3-butenamide) hydrogel. Colloid Surface B. 2007; 59: 158–163.

82. Park KH, Song SC. A thermosensitive poly(organophosphazene) hydrogel used as an extracellular matrix for artificial pancreas. J Biomater Sci Polym Ed. 2005; 16(11): 1421–1431.

83. Kang SI, Bae YH. A sulfonamide-based glucose-responsive hydrogel with covalently immobilized glucose oxidase and catalase. J Control Release. 2003; 86(1):115–121.

84. Pluta J, Karolewicz B. Hydrogels: properties and application in the technology of drug form I: the characteristics hydrogels. Polym Med. 2004; 34(2):3–19.

85. Eddington DT, Beebe DJ. Flow control with hydrogels. Adv Drug Deliv Rev. 2004; 56(2):199–210.

86. Lei M, Baldi A, Nuxoll E, Siegel RA, Ziaie B. A hydrogel-based implantable micromachined transponder for wireless glucose measurement. Diabetes Technol Ther. 2006; 8(1):112–122.

87. Kumar A, Lahiri SS, Singh H. Development of PEGDMA: MAA-based hydrogel microparticles for oral insulin delivery. Int J Pharm. 2006; 323(1–2):117–124.

88. Lee YJ, Pruzinsky SA, Braun PV. Glucose sensitive inverse opal hydrogels: analysis of optical diffraction response. Langmuir. 2004; 20(8):3096–3106.

89. Traitel T, Cohen Y, Kost J. Characterization of glucose-sensitive insulin release systems in simulated in-vivo conditions. Biomaterials. 2000; 21(16):1679–1687.

90. Kim JJ (1999). Phase-reversible glucose-sensitive hydrogels for modulated insulin delivery. PhD dissertations, Purdue University, Indiana, USA.

91. Obaidat AA, Park K. Characterization of protein release through glucose-sensitive hydrogel membranes. Biomaterials. 1997; 18:1801–1806.

92. Kim JJ, Park K. Modulated insulin delivery from glucose-sensitive hydrogel dosage forms. J Control Release. 2001; 77(1–2):39–47.

93. Yoshioka Y, Calvert P. Epoxy-based electroactive polymer gels. Exp Mech. 2002; 42: 404–408.

94. Tang M, Zhang R, Bowyer A, Eisenthal R, Hubble J. A reversible hydrogel membrane for controlling the delivery of macromolecules. Biotechnol Bioeng. 2003; 82(1):47–53.

95. Suzuki A, Tanaka T. Phase transition in polymer gels induced by visible light. Nature. 1990; 346:345–347.

96. Lam Y, Li H, Ng TY, Luo R. Modeling and stimulation of the deformation of multistate hydrogels subjected to electrical stimuli. Eng Anal Bound Elem. 2006; 30 (11): 1011–1017.

97. Zhang XZ, Lewis PJ, Chu CC. Fabrication and characterization of a smart drug delivery systems. Biomaterials. 2005; 26(16):3299–3309.

98. He H, Li L, Lee LJ. Photopolymerization and structure formation of methacrylic acid based hydrogels: the effect of light intensity. React Funct Polym. 2008; 68:13–113.

99. Akiyoshi K, Kobayashi S, Schichibe S, Mix D, Baudys M, Kim SW, Sunamoto J. Self-assembled hydrogel nanoparticle of cholesterol-bearing pullulan as a carrier of protein drugs: complexation and stabilization of insulin. J Control Release. 1998; 54(3): 313–320.

100. Kim IS, Jeong Y, Kim SH. Self-assembled hydrogel nanoparticles composed of dextran and poly(ethylene glycol) macromer. Int J Pharm. 2000; 205(1–2):109–116.

101. Bae YH, Okano T, Kim SW. On-off thermocontrol of solute transport II. Solute release from thermosensitive hydrogels. Pharm Res. 1991; 8(5):624–628.

102. Hennink WE, Franssen O, Wolthusis WNE, Talsma H. Dextran hydrogels for the controlled release of proteins. J Control Release. 1997; 48(2–3):107–114.

103. Gupta M, Gupta AK. In-vitro cytotoxicity studies of hydrogels pullulan nanoparticles prepared by AOT/n-hexane miceller system. J Pharm Sci. 2004; 7(1):38–46.

104. Chenguang L, Goud DK, Xiguang C, Jin PH. Preparation and characterization of self-assembled nanoparticles based on linolenic acid modified chitosan. J Ocean Univ China. 2007; 4(3):234–239.

105. Yamane S, Akiyoshi K. Nanogel-inorganic hybrid: synthesis and characterization of polysaccharide calcium phosphate nanomaterials. Eur Cells Mater. 2007; 14(3):113.

106. Langer R, Tirrell D. Designing materials for biology and medicine. Nature. 2004; 428(6982):487–492.

107. Charman W, Chan H, Finnin B, Charman S. Drug delivery: a key factor in realizing the full therapeutic potential of drugs. Drug Dev Res. 1999; 46(3–4):316–327.

108. Rosen H, Abribat T. The rise and rise of drug delivery. Nat Rev Drug Discov. 2005; 4(5): 381–385.

109. Hoffman A. Hydrogels for biomedical applications. Adv Drug Deliv Rev. 2002; 54(1): 3–12.

110. Hoare T, Kohane D. Hydrogels in drug delivery: progress and challenges. Polymer. 2008; 49(8):1993–2007.

111. Peppas N, Hilt J, Khademhosseini A, Langer R. Hydrogels in biology and medicine: from molecular principles to bionanotechnology. Adv Mater. 2006; 18(11):1345–1360.

112. Jeong B, Gutowska A. Lessons from nature: stimuli-responsive polymers and their biomedical applications. Trends Biotechnol. 2002; 20(7):305–311.

113. Qiu Y, Park K. Environment-sensitive hydrogels for drug delivery. Adv Drug Deliv Rev. 2001; 53(3): 321–339.

114. Schmaljohann D. Thermo- and pH-responsive polymers in drug delivery. Adv Drug Deliv Rev. 2006; 58(15):1655–1670.

115. Galaev I, Mattiasson B. "Smart" polymers and what they could do in biotechnology and medicine. Trends Biotechnol. 1999; 17(8):335–340.

116. Graham NB, Mc-Neil ME. Hydrogels for controlled drug delivery. Biomaterials. 1984; 5(1):27–36.

117. Bajpai SK, Sonkusley J. Hydrogels for oral drug delivery of peptides: synthesis and characterization. J Appl Polym Sci. 2002; 83:1717–1729.
118. Stastny M, Plocova D, Etrych T, Kova M, Ulbrich K, Richova B. HPMA-hydrogels containing static drugs kinetics of the drug release and in-vivo efficacy. J Control Release. 2002; 81:101–111.
119. Lowman AM, Peppas NA. (1991). Hydrogels. In: Mathiowitz E (Ed). Encyclopedia of Controlled Drug Delivery. Wiley, New York. pp. 397–418.
120. Peppas NA, Burer P, Leobandung W, Ichikawa H. Hydrogels in pharmaceutical formulations. Eur J Pharm Biopharm. 2000; 50:27–46.
121. Kim SW, Bae YH, Okano T. Hydrogels: swelling, drug loading, and release. Pharm Res. 1992; 9(3):283–290.
122. Yu L, Ding J. Injectable hydrogels as unique biomedical materials. Chem Soc Rev. 2008; 37(8):1473–1481.
123. Jeong B, Kim SW, Bae YH. Thermosensitive sol–gel reversible hydrogels. Adv Drug Deliv Rev. 2002; 54(1):37–51.
124. Klouda L, Mikos A. Thermoresponsive hydrogels in biomedical applications. Eur J Pharm Biopharm. 2008; 68(1):34–45.
125. Qiu Y, Park K. Environment-sensitive hydrogels for drug delivery. Adv Drug Deliv Rev. 2001; 53(3):321–339.
126. Bromberg LE, Ron ES. Temperature-responsive gels and thermogelling polymer matrices for protein and peptide delivery. Adv Drug Deliv Rev. 1998; 31(3):197–221.
127. Kamath KR, Park K. Biodegradable hydrogels in drug delivery. Adv Drug Deliv Rev. 1993; 11(1–2):59–84.
128. Leonard A, Blacher S, Crine M, Jomaa W. Evolution of mechanical properties and final textural properties of resorcinol formaldehyde xerogels during ambient air drying. J Non Cryst. 2008; 354:831–838.
129. Kim SW, Bae YH, Okano T. Hydrogels: swelling, drug loading, and release. Pharm Res. 1992; 9(3):283–290.
130. McNeill ME, Graham NB. Properties controlling the diffusion and release of water soluble solutes from poly(ethyloxide) hydrogels 1. Polymer composition. J Biomater Sci Polym Ed. 1993; 4(3):305–322.
131. Jhan MS, Andrade JD. Water and hydrogels. J Biomed Mater Res. 1973; 7(6):509–522.
132. Schellini SA, Zimmermann GPM, Hoyama E, Pellizon CH, Padovani CR, Selva D. Polyethylene gel in the subcutaneous tissue of rats: histopathologic and systemic evaluation. Orbit. 2008; 27:153–156.
133. Sharma G, Italia JL, Sonaje K, Tikoo K, Ravi Kumar MNV. Biodegradable in situ gelling system for subcutaneous administration of ellagic acid and ellagic acid loaded nanoparticles: evaluation of their antioxidant potential against cyclosporine induced nephrotoxicity in rats. J Control Release. 2007; 118:27–37.
134. Takahashi M, Heo YJ, Shibata H, Satou H, Kawanishi T, Okitsu T, Takeuchi S. Nanopatterned hydrogel reduced inflammatory effects in subcutaneous tissue. In: Satou H (Ed). Proceedings of the 2012 IEEE 25th International Conference on Micro Electro Mechanical Systems (MEMS), Paris, France, 29 January–2 February 2012; pp. 973–976.
135. Hou HY, Fu SH, Liu CH, Chen JP, Ray-Sea Hsu B. The graft survival protection of subcutaneous allogeneic islets with hydrogel grafting and encapsulated by CTLA4Ig and IL1ra. Polym J. 2014; 46:136–144.

136. Bae JH, Shrestha KR, Park YH, Kim IG, Piao S, Jung AR, Jeon SH, Park KD, Lee JY. Comparison between subcutaneous injection of basic fibroblast growth factor-hydrogel and intracavernous injection of adipose-derived stem cells in a rat model of cavernous nerve injury. Urology. 2014; 84:1248.

137. Halberstadt C, Austin C, Rowley J, Culberson C, Loebsack A, Wyatt S, Coleman S, Blacksten L, Burg K, Mooney D, Holder W. A hydrogel material for plastic and reconstructive applications injected into the subcutaneous space of a sheep. Tissue Eng. 2002; 8:309–319.

138. Markov PA, Khramova DS, Shumikhin KV, Nikitina IR, Beloserov VS, Martinson EA, Litvinets SG, Popov SV. Mechanical properties of the pectin hydrogels and inflammation response to their subcutaneous implantation. J Biomed Mater Res A. 2019; 107(9):2088–2098.

139. Khafagy ES, Morishita M, Onuki Y, Takayama K. Current challenges in non-invasive insulin delivery systems: a comparative review. Adv Drug Deliv Rev. 2007; 59:1521–1546.

140. Tulain UR, Ahmad M, Rashid A, Malik MZ, Iqbal FM. Fabrication of pH-responsive hydrogel and its in vitro and in vivo evaluation. Adv Polym Technol. 2018; 37:290–304.

141. Tan L, Xu X, Song J, Luo F, Qian Z. Synthesis, characterization, and acute oral toxicity evaluation of pH-sensitive hydrogel based on MPEG, poly ("-caprolactone), and itaconic acid. Biomed Res Int. 2013; 2013:239838.

142. Sharpe LA, Daily AM, Horava SD, Peppas NA. Therapeutic applications of hydrogels in oral drug delivery. Exp Opin Drug Deliv. 2014; 11:901–915.

143. Kim K, Kim K, Ryu JH, Lee H. Chitosan-catechol: a polymer with long-lasting mucoadhesive properties. Biomaterials. 2015; 52:161–170.

144. Xu J, Tam M, Samaei S, Lerouge S, Barralet J, Stevenson MM, Cerruti M. Mucoadhesive chitosan hydrogels as rectal drug delivery vessels to treat ulcerative colitis. Acta Biomater. 2017; 48:247–257.

145. Chakrabarti S, Islam J, Hazarika H, Mazumder B, Raju PS, Chattopadhyay P. Safety profile of silver sulfadiazine-bFGF-loaded hydrogel for partial thickness burn wounds. Cutan Ocul Toxicol. 2018; 37:258–266.

146. Wen APY, Halim AS, Saad AZM, Nor FM, Sulaiman WAW. A prospective study evaluating wound healing with sea cucumber gel compared with hydrogel in treatment of skin graft donor sites. Complement Ther Med. 2018; 41:261–266.

147. Fernandes R, Smyth NR, Muskens OL, Nitti S, Heuer-Jungemann A, Ardern-Jones MR, Kanaras AG. Interactions of skin with gold nanoparticles of different surface charge, shape, and functionality. Small. 2015; 11:713–721.

148. Basso J, Miranda A, Nunes S, Cova T, Sousa J, Vitorino C, Pais A. Hydrogel-based drug delivery nanosystems for the treatment of brain tumors. Gels. 2018; 4:62.

149. Zhao M, Danhier F, Bastiancich C, Joudiou N, Ganipineni LP, Tsakiris N, Gallez B, des Rieux A, Jankovski A, Bianco J, Préat V. Post-resection treatment of glioblastoma with an injectable nanomedicine-loaded photopolymerizable hydrogel induces long-term survival. Int J Pharm. 2018; 548:522–529.

150. Bastiancich C, Bianco J, Vanvarenberg K, Ucakar B, Joudiou N, Gallez B, Bastiat G, Lagarce F, Préat V, Danhier F. Injectable nanomedicine hydrogel for local chemotherapy of glioblastoma after surgical resection. J Control Release. 2017; 264:45–54.

151. Chen CH, Kuo CY, Chen SH, Mao SH, Chang CY, Shalumon KT, Chen JP. Thermosensitive injectable hydrogel for simultaneous intraperitoneal delivery of doxorubicin and prevention of peritoneal adhesion. Int J Mol Sci. 2018; 19:1373.

152. Yamashita K, Tsunoda S, Gunji S, Murakami T, Suzuki T, Tabata Y, Sakai Y. Intraperitoneal chemotherapy for peritoneal metastases using sustained release formula of cisplatin-incorporated gelatin hydrogel granules. Surg Today. 2019; 3:1–10.

153. Mandal A, Bisht R, Rupenthal ID, Mitra AK. Polymeric micelles for ocular drug delivery: from structural frameworks to recent preclinical studies. J Control Release. 2017; 248:96–116.

154. Bisht R, Jaiswal JK, Chen YS, Jin J, Rupenthal ID. Light-responsive in situ forming injectable implants for effective drug delivery to the posterior segment of the eye. Exp Opin Drug Deliv. 2016; 13:953–962.

155. Jacob JT. Biocompatibility in the development of silicone-hydrogel lenses. Eye Contact Lens. 2013; 39:12–18.

156. Hall BJ, Jones LW, Dixon B. Silicone allergies and the eye: fact or fiction? Eye Contact Lens. 2014; 40:51–57.

157. Jianyu Li, Mooney DJ. Designing hydrogels for controlled drug delivery. Nat Rev Mater. 2016; 1(12):16071.

158. Tiwari G, Tiwari R, Sriwastawa B, Bhati L, Pandey S, Pandey P, Bannerjee SK. Drug delivery systems: an updated review. Int J Pharm Investig. 2012; 2:2–11.

159. Bessa PC, Casal M, Reis R. Bone morphogenetic proteins in tissue engineering: the road from laboratory to clinic, part II (BMP delivery). J Tissue Eng Regen Med. 2008; 2:81–96.

160. Thorn R, Greeman J, Austin A. An in vitro study of antimicrobial activity and efficacy of iodine-generating hydrogel dressings. J Wound Care. 2006; 15:305.

161. Momoh FU, Boateng JS, Richardson SC, Chowdhry BZ, Mitchell JC. Development and functional characterization of alginate dressing as potential protein delivery system for wound healing. Int J Biol Macromol. 2015; 81:137–150.

162. Pandit A, Ashar R, Feldman D. The effect of TGF-β delivered through a collagen scaffold on wound healing. J Investig Surg. 1999; 12:89–100.

163. Jayakumar R, Prabaharan M, Kumar PS, Nair S, Tamura H. Biomaterials based on chitin and chitosan in wound dressing applications. Biotechnol Adv. 2011; 29:322–337.

164. Lee KY, Mooney DJ. Alginate: properties and biomedical applications. Prog Polym Sci. 2012; 37:106–126.

165. Tellechea A, Silva EA, Min J, Leal EC, Auster ME, Nabzdyk LP, Shih W, Mooney DJ, Veves A. Alginate and DNA gels are suitable delivery systems for diabetic wound healing. Int J Low Extrem Wounds. 2015; 14:146–153.

166. Zhang L, Chen J, Han C. A multicenter clinical trial of recombinant human GM-CSF hydrogel for the treatment of deep second-degree burns. Wound Repair Regen. 2009; 17:685–689.

167. Silva EA, Mooney DJ. Spatiotemporal control of vascular endothelial growth factor delivery from injectable hydrogels enhances angiogenesis. J Thromb Haemost. 2007; 5:590–598.

168. Silva EA, Kim ES, Kong HJ, Mooney DJ. Material-based deployment enhances efficacy of endothelial progenitor cells. Proc Natl Acad Sci USA. 2008; 105:14347–14352.

169. Hiemstra C, Zhong Z, van Tomme SR, van Steenbergen MJ, Jacobs JJL, Otter WD, Hennink WE, Feijen J. In vitro and in vivo protein delivery from in situ forming poly(ethylene glycol)–poly(lactide) hydrogels. J Control Release. 2007; 119:320–327.

170. Jin R, Teixeira LSM, Krouwels A, Dijkstra PJ, van Blitterswijk CA, Karperien M, Feijen J. Synthesis and characterization of hyaluronic acid-poly(ethylene glycol) hydrogels via

Michael addition: an injectable biomaterial for cartilage repair. Acta Biomater. 2010; 6:1968–1977.

171. Lim DW, Nettles DL, Setton LA, Chilkoti A. Rapid cross-linking of elastin-like polypeptides with (hydroxymethyl) phosphines in aqueous solution. Biomacromolecules. 2007; 8:1463–1470.

172. Wieduwild R, Tsurkan M, Chwalek K, Murawala P, Nowak M, Freudenberg U, Neinhuis C, Werner C, Zhang Y. Minimal peptide motif for non-covalent peptide-heparin hydrogels. J Am Chem Soc. 2013; 135:2919–2922.

173. Kiick KL. Peptide- and protein-mediated assembly of heparinized hydrogels. Soft Matter. 2008; 4:29–37.

174. Ishii S, Kaneko J, Nagasaki Y. Development of a long-acting, protein-loaded, redox-active, injectable gel formed by a polyion complex for local protein therapeutics. Biomaterials. 2016; 84:210–218.

175. Desai RM, Koshy ST, Hilderbrand SA, Mooney DJ, Joshi NS. Versatile click alginate hydrogels cross-linked via tetrazine–norbornene chemistry. Biomaterials. 2015; 50:30–37.

176. Jewett JC, Bertozzi CR. Cu-free click cycloaddition reactions in chemical biology. Chem Soc Rev. 2010; 39:1272–1279.

177. Deforest CA, Anseth KS. Cytocompatible click-based hydrogels with dynamically tunable properties through orthogonal photoconjugation and photocleavage reactions. Nat Chem. 2011, 3:925–931.

178. Guvendiren M, Lu HD, Burdick JA. Shear-thinning hydrogels for biomedical applications. Soft Matter. 2012; 8:260–272.

179. Altunbas A, Lee SJ, Rajasekaran SA, Schneider JP, Pochan DJ. Encapsulation of curcumin in self-assembling peptide hydrogels as injectable drug delivery vehicles. Biomaterials. 2011; 32:5906–5914.

180. Rajagopal K, Schneider JP. Self-assembling peptides and proteins for nanotechnological applications. Curr Opin Struct Biol. 2004; 14:480–486.

181. Haines-Butterick L, Rajagopal K, Branco M, Salick D, Rughani R, Pilarz M, Lamm MS, Pochan DJ, Schneider JP. Controlling hydrogelation kinetics by peptide design for three-dimensional encapsulation and injectable delivery of cells. Proc Natl Acad Sci USA. 2007; 104:7791–7796.

182. Yan C, Altunbas A, Yucel T, Nagarkar RP, Schneider JP, Pochan DJ. Injectable solid hydrogel: mechanism of shear-thinning and immediate recovery of injectable β-hairpin peptide hydrogels. Soft Matter. 2010; 6:5143–5156.

183. Haines-Butterick LA, Salick DA, Pochan DJ, Schneider JP. In vitro assessment of the pro-inflammatory potential of β-hairpin peptide hydrogels. Biomaterials. 2008; 29: 4164–4169.

184. Micklitsch CM, Knerr PJ, Branco MC, Nagarkar R, Pochan DJ, Schneider JP. Zinc-triggered hydrogelation of a self-assembling β-hairpin peptide. Angew Chem Int Ed Engl. 2011; 123:1615–1617.

185. Silva EA, Mooney DJ. Spatiotemporal control of vascular endothelial growth factor delivery from injectable hydrogels enhances angiogenesis. J Thromb Haemost. 2007; 5:590–598.

186. Silva EA, Kim ES, Kong HJ, Mooney DJ. Material-based deployment enhances efficacy of endothelial progenitor cells. Proc Natl Acad Sci USA. 2008; 105:14347–14352.

187. Alexis F, Pridgen E, Molnar LK, Farokhzad OC. Factors affecting the clearance and biodistribution of polymeric nanoparticles. Mol Pharm. 2008; 5:505–515.

188. Mitragotri S, Lahann J. Physical approaches to biomaterial design. Nat Mater. 2009; 8:15–23.

189. Euliss LE, DuPont JA, Gratton S, DeSimone J. Imparting size, shape, and composition control of materials for nanomedicine. Chem Soc Rev. 2006; 35:1095–1104.

190. Gratton SEA, Ropp PA, Pohlhaus PD, Luft JC, Madden VJ, Napier ME, DeSimone JM. The effect of particle design on cellular internalization pathways. Proc Natl Acad Sci U S A. 2008; 105:11613–11618.

191. Merkel TJ, Chen K, Jones SW, Pandya AA, Tian S, Napier ME, Zamboni WE, DeSimone JM. The effect of particle size on the biodistribution of low-modulus hydrogel PRINT particles. J Control Release. 2012; 162:37–44.

192. Ginn SL, Alexander IE, Edelstein ML, Abedi MR, Wixon J. Gene therapy clinical trials worldwide to 2012—an update. J Gene Med. 2013; 15:65–77.

193. Vinogradov SV, Bronich TK, Kabanov AV. Nanosized cationic hydrogels for drug delivery: preparation, properties, and interactions with cells. Adv Drug Deliv Rev. 2002; 54:135–147.

194. Vicent MJ, Duncan R. Polymer conjugates: nanosized medicines for treating cancer. Trends Biotechnol. 2006; 24:39–47.

195. Li J, Zheng C, Cansiz S, Wu C, Xu J, Cui C, Liu Y, Hou W, Wang Y, Zhang L, Teng T, Yang HH, Tan W. Self-assembly of DNA nanohydrogels with controllable size and stimuli-responsive property for targeted gene regulation therapy. J Am Chem Soc. 2015; 137:1412–1415.

196. Oh JK, Drumright R, Siegwart DJ, Matyjaszewski K. The development of microgels/nanogels for drug delivery applications. Prog Polym Sci. 2008; 33:448–477.

197. Rolland JP, Maynor BW, Euliss LE, Exner AE, Denison GM, DeSimone JM. Direct fabrication and harvesting of monodisperse, shape-specific nanobiomaterials. J Am Chem Soc. 2005; 127:10096–10100.

198. Perry JL, Reuter KG, Kai MP, Herlihy KP, Jones SW, Luft JC, Napier M, Bear JE, DeSimone JM. PEGylated PRINT nanoparticles: the impact of PEG density on protein binding, macrophage association, biodistribution, and pharmacokinetics. Nano Lett. 2012; 12:5304–5310.

199. Dunn SS, Tian ST, Blake S, Wang J, Galloway AL, Murphy A, Pohlhaus PD, Rolland JP, Napier ME, DeSimone JM. Reductively responsive siRNA-conjugated hydrogel nanoparticles for gene silencing. J Am Chem Soc. 2012; 134:7423–7430.

200. Xu J, Wong DHC, Byrne JD, Chen K, Bowerman C, DeSimone JM. Future of the particle replication in nonwetting templates (PRINT) technology. Angew Chem Int Ed Engl. 2013; 52(26):6580–6589.

201. Kaurav H. Mucoadhesive microspheres as carriers in drug delivery: a review. Int J Drug Dev Res. 2012; 4(2):21–34.

202. Lin HA, Varma DM, Hom WW, Cruz MA, Nasser PR, Phelps RG, Iatridis JC, Nicoll, SB. Injectable cellulose-based hydrogels as nucleus pulposus replacements: assessment of in vitro structural stability, ex vivo herniation risk, and in vivo biocompatibility. J Mech Behav Biomed Mater. 2019; 96:204–213.

203. Hyun H, Kim YH, Song IB, Lee JW, Kim MS, Khang G, Park K, Lee HB. In vitro and in vivo release of albumin using a biodegradable MPEG-PCL diblock copolymer as an in situ gel-forming carrier. Biomacromolecules. 2007; 8:1093–1100.

204. Wang Y, Chen L, Tan L, Zhao Q, Luo F, Wei Y, Qian Z. PEG–PCL-based micelle hydrogels as oral docetaxel delivery systems for breast cancer therapy. Biomaterials. 2014; 35: 6972–6985.

205. Ramadan AA, Elbakry AM, Esmaeil AH, Khaleel SA. Pharmaceutical and pharmacokinetic evaluation of novel rectal mucoadhesive hydrogels containing tolmetin sodium. J Pharm Investig. 2018; 48:673–683.

206. Bhaskar K, Mohan CK, Lingam M, Mohan SJ, Venkateswarlu V, Rao YM, Bhaskar K, Anbu J, Ravichandran V. Development of SLN and NLC enriched hydrogels for transdermal delivery of nitrendipine: in vitro and in vivo characteristics. Drug Dev Ind Pharm. 2009; 35:98–113.

207. Wu Q, Wang N, He T, Shang J, Li L, Song L, Yang X, Li X, Luo N, Zhang W, Gong C. Thermosensitive hydrogel containing dexamethasone micelles for preventing postsurgical adhesion in a repeated-injury model. Sci Rep. 2015; 5:13553.

208. Ohta S, Hiramoto S, Amano Y, Emoto S, Yamaguchi H, Ishigami H, Kitayama J, Ito T. Intraperitoneal delivery of cisplatin via a hyaluronan-based nanogel/in situ cross-linkable hydrogel hybrid system for peritoneal dissemination of gastric cancer. Mol Pharm. 2017; 14:3105–3113.

209. Hosny KM. Ciprofloxacin as ocular liposomal hydrogel. AAPS Pharm Sci Tech. 2010; 11:241–246.

210. Kong HJ, Kaigler D, Kim K, Mooney DJ. Controlling rigidity and degradation of alginate hydrogels via molecular weight distribution. Biomacromolecules. 2004; 5:1720–1727.

211. Boontheekul T, Kong HJ, Mooney DJ. Controlling alginate gel degradation utilizing partial oxidation and bimodal molecular weight distribution. Biomaterials. 2005; 26:2455–2465.

212. O'Shea TM, Aimetti AA, Kim E, Yesilyurt V, Langer R. Synthesis and characterization of a library of *in-situ* curing, non-swelling ethoxylated polyolthioffene hydrogels for tailorable macromolecule delivery. Adv Mater. 2015; 27:65–72.

213. Ishihara M, Obara K, Ishizuka T, Fujita M, Sato M, Masuoka K, Saito Y, Yura H, Matsui T, Hattori H, Kikuchi M, Kurita A. Controlled release of fibroblast growth factors and heparin from photocrosslinked chitosan hydrogels and subsequent effect on in vivo vascularization. J Biomed Mater Res A. 2003; 64:551–559.

214. Lutolf M, Lauer-Fields JL, Schmoekel HG, Metters AT, Weber FE, Fields GB, Hubbell JA. Synthetic matrix metalloproteinase-sensitive hydrogels for the conduction of tissue regeneration: engineering cell-invasion characteristics. Proc Natl Acad Sci U S A. 2003; 100:5413–5418.

215. Um SH, Lee JB, Park N, Kwon SY, Umbach CC, Luo D. Enzyme-catalyzed assembly of DNA hydrogel. Nat Mater. 2006; 5:797–801.

216. Purcell BP, Lobb D, Charati MB, Dorsey SM, Wade RJ, Zellars KN, Doviak H, Pettaway S, Logdon CB, Shuman JA, Freels PD, Gorman JH, Gorman RC, Spinale FG, Burdick JA. Injectable and bioresponsive hydrogels for on-demand matrix metalloproteinase inhibition. Nat Mater. 2014; 13:653–661.

217. Fischel-Ghodsian F, Brown L, Mathiowitz E, Brandenburg D, Langer R. Enzymatically controlled drug delivery. Proc Natl Acad Sci U S A. 1988; 85:2403–2406.

218. Podual K, Doyle FJ, Peppas NA. Glucose-sensitivity of glucose oxidase-containing cationic copolymer hydrogels having poly(ethylene glycol) grafts. J Control Release. 2000; 67:9–17.

219. Maitz MF, Freudenberg U, Tsurkan MV, Fischer M, Beyrich T, Werner C. Bioresponsive polymer hydrogels homeostatically regulate blood coagulation. Nat Comm. 2013; 4:2168.

220. Lin KY, Lo JH, Consul N, Kwong GA, Bhatia SN. Self-titrating anticoagulant nanocomplexes that restore homeostatic regulation of the coagulation cascade. ACS Nano. 2014; 8:8776–8785.

221. Zhang Y, Wang R, Hua Y, Baumgartner R, Cheng J. Trigger-responsive poly(β-amino ester) hydrogels. ACS Macro Lett. 2014; 3:693–697.
222. Tibbett MW, Han BW, Klaxon AM, Ansett KS. Synthesis and application of photodegradable microspheres for spatiotemporal control of protein delivery. J Biomed Mater Res A. 2012; 100:1647.
223. Yan B, Boyer JC, Habault D, Branda NR, Zhao Y. Near infrared light triggered release of biomacromolecules from hydrogels loaded with up conversion nanoparticles. J Am Chem Soc. 2012; 134:16558–16561.
224. Brannonpeppas L, Peppas NA. Equilibrium swelling behavior of pH-sensitive hydrogels. Chem Eng Sci. 1991; 46:715–722.
225. Hong W, Zhao X, Zhou J, Suo Z. A theory of coupled diffusion and large deformation in polymeric gels. J Mech Phys Solids. 2008; 56:1779–1793.
226. Hirokawa Y, Tanaka T. Volume phase-transition in a nonionic gel. J Chem Phys. 1984; 81:6379–6380.
227. Obaidat AA, Park K. Characterization of protein release through glucose-sensitive hydrogel membranes. Biomaterials. 1997; 18:801–806.
228. Kokufata E, Zhang YQ, Tanaka T. Saccharide-sensitive phase transition of a lectin-loaded gel. Nature. 1991; 351:302–304.
229. Zhang S, Bellinger AM, Glettig DL, Barman R, Lee YAL, Zhu J, Cleveland C, Montgomery VA, Gu L, Nash LD, Maitland DJ, Langer R, Traverso G. A pH-responsive supramolecular polymer gel as an enteric elastomer for use in gastric devices. Nat Mater. 2015; 14(10):1065–1071.
230. Ohmine I, Tanaka T. Salt effects on the phase-transition of ionic gels. J Chem Phys. 1982; 77:5725–5729.
231. Murdan S. Electroresponsive drug delivery from hydrogels. J Control Release. 2003; 92:1–17.
232. Mumper RJ, Huffman AS, Puolakkainen PA, Bouchard LS, Gombotz WR. Calcium-alginate beads for the oral delivery of transforming growth factor-β1 (TGF-β1): stabilization of TGF-β1 by the addition of polyacrylic acid within acid-treated beads. J Control Release. 1994; 30:241–251.
233. Kanamala M, Wilson WR, Yang M, Palmer BD, Wu Z. Mechanisms and biomaterials in pH-responsive tumor targeted drug delivery: a review. Biomaterials. 2016; 85:152–167.
234. Shirakura T, Kelson TJ, Ray A, Malyarenko AE, Kopelman R. Hydrogel nanoparticles with thermally controlled drug release. ACS Macro Lett. 2014; 3:602–606.
235. Huebsch N, Kearney CJ, Zhao X, Kim J, Cezar CA, Suo Z, Mooney DJ. Ultrasound-triggered disruption and self-healing of reversibly cross-linked hydrogels for drug delivery and enhanced chemotherapy. Proc Natl Acad Sci U S A. 2014; 111:9762–9767.
236. Brudno Y, Mooney DJ. On-demand drug delivery from local depots. J Control Release. 2015; 219:8–17.
237. Lee KY, Peters MC, Anderson KW, Mooney DJ. Controlled growth factor release from synthetic extracellular matrices. Nature. 2000; 408:998–1000.
238. Liu TY, Hu SH, Liu TY, Liu DM, Chen SY. Magnetic-sensitive behavior of intelligent ferrogels for controlled release of drug. Langmuir. 2006; 22:5974–5978.
239. Hu SH, Liu TY, Liu DM, Chen SY. Nano-ferrosponges for controlled drug release. J Control Release. 2007; 121:181–189.
240. Zhao X, Kim J, Cezar CA, Huebsch N, Lee K, Bouhadir K, Mooney DJ. Active scaffolds for on-demand drug and cell delivery. Proc Natl Acad Sci U S A. 2011; 108:67–72.

241. Mitragotri S. Healing sound: the use of ultrasound in drug delivery and other therapeutic applications. Nat Rev Drug Dis. 2005; 4:255–260.
242. Mitragotri S, Blankschtein D, Langer R. Ultrasound-mediated transdermal protein delivery. Science. 1995; 269:850–853.
243. Mann BK, Schmedlen RH, West JL. Tethered-TGF-β increases extracellular matrix production of vascular smooth muscle cells. Biomaterials. 2001; 22:439–444.
244. Kolate A, Baradia D, Patil S, Vhora I, Kore G, Misra A. PEG—a versatile conjugating ligand for drugs and drug delivery systems. J Control Release. 2014; 192:67–81.
245. Shah NJ, Hyder N, Quadir MA, Courchesne NMD, Seeherman HJ, Nevins M, Spector M, Hammond PT. Adaptive growth factor delivery from a polyelectrolyte coating promotes synergistic bone tissue repair and reconstruction. Proc Natl Acad Sci U S A. 2014; 111:12847–12852.
246. Macdonald ML, Samuel RE, Shah NJ, Padera RF, Beben YM, Hammond PT. Tissue integration of growth factor-eluting layer-by-layer polyelectrolyte multilayer coated implants. Biomaterials. 2011; 32:1446–1453.
247. Silva EA, Mooney DJ. Effects of VEGF temporal and spatial presentation on angiogenesis. Biomaterials. 2010; 31:1235–1241.
248. Kolambkar YM, Dupont KM, Boerckel JD, Huebasch N, Mooney DJ, Hutmacher DW, Guldberg RE. An alginate-based hybrid system for growth factor delivery in the functional repair of large bone defects. Biomaterials. 2011; 32:65–74.
249. Martino MM, Briquez PS, Güç E, Tortelli F, Kilarski WW, Metzger S, Rice JJ, Kuhn GA, Müller R, Swartz MA, Hubbell JA. Growth factors engineered for super-affinity to the extracellular matrix enhance tissue healing. Science. 2014; 343:885–888.
250. Pike DB, Cai S, Pomraning KR, Firpo MA, Fisher RJ, Shu XZ, Prestwich GD, Peattie RA. Heparin-regulated release of growth factors in vitro and angiogenic response in vivo to implanted hyaluronan hydrogels containing VEGF and bFGF. Biomaterials. 2006; 27:5242–5251.
251. Freeman I, Kedem A, Cohen S. The effect of sulfation of alginate hydrogels on the specific binding and controlled release of heparin-binding proteins. Biomaterials. 2008; 29:3260–3268.
252. Freudenberg U, Zieris A, Chwalek K, Tsurkan MV, Maitz MF, Atallah P, Levental KR, Eming SA, Werner C. Heparin desulfation modulates VEGF release and angiogenesis in diabetic wounds. J Control Release. 2015; 220:79–88.
253. Thatiparti TR, Shoffstall AJ, von Recum HA. Cyclodextrin-based device coatings for affinity-based release of antibiotics. Biomaterials. 2010; 31:2335–2347.
254. Zhang P, Cheetham AG, Lin YA, Cui H. Self-assembled Tat nanofibers as effective drug carrier and transporter. ACS Nano. 2013; 7:5965–5977.
255. Soukasene S, Toft DJ, Moyer TJ, Lu H, Lee HK, Standley SM, Cryns VL, Stupp SI. Antitumor activity of peptide amphiphile nanofiber-encapsulated camptothecin. ACS Nano. 2011; 5:9113–9121.
256. Jensen BE, Dávila I, Zelikin AN. Poly(vinyl alcohol) physical hydrogels: matrix-mediated drug delivery using spontaneously eroding substrate. J Phys Chem B. 2016; 120(26):5916–5926.
257. Mateen R, Hoare T. Injectable, in situ gelling, cyclodextrin–dextran hydrogels for the partitioning-driven release of hydrophobic drugs. J Mater Chem B. 2014; 2:5157–5167.
258. Kearney CJ, Mooney DJ. Macroscale delivery systems for molecular and cellular payloads. Nat Mater. 2013; 12:1004–1017.

259. Alconcel SN, Baas AS, Maynard HD. FDA-approved poly(ethylene glycol)–protein conjugate drugs. Polym Chem. 2011; 2:1442–1448.
260. Fishburn CS. The pharmacology of PEGylation: balancing PD with PK to generate novel therapeutics. J Pharm Sci. 2008; 97:4167–4183.
261. Lee S, Greenwald RB, McGuire J, Yang K, Shi C. Drug delivery systems employing 1, 6-elimination: releasable poly(ethylene glycol) conjugates of proteins. Bioconjugate Chem. 2001; 12:163–169.

CHAPTER 15

Polymeric Nanoparticles for Drug Delivery

R. SHELMA

Department of Chemistry and Polymer Chemistry, KSMDB College, Kollam, Kerala, India

*Corresponding author. E-mail: shelma82@gmail.com

ABSTRACT

The possibilities of using polymers as drug carriers were brought to the attention of many scientists decades ago. Polymeric nanoparticles are increasingly being used for different applications, including drug carrier systems and the blood–brain barrier to pass organ barriers because of their unique properties. Of these many nanoparticles are receiving a lot of attention for potential use in drug discovery. The application of nanotechnology in drug delivery is set to spread rapidly. Currently, polymeric substrates are analyzed for drug delivery and more explicitly, in cancer therapies. Pharmaceutical sciences use polymeric nanoparticles for reducing the toxicity and to prevent the side effects of drugs and also to enhance solubility and bioavailability. This chapter addresses recent work utilizing polymeric nanoparticles for controlled drug delivery applications.

15.1 INTRODUCTION

Some therapeutic agents have limitations like low aqueous solubility and short half-life and hence it is necessary to design a delivery system to deliver a drug efficiently. Nowadays polymeric nanoparticles such as micelles, dendrimers, nanoparticles, nanogels, nanocapsules, nanovesicles, etc., are gaining much more attention toward drug delivery applications as it offers a platform to amend the basic properties of drug molecules, namely, solubility, half-life, biocompatibility, and its release. Such carriers usually exhibit the properties of the chosen polymers that respond to a stimulus or their environment like changes in temperature, pH, light, etc., useful to release the drugs [1, 2]. Nowadays scientific researchers are focusing on the realization of efficient vectors for the controlled release at their desired action site [3–5]. Most polymeric materials are described as a carrier for the drug owing to its potential toward the surface modification through chemical and physical methods and can easily achieve the desired drug loading and thus bioavailability enhancement and controlled-targeted release to a specific site with the suitable functionalization of polymeric nanomaterials [6, 7]. Polymeric nanocarriers such as dendrimers, micelles, polymeric nanoparticles, nanogels, nanocapsules, vesicles are used for their easy surface modulation as drug delivery carriers.

15.2 DENDRIMERS

Dendrimers are highly branched nanostructures. The drug is incorporated both in the interior core as well as attached on the branched surface either covalently or by ionically. The physical characteristics like monodispersity, water-solubility, encapsulation efficiency, presence of a large number of functionalizable peripheral groups, multivalency, well-defined molecular weight, series of branches, and globular structure with controlled surface functionality make these dendrimers appropriate candidates for evaluation as drug delivery vehicles. Dendrimers have been explored for the encapsulation of hydrophobic therapeutic compounds like anticancer drugs. There are mainly three approaches to making drugs incorporated by dendrimers. The very first approach is the covalent bonding of the drug to the periphery of the dendrimer to form dendrimer prodrugs, secondly, the drug is ionically coordinated to the outer functional groups, and the final approach is the formation of a unimolecular micelle of the dendrimer-drug supramolecular assembly after the encapsulation of drug to the dendrimer. It has been widely explored for the delivery of antiretroviral bioactives because of its inherent antiretroviral activity.

Some of the major advantages are their increased half-life, increased solubility, stability, and permeability of drugs, the capability to deliver a variety of drugs, reduced macrophage uptake, targeting ability, improved delivery efficiency, reduced side effects by targeted delivery, facile passage across biological barriers, rapid cellular entry, etc. [8–11]. Most of the drug delivery reported based on the carrier polymers like polyamidoamine (PAMAM), polypropyleneimine, polyarylether, etc., are in the nano range especially below

10 nm [12–17]. But earlier reports have shown several limitations such as poor/unstable hydrophobic drug loadings, the inefficient release of drugs at targeting using the above-mentioned carriers [18]. This limitation could be overcome to some extent either by developing a new class of molecules called dendronized polymers, linear polymers that bear dendrons at each repeat unit [19], or by using dendrimers incorporating a degradable link that can be further used to control the release of the drug. By using this concept, Chang et al. prepared a drug release system based on folic acid conjugated to poly(ethylene glycol) (PEG)-modified dendrimers (PAMAM) with doxorubicin (DOX) and superparamagnetic iron oxide [20].

15.3 MICELLES

Generally, a micelle in an aqueous solution forms an aggregate that will have hydrophobic single-tail regions in the micelle center and hydrophilic head regions in contact with the surrounding solvent. Amphiphilic polymeric molecules form micelle in aqueous medium forming polymeric micelles. Hydrophobic drugs can be encapsulated in the core of the polymeric micelle and its multifunctionality should lead to more developments regarding biomedical applications. Due to their nanoscopic size, ability to solubilize hydrophobic drugs in large amounts, polymeric micelles have gained attention as a multifunctional nanotechnology-based delivery system for poor water-soluble drugs, and achieve site-specific delivery thus enhance their bioavailability [21].

In general, polymeric micelles are formed from amphiphilic polymers and most of them are found to be stable in physiological solutions: the inner core of a micelle is hydrophobic while the surface corona is hydrophilic which reducing its interaction with serum proteins and prolonging their circulation time in the blood [22, 23]. Because of the enhanced permeability and retention effect of tumor tissues, polymeric micelles have been extensively used for passive targeting [24, 25]. But its major disadvantages are that micelles are not stable and they may dissociate upon dilution and limited targeting ability due to low drug loading and its low drug incorporation stability that causes the drug release before getting to the active site [26, 27].

Researchers then focused on the crosslinking approaches to improve the stability of micelles [28, 29] but resulted in extremely slow drug release when they are at the target sites. Then the crosslinking with degradable linkages would facilitate the drug release. Micelles are very promising toward stimuli and can achieve sudden drug release with an environmental stimulus such as temperature [30], pH [31], light [32, 33], and redox [34, 35].

15.4   POLYMERIC NANOPARTICLES

Generally, polymeric nanoparticles are colloidal soft particles of spherical, branched, or shell structures with a size range of 1–1000 nm. These nanoparticles may develop from biodegradable and nonbiodegradable polymers and their small sizes enable them to penetrate and to be taken up by cells, thereby increasing the accumulation of drugs at target sites. Advantages are improved bioavailability by enhancing aqueous solubility, increasing resistance time in the body, and its target-specific drug delivery location in the body (its site of action). The abovementioned properties help in reducing the quantity of the therapeutic drug required and dosage toxicity which enable the safe delivery of toxic therapeutic drugs and protection of nontarget tissues and cells from severe side effects [36]. The drug is incorporated into polymeric nanoparticles by dissolution, precipitation, adsorption, or attachment [37–39]. In general, nanoparticles used as drug carriers should have at least the following important components: the constituent material, the therapeutic molecules, and the biological surface modifiers, which improve the biodistribution and tumor targeting of the nanoparticles [40]. Polymeric nanoparticles are widely used as drug carriers because of their sustained release of drugs for longer periods. The therapeutic drug can be coupled to macromolecules or conjugated to a tissue or cell-specific ligand for the site-specific action that reaches the target organs [41, 42]. Some of the main applications of polymeric nanoparticles used for the purposes are brain drug targeting for neurodegenerative disorders such as Alzheimer's disease [43, 44], topical administration to enhance penetration, and distribution in and across the skin barrier [45], and pH-sensitive polymeric nanoparticles to improve oral bioavailability of drugs [46, 47]. Biodegradable polymers such as chitosan, alginate, albumin, gelatin, polyacrylates, polycaprolactones, poly(D,L-lactide-*co*-glycolide), poly(D,L-lactide), etc., have been reported.

15.5   DRUG LOADING ON TO THE POLYMERIC NANOPARTICLES

A drug delivery system may be termed as successful when it has a high loading capacity to reduce the quantity of the carrier required for administration. Drug loading onto nanoparticle carrier is achieved by two methods: one, "in situ" method that is by incorporating the drug at the time of nanoparticle production, or secondly, by physisorption method, that is, the drug is adsorbed after the formation of nanoparticles by incubating them in the drug solution. The former method of incorporation enables a larger amount of drug entrapment than the latter method of adsorption.

15.6   MECHANISM OF DRUG RELEASE

Diffusion, degradation, or swelling followed by diffusion are the three mechanisms by which a drug can be released from a delivery system. In diffusion, a drug or other active agent passes through the polymer that forms the controlled-release device. The diffusion may possible on a macroscopic scale through pores in the polymer matrix or on a molecular level, by passing between polymer chains. In the swelling mechanism, the drug-controlled release systems absorb water or other body fluids and then swell when placed in the body. This swelling within the system enabling the drug to diffuse through the swollen network into the external environment. The degradation normally takes place in two ways, namely bulk erosion and surface erosion. Polymer degradation is much faster than the water imbibition into the polymer bulk in the surface erosion method. Therefore, degradation occurs predominantly within the outermost polymer layers hence erosion affects only the surface and not the core of the system. But the bulk eroding polymers degrade more slowly and the water uptake is much faster than the degradation of the polymer. These polymers easily get wet and the polymer chain cleavage occurs throughout the system and erosion is not restricted to the polymer surface only. Generally, it can be said that polymers with less reactive functional groups tend to be bulk eroding, and polymers with very reactive functional groups tend to degrade fast and tend to be surface eroding.

For using polymers in drug delivery applications, a polymer should be biocompatible which forms harmless by products, such as nontoxic alcohols, acids, and other easily eliminated low molecular weight products on erosion/degradation with the diffusion of drug through the polymeric material.

The drug encapsulated polymer releases the drug by controlled diffusion or erosion from the core across the polymeric membrane or matrix. Solubility and diffusivity of drugs in polymer membrane turn out to be the determining factor in drug release as the membrane coating acts as a barrier to release the drug. The drug release can be made very controlled or almost to no burst release by the formation of less water-soluble complex with the drug and the other auxiliary ingredients [48]. For the effective drug delivery system, both drug release and polymer biodegradation are important factors for consideration. The drug release rate depends on many factors such as solubility of the drug, desorption of the surface-bound/adsorbed drug, diffusion through nanoparticle matrix, erosion/degradation of nanoparticle matrix, a combination of erosion/diffusion process [49].

Smart or stimulus-responsive polymers are gaining interest as drug delivery systems and they exhibit large, sharp changes in response to physical stimuli, such as temperature, solvents, light, or to chemical stimuli like reactants, ions in solution, pH, or chemical recognition. Various responses shown depending on the stimulus applied and may change in volume, shape, mechanical properties, or permeation rates.

A large number of polymeric nanoparticles are widely used in drug delivery applications.

The most engaged polymer for drug delivery applications is the saturated poly(α-hydroxy esters) like poly(lactic acid) (PLA), poly(glycolic acid), and poly(lactic-*co*-glycolide) (PLGA) copolymers. For their excellent safety profile, worthy biocompatibility, low levels of immunogenicity and toxicity, and the favorable rate of biodegradation in vivo, these polymers have been accepted as effective carriers for drug delivery in humans.

The biodegradability of polyhydroxyesters is based on hydrolytic degradation through de-esterification to generate the monomeric components, which are metabolized and removed by the body by natural pathways (such as the Krebs cycle). Their mechanical and physicochemical properties can be altered via the selection of the polymer molecular weight, degree of copolymerization, and functionalization. Polyethylene glycol is the apt hydrophilic polymer for surface modification of both (hydrophobic) PLA and PLGA to form an amphiphilic block copolymer [50, 51]. These types of amphiphilic block copolymeric nanoparticles, micelles, and hydrogels have been applied for drug delivery systems although the hydrophilic PEG shell prevents the adsorption of proteins and phagocytes but the hydrophobic PLGA/PLA core can efficiently encapsulate many therapeutic agents, thus extending the blood circulation periods [52].

Several studies indicate the nanocarrier use of PEG-PLGA for the encapsulation of proteins and peptide drugs like calcitonin, insulin, and DNA. A PLGA-PEG-folate theranostic system was combined with dual imaging tracers like near-infrared and 19F magnetic resonance imaging with the chemotherapeutic agent doxorubicin DOX. The folate-targeted PLGA-PEG nanoparticles were found to be able to kill cancer cells more efficiently than nonfolate conjugated particles on in vitro cytotoxicity assay [53].

Doxorubicin (DOX-) conjugated PLGA/PEG micellar nanocarriers with a higher DOX loading have been demonstrated by researchers to display sustained drug release behavior when compared with physically incorporated DOX in PEG/PLGA micelles. Release of the drug, up to 50% from the matrix conjugated DOX-PLGA/PEG micelles was obtained over 2 weeks when a total release of physically entrapped PEGPLGA micelles took only 3 days [54].

Moreover, preliminary animal studies have displayed the potential of these polymers PLA- and PLGA-based nanocarriers in the treatment of diseases like diabetes, cancer, cardiac disorder, bacterial, viral infection, autoimmune diseases, and cartilage damage [55–59].

Chitosan is a natural polymer that possesses distinguishing properties with biocompatibility and the presence of functional groups [60]. Chitosan and its derivatives are used in the encapsulation or coating of various types of drugs. Self-assembled amphiphilic chitosan is used as carriers of paclitaxel (PTX) to improve its intestinal pharmacokinetic profile [61]. Experimental results indicate that chemical modification of chitosan nanoparticles improves their targeting and bioavailability and recent advances highlight the use of chitosan nanoparticles for tumor targeting [62].

The intestinal absorption of antioxidant flavonoids like catechin and epigallocatechin gallate can be improved by encapsulating them in chitosan nanoparticles [63]. Permeation of orally given anticancer drug tamoxifen across the intestinal epithelium is increased by formulating tamoxifen into lecithin-chitosan nanoparticles through a paracellular pathway [64]. Feng et al. prepared nanoparticles of doxorubicin hydrochloride (DOX) with chitosan and the carboxymethyl chitosan was found to enhance the intestinal absorption of DOX throughout the small intestine [65]. The direct oral insulin is not favored as the harsh conditions of the gastrointestinal tract denature proteins. In one example of insulin-loaded lauroyl chitosan nanoparticles, the modified chitosan was crosslinked with tripolyphosphate. The particle uptake is found to be significant in the intestine epithelium [66]. The solubility and oral bioavailability of the active inhibitor of hepatitis B virus Bay 41-4109 are improved after the formulation with chitosan [67].

Carboxymethyl chitosan nanoparticles for carbamazepine, a drug for the treatment of epilepsy have been found to enhance bioavailability and brain targeting via the nasal route [68]. The bioavailability of prostate cancer drug leuprolide is found to be increased when formulated as thiolated-chitosan nanoparticles and a 25-fold increase in drug transport across porcine nasal mucosa is also observed [69].

Chitosan nanoparticle when incorporated with the antitubercular drug rifampicin has shown sustained drug release until 24 h and no toxicity at both cell and organ [70]. The aerosolization properties of antifungal drug itraconazole were found to be significantly improved by formulating the drug in spray-dried chitosan nanoparticles with lactose, mannitol, and leucine. The pulmonary deposition of itraconazole is shown to be increased [71].

Among the most versatile biopolymers, alginates are getting established as they are widely used in a range of applications including, as an excipient in drug products owing to their thickening, gel-forming, and stabilizing properties. The need for prolonged and improved control of drug administration has led to a significant role in the design of a controlled-release product.

Curcumin-loaded magnetic alginate/chitosan nanoparticles with sizes ranging from 120 to 200 nm are found to improve the bioavailability, uptake efficiency, and cytotoxicity of curcumin to Human Caucasian Breast Adenocarcinoma cells. These nanoparticles, for their sustained release profiles, enhanced uptake efficiency, and cytotoxicity to cancer cells, as well as directed targeting, have become a promising candidates for cancer therapy [72]. The application of the curcumin-loaded calcium alginate-based nanoparticles on excised human skin showed a significant accumulation of the active molecules in the upper layers of the skin proving the potential of these nanocarriers in active pharmaceutical and cosmetic ingredients topical delivery [73]. Eight doses of econazole-loaded alginate nanoparticles showed a similar antibacterial effect of 112 twice-a-day doses of the free drug due to the ability of alginate nanoparticles to cross the intestinal barrier and reach the bloodstream, as opposed to microparticles that are mainly retained in the gut mucosa [74]. The same reason is observed for the enhancement of mucopenetrating alginate/chitosan nanoparticles for the release of amoxicillin in the treatment of the infection by Helicobacter pylori, a pathogen that colonizes the deep gastric mucosa lining [75]. These carriers showed greater mucopenetration than pure chitosan. The same observations of enhanced permeation of bovine serum albumin-loaded N-trimethyl chitosan nanoparticles across Caco2 cell monolayers, when modified with alginate were studied by Chen et al. [76].

Hyaluronic acid is a biocompatible, biodegradable, high viscoelastic linear macromolecular mucopolysaccharide composed of alternatingly linked two saccharide units of glucuronic acid and N-acetylglucosamine [77, 78]. Due to the explicit binding of hyaluronic acid to the receptors on the surface of cancer cells, this can be used in the targeted drug delivery of anticancer drugs. It can be reacted with drugs to form conjugates and will exhibit controlled release and targeted effect aiding in the delivery of multiple drugs to various pathological sites, to achieve the purpose of timing, and directional release [79]. The amphipathic vector hyaluronic acid-PEI has been synthesized for gene delivery by periodic acid oxidation of hyaluronic acid and PEI and protected DNA from nuclease degradation well and isolated DNA from the complex. This vector can overcome the nonspecific transfection shortcomings of PEI and has a high transfection rate in HepG2 cells thus promotes cell uptake more effectively [80]. The transfection efficiency of encapsulated DNA is improved by using Hyaluronic acid-spermine conjugate [81]. Hyaluronic acid-paclitaxel conjugate showed an inhibiting effect on head and neck squamous cell carcinoma cell lines OSC-19 and HN5 and it increased the survival rate of mice and expressively reduced the density of microvessels in tumor tissues, and effectively inhibited the growth of tumors [82].

15.7 CONCLUSIONS

Polymer-based nanoparticles used as drug carriers hold great potential to efficiently target drugs that overcome some of the problems like poor bioavailability, drug resistance, and to facilitate the movement of drugs across barriers. The low efficiency in drug delivery leads to the low drug concentrations to the active site and the very short drug residence time in the cellular and anatomical sites. This defect requires research in the field of novel drug delivery systems. Smart polymeric nanodelivery systems have shown notable ability in overcoming many of the anatomical and physiological barriers and deliver drugs locally to sites of interest thus improving therapy. The current focus in the pharmaceutical industry is moving toward the drug delivery system which increases the effectiveness and decreases the toxicity of drugs.

CONFLICT OF INTERESTS

The author declares that there is no conflict of interest regarding the publication of this paper.

KEYWORDS

- **drug delivery**
- **nanoparticles**
- **biodegradable polymer**
- **cancer**

REFERENCES

1. Sagadevan, S., Periasamy, M., 2014. A review on role of nanostructures in drug delivery systems. Rev. Adv. Mater. Sci. 36, 112–117.
2. Hruby, M., Filippov, S.K., Stepanek, P., 2015. Smart polymers in drug delivery systems On crossroads: which way deserves following? Eur. Polym. J. 65, 82–97.
3. Chithrani, B.D., Ghazani, A.A., Chan, W.C., 2006. Determining the size and shape dependence of gold nanoparticle uptake into mammalian cells. Nano Lett. 6, 662.
4. Bessar, H., Venditti, I., Fratoddi, I., Benassi, L., Vaschieri, C., Azzoni, P., Pellacani, G., Magnoni, C., Botti, E., Casagrande, V., Federici, M., Costanzo, A., Fontana, L., Testa, G., Mostafa, F.F., Ibrahim, S.A., Russo, M.V., 2016. Functionalized gold nanoparticles for topical delivery of Methotrexate for the possible treatment of psoriasis. Colloids Surf., B: Biointerfaces 141, 141–147.
5. Porcaro, F., Battocchio, C., Antoccia, A., Fratoddi, I., Venditti, I., Moreno, S., Luisetto, I., Russo, M.V., Polzonetti, G., 2016. Synthesis of functionalized gold nanoparticles capped with 3-mercapto-1-propansulfonate and 1-thiolglucose mixed thiols and in vitro bioresponse. Colloids Surf. B: Biointerfaces 142, 408–416.
6. Couvreur, P., 2013. Nanoparticles in drug delivery: past, present and future. Adv. Drug Delivery Rev. 65, 21–23.
7. Jia, F., Liu, X., Li, L., Mallapragada, S., Narasimhan, B., Wang, Q., 2013. Multifunctional nanoparticles for targeted delivery of immune activating and cancer therapeutic agents. J. Controlled Release 172, 1020–1034.
8. Nowacek, A., Gendelman, H.E., 2009. NanoART, neuroAIDS and CNS drug delivery. Nanomedicine 4, 557–574.
9. Najlah, M., Freeman, S., Attwood, D., D'Emanuele, A., 2007. In vitro evaluation of dendrimer prodrugs for oral drug delivery. Int. J. Pharm. 336, 183–190.
10. Najlah, M., D'Emanuele, A., 2006. Crossing cellular barriers using dendrimer nanotechnologies. Curr. Opin. Pharmacol. 6, 522–527.
11. Wong, H.L., Wu, X.Y., Bendayan, R., 2012. Nanotechnological advances for the delivery of CNS therapeutics. Adv. Drug Delivery Rev. 64, 686–700.
12. Zhao, Y., Li, Y., Song, Y., Jiang, W., Wu, Z., Wang, Y.A., Sun, J., Wang, J., 2009. Architecture of stable and water-soluble CdSe/ZnS core-shell Dendron nanocrystals via ligand exchange. J. Colloid Interface Sci. 339, 336–343.
13. Eichman, J., Bielinska, A., Kukowska-Latallo, J., Donovan, B., Baker, J., 2001. Dendrimers and Other Dendritic Polymers. Wiley: Chichester, pp. 441–462.

14. Newkome, G.R., Shreiner, C.D., 2008. Poly(amidoamine), polypropylenimine, and related dendrimers and dendrons possessing different 1® 2 branching motifs: an overview of the divergent procedures. Polymer 49, 1–173.

15. Kim, T., Baek, J., Bai, C.Z., Park, J., 2007. Arginine-conjugated polypropylenimine dendrimer as a non-toxic and efficient gene delivery carrier biomaterials. Biomaterials 28, 2061–2067.

16. Murugan, E., Geetha Rani, D.P., Yogaraj, V., 2014. Drug delivery investigations of quaternised poly(propylene imine) dendrimer using nimesulide as a model drug. Colloids Surf. B. 114, 121–129.

17. Ponnapati, R., Felipe, M.J., Advincula, R., 2011. Electropolymerizable terthiophene-terminated poly(aryl ether) dendrimers with naphthalene and perylene cores. Macromolecules 44, 7530–7537.

18. Bugno, J., Hsu, H.-J., Hong, S., 2015. Tweaking dendrimers and dendritic nanoparticles for controlled nano-bio interactions: potential nanocarriers for improved cancer targeting. J. Drug Target. 23, 642–650.

19. Tomalia, D.A., Christensen, J.B., Boas, U., 2012. Dendrimers, Dendrons, and Dendritic Polymers: Discovery, Applications, and the Future. Cambridge University Press: Cambridge.

20. Chang, Y., Liu, N., Chen, L., Meng, X., Liu, Y., Li, Y., Wang, J., 2012. Synthesis and characterization of DOX-conjugated dendrimer-modified magnetic iron oxide conjugates for magnetic resonance imaging, targeting, and drug delivery. J. Mater. Chem. 22, 9594–9601.

21. Ale, E.C., Maggio, B., Fanani, M.L., 2012. Ordered-disordered domain coexistence in ternary lipid monolayers activates sphingomyelinase by clearing ceramide from the active phase. Biochim. Et Biophys. Acta-Biomembr. 1818, 11, 2767–2776.

22. Jiang, X., Sha, X., Xin, H., Chen, L., Gao, X., Wang, X., Law, K., Gu, J., Chen, Y., Jiang, Y., Ren, X., Ren, Q., Fang, X., 2011. Self-aggregated pegylated poly (trimethylene carbonate) nanoparticles decorated with c(RGDyK) peptide for targeted paclitaxel delivery to integrin-rich tumors. Biomaterials 32, 9457–9469.

23. Lai, Y.S., Long, Y.Y., Lei, Y., Deng, X., He, B., Sheng, M.M., Li, M., Gu, Z.W., 2012. A novel micelle of coumarin derivative monoend-functionalized PEG for antitumor drug delivery: in vitro and in vivo study. J. Drug Target. 20, 246–254.

24. Bae, Y., Kataoka, K., 2009. Intelligent polymeric micelles from functional poly(ethylene glycol)-poly(amino acid) block copolymers. Adv. Drug Delivery Rev. 61, 768–784.

25. Tyrrell, Z.L., Shen, Y.Q., Radosz, M., 2010. Fabrication of micellar nanoparticles for drug delivery through the self-assembly of block copolymers. Prog. Polym. Sci. 35, 1128–1143.

26. Yamamoto, T., Yokoyam, M., Opanasopit, P., Hayama, A., Kawano, K., Maitani, Y., 2007. What are determining factors for stable drug incorporation into polymeric micelle carriers? Consideration on physical and chemical characters of the micelle inner core. J. Controlled Release 123, 11–18.

27. Seow, W.Y., Xue, J.M., Yang, Y.-Y., 2007. Targeted and intracellular delivery of paclitaxel using multi-functional polymeric micelles. Biomaterials 28, 1730–1740.

28. Read, E.S., Armes, S.P., 2007. Recent advances in shell cross-linked micelles. Chem. Commun. 7, 3021–3035.

29. Li, Y.T., Lokitz, B.S., Armes, S.P., McCormick, C.L., 2006. Synthesis of reversible shell cross-linked micelles for controlled release of bioactive agents. Macromolecules 39, 2726–2728.

30. Fujimori, J., Yoshihashi, Y., Yonemochi, E., Terada, K., 2005. Application of Eudragit RS to thermo-sensitive drug delivery systems: II. Effect of temperature on drug permeability through membrane consisting of Eudragit RS/PEG 400 blend polymers. J. Control. Release 102, 49–57.

31. Chan, Y., Wong, T., Byrne, F., Kavallaris, M., Bulmus, V., 2008. Acid-labile core crosslinked micelles for pH-triggered release of antitumor drugs. Biomacromolecules 9, 1826–1836.

32. Patnaik, S., Sharma, A.K., Garg, B.S., Gandhi, R.P., Gupta, K.C., 2007. Photoregulation of drug release in azo-dextran nanogels. Int. J. Pharm. 342, 184–193.

33. Dai, J., Lin, S., Cheng, D., Zou, S., Shuai, X., 2011. Interlayer-crosslinked micelle with partially hydrated core showing reduction and pH dual sensitivity for pinpointed intracellular drug release. Angew. Chem. Int. Ed. 50, 9404–9408.

34. Song, N., Liu, W., Tu, Q., Liu, R., Zhang, Y., Wang, J., 2011. Preparation and in vitro properties of redox-responsive polymeric nanoparticles for paclitaxel delivery. J. Colloids Surf. B 87, 454–563.

35. Li, Y., Xiao, K., Luo, J., Xiao, W., Lee, J.S., Gonik, A.M., Kato, J., Dong, T.A., Lam, K.S., 2011. Well-defined, reversible disulfide cross-linked micelles for on-demand paclitaxel delivery. Biomaterials 32, 6633–6645.

36. Irving, B., 2007. Nanoparticle drug delivery systems. Inno. Pharm. Biotechnol. 24, 58–62.

37. Kumari, A., Yadav, S.K., Yadav, S.C., 2010. Biodegradable polymeric nanoparticles based drug delivery systems. Colloids Surf. B 75, 1–18.

38. Tang, L., Azzi, J., Kwon, M., Mounayar, M., Tong, R., Yin, Q., Moore, R., Skartsis, N., Fan, T.M., Abdi, R., Cheng, J., 2012. Immunosuppressive activity of sizecontrolled PEG-PLGA nanoparticles containing encapsulated cyclosporine A. J. Transplantation, 2012, 896141.

39. Reis, C.P., Neufeld, R.J., Ribeiro, A.J., Veiga, F., 2006. Nanoencapsulation I. Methods for preparation of drug-loaded polymeric nanoparticles. Nanomed. Nanotechnol. Biol. Med. 2, 8–21.

40. Ferrari, M., 2005. Cancer nanotechnology: opportunities and challenges. Nat. Rev. Cancer 5, 161–171.

41. Guicun, W., Fang, Z., Linfu, G., Ximin, L., Fansheng, K., 2012. Novel Mannan-PEG-PE Modified Bioadhesive PLGA nanoparticles for targeted gene delivery. J. Nanomater., 1–9.

42. Laganà, A., Venditti, I., Fratoddi, I., Capriotti, A.L., Caruso, G., Battocchio, C., Polzonetti, G., Acconcia, F., Marino, M., Russo, M.V., 2011. Nanostructured functional copolymers bioconjugate integrin inhibitors. J. Colloids Interfaces Sci. 361, 465–471.

43. Masserini, M., 2013. Nanoparticles for brain drug delivery. ISRN Biochem., 1–18.

44. Mittal, G., Carswell, H., Brett, R., Currie, S., Kumar, M.N., 2011. Development and evaluation of polymer nanoparticles for oral delivery of estradiol to rat brain in a model of Alzheimer's pathology. J. Control Release 10, 220–228.

45. Schneider, M., Stracke, F., Hansen, S., Schaefer, U.F., 2009. Nanoparticles and their interactions with the dermal barrier. Dermatoendocrinol. 1, 197–206.

46. Shelma, R., Sharma, C.P., 2013. *In vitro and in vivo* evaluation of curcumin loaded lauroyl sulphated chitosan for enhancing bioavailability, Carbohydr. Polym. 95, 441–448.

47. Wagh, V.D., Dipak, U., 2014. Cyclosporine loaded PLGA nanoparticles for dry eye disease: in vitro characterization studies. J. Nanotechnol. 2014, 683153.

48. Chen, Y., McCulloch, R.K., Gray, B.N., 1994. Synthesis of albumindextransulfate microspheres possessing favourable loading and release characteristics for the anti-cancer drug doxorubicin. J. Control Release 31, 1, 49–54.

49. Mohanraj, V.J., Chen, Y., 2006. Nanoparticles: a review. Trop. J. Pharm. Res. 5, 1, 561–573.

50. Tyler, B., Gullotti, D., Mangraviti, A., Utsuki, T., Brem, H., 2016. Polylactic acid (PLA) controlled delivery carriers for biomedical applications, Adv. Drug Delivery Rev., 107, 163–175.

51. Wang, J., Li, S., Han, Y., et al., 2018, Poly(ethylene glycol)–polylactide micelles for cancer therapy, Front. Pharmacol. 9, 202.

52. Tang, K.X., Zhang, J., et al., 2014. PEG-PLGA copolymers: their structure and structure-influenced drug delivery applications, J. Controlled Release 183, 10, 77–86.

53. Yoo, H.S., Park, T.G., 2001, Biodegradable polymeric micelles composed of doxorubicin conjugated PLGA–PEG block copolymer, J. Controlled Release 70, 1-2, 63–70.

54. Tyler, B., Gullotti, D., Mangraviti, A., Utsuki, T., Brem, H., 2016, Polylactic acid (PLA) controlled delivery carriers for biomedical applications, Adv. Drug Delivery Rev., 107, 163–175.

55. Wang, J., Li, S., Han, Y., et al., 2018, Poly(ethylene glycol)–polylactide micelles for cancer therapy, Front. Pharmacol., 9, 202, 2018.

56. Ding, D., Zhu, Q., 2018, Recent advances of PLGA micro/nanoparticles for the delivery of biomacromolecular therapeutics, Mater. Sci. Eng.: C, 92, 1041–1060.

57. Tang, K.X., Zhang, J., et al., PEG-PLGA copolymers: their structure and structure-influenced drug delivery applications, J. Controlled Release 183, 10, 77–86, 201.

58. Cho, H., Gao, J., Kwon, G.S., 2016, PEG-b-PLA micelles and PLGA-b-PEG-b-PLGA sol–gels for drug delivery, J. Controlled Release 240, 28, 191–201.

59. Shelma, R., Sharma, C.P., 2013, *In vitro* cell culture evaluation and *in vivo* efficacy of amphiphilic chitosan for oral insulin delivery, J. Biomed. Nanotech. 9, 2, 167–176.

60. Vu-Quang, H., Vinding, M.S., Nielsen, T., Ullisch, M.G., Nielsen, N.C., Kjems, J., 2016, Theranostic tumor targeted nanoparticles combining drug delivery with dual near infrared and 19F magnetic resonance imaging modalities, Nanomed.: Nanotechnol., Biol. Med. 12, 7, 1873–1884.

61. Din, F.U., Aman, W., Ullah, I., et al., 2017, Effective use of nanocarriers as drug delivery systems for the treatment of selected tumors, Int. J. Nanomed. 12, 7291–7309.

62. Dube, A., Nicolazzo, J.A., Larson, I., 2010, Chitosan nanoparticles enhance the intestinal absorption of the greentea catechins (+)-catechin and (−)-epigallocatechin gallate. Eur. J. Pharm. Sci. 41, 219–225.

63. Barbieri, S., Buttini, F., Rossi, A., Bettini, R., Colombo, P., Ponchel, G., Sonvico, F., 2015, Ex vivo permeation oftamoxifen and its 4-OH metabolite through rat intestine from lecithin/chitosan nanoparticles. Int. J. Pharm. 491, 99–104.

64. Feng, C., Wang, Z., Jiang, C., Kong, M., Zhou, X., Li, Y., Cheng, X., Chen, X., 2013, Chitosan/o-carboxymethylchitosan nanoparticles for efficient and safe oral anticancer drug delivery: in vitro and in vivo evaluation. Int. J. Pharm.,457, 158–167.

65. Rekha, M.R., Sharma, C.P., 2009, Synthesis and evaluation of lauryl succinyl chitosan particles towards oral insulin delivery and absorption, J. Controlled Release 135, 2, 144–151.

66. Xue, M., Hu, S., Lu, Y., Zhang, Y., Jiang, X., An, S., Guo, Y., Zhou, X., Hou, H., Jiang, C., 2015, Development of chitosan nanoparticles as drug delivery system for a prototype capsid inhibitor. Int. J. Pharm. 495, 771–78.

67. Liu, S., Yang, S., Ho, P.C., 2017, Intranasal administration of carbamazepine-loaded carboxymethyl chitosan nanoparticles for drug delivery to the brain. Asian J. Pharm. Sci. 13(1), 72–81.

68. Lisbeth, I. 2003, Nasal drug delivery—possibilities, problems and solutions.J. Control. Release, 87, 187–198.

69. Rawal, T., Parmar, R., Tyagi, R.K., Butani, S., 2017, Rifampicin loaded chitosan nanoparticle dry powder presents an improved therapeutic approach for alveolar tuberculosis. Colloids Surf. B Biointerfaces, 154, 321–330.

70. Jafarinejad, S., Gilani, K., Moazeni, E., Ghazi-Khansari, M., Najafabadi, A.R., Mohajel, N., 2012, Development of chitosan-based nanoparticles for pulmonary delivery of itraconazole as dry powder formulation. Powder Technol. 222, 65–70.

71. Wenxing, S., Xing, S., David, A.G., Wei, L., Zhiqiang, C., Xiubo, Z., 2018, Magnetic alginate/chitosan nanoparticles for targeted delivery of curcumin into human breast cancer cells, Nanomaterials 8, 907–930.

72. Tønnesen, H.H., Karlsen, J., 2002, Alginate in drug delivery systems, Drug Dev. Ind. Pharm. 28, 6, 621–30.

73. Ahmad, Z., Sharma, S., Khuller, G.K., 2007, Chemotherapeutic evaluation of alginate nanoparticle-encapsulated azole antifungal and antitubercular drugs against murine tuberculosis, Nanomed. Nanotechnol., Biol., Med., 3, 3, 239–243.

74. Arora, S., Gupta, S., Narang, R.K., Budhiraja, R.D., 2011, Amoxicillin loaded chitosan-alginate polyelectrolyte complex nanoparticles as mucopenetrating delivery system for H. pylori, Sci. Pharm. 79, 3, 673–694.

75. Chen, F., Zhang, Z.-R., Yuan, F., Qin, X., Wang, M., Huang, Y., 2008, In vitro and in vivo study of N-trimethyl chitosan nanoparticles for oral protein delivery, Int. J. Pharm. 349, 1-2, 226–233.

76. Alaniz, L., Cabrera, P.V., Blanco, G., et al., 2016. Interaction of CD44 with different forms of hyaluronic acid. Its role in adhesion and migration of tumor cells. Cell Commun. Adhes. 9, 117–30.

77. Widjaja, L.K., Bora, M., Chan, P.N., et al., 2014. Hyaluronic acid-based nano-composite hydrogels for ocular drug delivery applications. J. Biomed. Mater. Res. A. 102, 3056–3065.

78. Chen, B., Miller, R.J., Dhal, P.K., 2014. Hyaluronic acid-based drug conjugates: state-of-the-art and perspectives. J. Biomed. Nanotechnol. 10, 4–16.

79. Yao, J., Fan, Y., Du, R., et al., 2010. Amphoteric hyaluronic acid derivative for targeting gene delivery. Biomaterials 31, 9357–9365.

80. Xu, P., Kc, R.B., 2016. Ternary gene delivery system for gene therapy and methods of its use. US 20160008289 A1.

81. Lee, S.J., Ghosh, S.C., Han, H.D., et al., 2012. Metronomic activity of CD44-targeted hyaluronic acid-Paclitaxel in ovarian carcinoma. Clin. Cancer Res. 18, 4114–4121.

Index

For Product Safety Concerns and Information please contact our EU
representative GPSR@taylorandfrancis.com
Taylor & Francis Verlag GmbH, Kaufingerstraße 24, 80331 München, Germany